Ethnodramatherapy

W0112840

Ethnodramatherapy explores the integration of the performance ethnography method, known as ethnodrama, with the principles and practices of drama therapy to establish a sound theoretical formulation for ethnodramatherapy, and considers its use as art, as therapy, as research and as a vehicle for social justice.

The book begins by defining ethnodramatherapy – an original synthesis created by the author through deep study and practice of Mienczakowski's ethnodrama, combined with 35 years of his own practice and research in drama therapy, creative arts therapies and therapeutic theatre. The book describes the origins of ethnodramatherapy, along with its evolution and method. It then delves into applications of the practice highlighted by five case studies with different audiences in different settings. Subjects include adults with developmental disabilities, female adolescents in youth protection, caregivers for loved ones with mental illnesses and Chinese students exploring controversial issues of oppression in China. Complex ethical issues are reviewed and suggestions are made on how to deal with some of the challenging ethical situations that are likely to arise in the ethnodramatherapy process. What emerges is a powerful tool that harnesses theatrical art, ethnographic research and the clinical techniques of drama therapy to create a potential for emancipatory experience for both performers and audiences.

This exciting and dynamic synthesis of drama therapy, performance ethnography, theatrical art and social activism will be of interest to the whole community of theatre practitioners and scholars who use theatre to effect individual and social change, including the disciplines of applied theatre, theatre education, experimental theatre, performance studies and, of course, drama therapy, psychodrama and the other creative arts therapies.

Stephen Snow, Ph.D., RDT-BCT, is a drama therapist, a performance theorist and a theatre practitioner. He is Emeritus Professor of Drama Therapy at Concordia University, where he co-founded the Centre for the Arts in Human Development (1996) and the Graduate Drama Therapy Program (1997). Dr. Snow has received research awards from Concordia University, the North American Drama Therapy Association, the American Association for Intellectual and Developmental Disabilities and AMI-Québec Action on Mental Illness. His most recent work is in developing an integrative approach called ethnodramatherapy (EDT). His documentary on this work can be found on psychotherapy.net.

Ethnodramatherapy

Integrating Research, Therapy, Theatre and Social Activism into One Method

Stephen Snow

Forewords by Renée Emunah, Jim Mienczakowski and Eric Mongerson

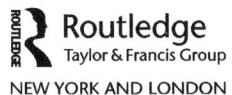
Routledge
Taylor & Francis Group

NEW YORK AND LONDON

First published 2022
by Routledge
605 Third Avenue, New York, NY 10158

and by Routledge
2 Park Square, Milton Park, Abingdon, Oxon, OX14 4RN

Routledge is an imprint of the Taylor & Francis Group, an informa business

© 2022 Stephen Snow

The right of Stephen Snow to be identified as author of this work has been asserted by him in accordance with sections 77 and 78 of the Copyright, Designs and Patents Act 1988.

All rights reserved. No part of this book may be reprinted or reproduced or utilised in any form or by any electronic, mechanical, or other means, now known or hereafter invented, including photocopying and recording, or in any information storage or retrieval system, without permission in writing from the publishers.

Trademark notice: Product or corporate names may be trademarks or registered trademarks, and are used only for identification and explanation without intent to infringe.

Library of Congress Cataloging-in-Publication Data
Names: Snow, Stephen, author. | Emunah, Renee, writer of foreword. | Mienczakowski, Jim, writer of foreword. | Mongerson, Eric, writer of foreword.
Title: Ethnodramatherapy : integrating research, therapy, theatre and social activism into one method / Stephen Snow ; forewords by Renée Emunah, Jim Mienczakowski and Eric Mongerson.
Description: New York, NY : Routledge, 2022. | Includes bibliographical references and index.
Identifiers: LCCN 2021020458 (print) | LCCN 2021020459 (ebook) | ISBN 9780367539481 (hardback) | ISBN 9780367539474 (paperback) | ISBN 9781003083818 (ebook)
Subjects: LCSH: Drama—Therapeutic use. | Theater—Anthropological aspects. | Ethnology—Methodology. | Ethnology in literature.
Classification: LCC RC489.P7 S66 2022 (print) | LCC RC489.P7 (ebook) | DDC 616.89/1523—dc23
LC record available at https://lccn.loc.gov/2021020458
LC ebook record available at https://lccn.loc.gov/2021020459

ISBN: 978-0-367-53948-1 (hbk)
ISBN: 978-0-367-53947-4 (pbk)
ISBN: 978-1-003-08381-8 (ebk)

DOI: 10.4324/9781003083818

Typeset in Goudy
by codeMantra

This book is dedicated to all my clients and students of the past 35 years. I have learned so very much from all of you. My interface with you has helped me to grow as a person. Thank you.

Contents

Illustrations and Tables

Figures

Tables

Foreword

A Drama Therapy Perspective

Renée Emunah, Ph.D., RDT-BCT

Founder/Director/Professor, Drama Therapy Program,
California Institute of Integral Studies, San Francisco

Combining his decades-long experience in drama therapy and therapeutic theatre with his extensive training in performance ethnography, Dr. Stephen Snow offers a broad and scholarly exploration of the intersections of these fields, as well as close-up and concrete descriptions of his numerous collaborative productions. Infused with his natural skill at synthesizing, the book is inherently integrative, as is the form, ethnodramatherapy.

The work of Dr. Jim Mienczakowski, who initiated ethnodrama, is featured, given its immense influence on Stephen Snow. Dr. Snow is particularly drawn to Mienczakowski's concept of emancipation, which was in part inspired by Augusto Boal's "emancipatory pedagogy." Emancipation is a relevant concept to drama therapy. The freedom inherent in acting – to safely express any emotion or try on new roles or experience different realities – holds liberatory potential that is central to the psychological healing drama therapy can offer. But the field of drama therapy is not geared solely toward personal psychological healing and growth. Liberation ultimately involves not only individual but also social spheres of change. Performance- and social justice-oriented drama therapy extend possibilities for emancipation. In addition to the agency performers experience onstage, productions which incite audiences to be agents of change – by questioning preconceived attitudes, awakening to injustices and taking action – expand our ever-evolving drama therapy field. Inspired by Boal and Brecht, and the many feminist and BIPOC theatre artists who have over decades produced performances that challenge the status quo and *visibilize* harm induced by oppressive forces, drama therapists have developed such efforts and have also added complexity by inviting people – whose voices have been squelched and who have often been perceived in limited ways that obscure their full humanity – to be center stage.

I say *added complexity* because when it comes to performances by people who have been stigmatized, and facilitated/directed by professional drama therapists, the issues are not simple. The very aims of de-stigmatization and fostering social justice can paradoxically backfire. There are the power dynamics between a troupe that is "on the inside" and a drama therapist that is "on the outside." There can be mismatches between intentions and impact, between overt and covert messages, and there is the dignity of the performers to be unquestionably upheld – all of which are delicate matters, not to be assumed but rather to be consciously considered if not scrutinized. Stephen Snow does not shy away from these and other ethical considerations; some chapters even include criticisms and challenging questions raised by others in the field. Chapter 8, "Ethical Challenges in Ethnodramatherapy," is in fact core to the book. I predict such issues will propel lively discourse in the drama therapy field. Through reflection, dialogue, play and (openness to) feedback, these questions should be kept alive, which will help all performative forms of drama therapy to healthfully evolve and thrive.

The author describes four roles that the ethnodramatherapist juggles: theatre artist, drama therapist, researcher and social activist. Such role-juggling – at least between theatre artist and drama therapist – is familiar to drama therapists using therapeutic theatre, which has long been a part of, and an option within, the field of drama therapy. While reading the book I could not help reflecting on a performance troupe I created and directed early in my own career. The troupe was composed of people who had been in psychiatric facilities but had newly transitioned to independent living. Our home – for workshop sessions and performances – was a San Francisco theatre; the intention was to take people far from psychiatric institutions and close to the heart of the local artistic community. While Beyond Analysis (the name we came up with) was among my most rewarding projects, it was also one of the most challenging – largely because of the juggling of these roles. The theatre artist in me cared deeply about the quality of the productions. The drama therapist in me cared deeply about the quality of the therapeutic journey for the troupe members. The social activist in me wanted to de-stigmatize mental illness, and to have audiences resonate with the actors and their struggles, rather than marginalize them. I didn't call my client–actors "informants" (a term used in ethnodramatherapy), but it was their stories that were elicited and performed, and creating truthful and meaningful representations of their experiences was of utmost importance. The researcher in me was latent, but still I wanted to reflect on and analyze the process, in part so that other drama therapists might benefit from the dilemmas I grappled with and methods I designed. But over the decades not many in the field took on such projects. Most drama therapists who engaged in performance projects worked inside institutions, and many more focused on process-oriented or private practice work. Stephen Snow though, over nearly 20 years, continuously produced full-scale performances, largely working with people who have developmental disabilities, all the while engaging teams of creative arts therapists at Concordia University and contributing to the training of emergent drama therapists.

The role of researcher in ethnodramatherapy is unique, and its presence creates a new potential emphasis or way of working within the field of drama therapy. The idea is to delve into an issue by working drama therapeutically with the people who know that issue or domain from the inside; they are the "informants," and typically though not necessarily the performers. The issues – which tend to be ones that are in need of societal attention – are explored and understood from the informants' perspectives. There is a carefully considered protocol in Snow's ethnodramatherapy, including the informants' validation of the script.

The juggling of multiple roles in ethnodramatherapy and other performance-oriented forms within the field of drama therapy, including simultaneously holding high standards for both process and product, can be intense but also incredibly generative, especially when some of the seemingly contradictory goals in fact collide in ways that enhance each other. For example, what a scene or theatre piece may need from an aesthetic perspective is often what would infuse greater therapeutic depth or clarity, or directions from a therapeutic lens may further layer a piece theatrically. Directions from both perspectives often lead to more compelling theatre and more impactful therapy. And when the performers are not only mastering an artistic production but are also advocating for and instigating needed reform, their sense of agency and experience of engaging in meaningful work are rightfully magnified. Through their stories and creativity and talents, audiences are moved to revisit their perspectives and activated to make changes – not only inwardly, but in systems and structures that are oppressive or reductionistic. Such is the case with the melding of theatre/therapy/activism/research – ethnodramatherapy! – which is so comprehensively examined in this book.

Foreword

An Ethnodrama Perspective

Jim Mienczakowski, Ph.D.
Emeritus Professor, Curtin University

Creator, Critical Ethnodrama Method

There is sometimes something special and rare – which Paulo Freire (1994) once described as an "intellectual kinship" or "the sensation of an old, very old camaraderie" – between people who have never met but who have shared similar, deeply motivating experiences and who have, by coincidence, explored convergent intellectual trajectories. This "kinship" is certainly something I immediately felt when learning of Stephen Snow's academic journey and his development of ethnodramatherapy (EDT).

In *Ethnodramatherapy*, Snow opens the doors to a potent world of research, performance, therapy and social activism in the hope of producing positive critical action on behalf of his informants and their audiences. And Dr. Snow is profoundly aware of the fine line along which his research performances will sometimes teeter in respect to transgressing the ethical boundaries embedded in any research-driven theatre involving vulnerable and sensitive informants in its performances. Consequently, he engages a particular and necessary lens through which he can balance his production work in order to meet the all too important ambition of "doing no harm." Here in, the diamond of ethnodramatherapy (see Figure 1.4 in Chapter 1) is introduced as a procedural means for analyzing and balancing the veracity, import and ethicality of his research. It embeds what Kathy Bishop (2014) has described as "a moral compass" to his overall project.

This diamond lens is a vital tool to possess in an academic and cultural environment in which the waters between disciplines are being forded and, sometimes, bridged through multidisciplinary approaches such as EDT. In *Ethnodramatherapy* Snow authoritatively and competently guides the reader through key areas of the troubled discipline terrain as he explains his decision-making processes for the progression of his wider project. The most

prevalent concerns posed, in respect to the trade-offs between accurate ethnographic reporting and the "aesthetics of making theatre," are covered in
Chapter 8, "Ethical Challenges in Ethnodramatherapy." The urge to *fiction-
alize* and "round off" research narratives to fit audience expectations and aesthetic conventions is powerful and is a natural part of human storytelling
in literature and the arts and, thus, its pervasive nature cannot be under-
estimated. Snow brings insight and balance to this discussion by using real,
heartfelt examples of his own exploration and experiences of meeting ethical
challenges during production work as well as discussions with others from
related fields. What we gain is a strong sense of the commitment and dedi-
cation required to work in this very structured way. Its *learning by doing* with
constraints seldom applied to commercial theatre or public performance
works. That's also one reason why it's so special.

Freire mooted that the necessity of *intellectual kinship* entailed the development of tolerance in the hope that academics might overcome unnecessary
(unimportant) boundary conflicts and dissention (academic difference) in
order to collectively derive more important social outcomes. And Snow's
work is situated amidst some very contested and, frequently, marginalized
academic discipline territories – but the project of ethnodramatherapy, in
its theoretical and methodological construction, and in its voicing and expression of the lived realities of his health informants, overcomes nay saying.
It is a clear manifestation and undertaking of shared, positive social action.

In its earliest days, ethnodrama came close to working with informant actors
and therapists, in the way that Stephen has achieved, when a young graduate
student, Paul Appleby, took his ethnodrama production "A Good Smack in
the Head" and worked with a group of informants who had acquired brain
injuries, using them as both his informants and performers. I could see at that
moment the huge therapeutic potential such theatre work could have, but,
for a number of reasons, important at that time, our ethnodrama construct
intentionally did not benefit from health consumers as actors in their own
stories. Snow has now completed the circle and bought forward not only rec-
ognition of the importance and power of performance advocacy work with
health consumer groups, but he has also demonstrated the validity of EDT's
ethnographic research approach and its therapeutic strengths.

References

Bishop, K. (2014). Six perspectives in search of an ethical solution: Utilizing a moral imperative with a multiple ethics paradigm to guide research-based theatre/applied theatre. *The Journal of Applied Theatre and Performance, 19*(1), 64–75.

Freire, P. (1994). *Preface* to McLaren, P. (1995) *Critical pedagogy and predatory culture: Oppositional politics in a postmodern era*. Routledge.

Foreword

A Theatre Arts Perspective

Eric Mongerson, MFA
Emeritus Professor and Former Chair, Department of
Theatre, Concordia University

I have worked with Stephen Snow for many years as a designer (sets and lights) and technical director. My background is in scenography and theatre technology not drama therapy or performance ethnography.

What follows is a fascinating look at the development of ethnodramatherapy. This is also a "how to" book benefiting from years of Stephen's experience and skill. Somehow every production was successful and nearly sold out. I soon learned that the risks were just too high to allow failure when working with participants with developmental challenges or adolescent females in youth protection.

During this time, I was working as a lighting and set designer professionally. In that situation, great risks were often taken. However, the main thing to be lost or won was money. In the case of the ethnodramas the risk was to the participants; their self-esteem was often low to begin with and could be easily damaged.

After working on several therapeutic theatre productions usually centered around fairy tales, Stephen had the idea to go off in a new direction. We were not going to do drama therapy. It was to be ethnodrama. He gave me Jim Mienczakowski's thesis to explain what that was. Furthermore, the cast was to include some participants from earlier drama therapy projects.

It became very clear to me after a few rehearsals that the therapy had not gone anywhere as it crept back into the modus operandi of the production (*It's a Wonderful World*). The fairy tales were gone and the method of developing the script improved.

It seemed to me that there was a great symbiotic relationship developing. The performers received much appreciated therapy, and the production received their amazing skills as actors. I recall professional actors coming to watch the shows just to see the participants work. What the performers were missing in technical ability they more than made up with charisma and their ability to make the audience very clearly feel their emotions. There were almost always full houses with standing ovations.

Stephen as theatre director, drama therapist, researcher or social activist was exceptionally good at changing hats and watching out for the wellbeing of the participants. There were often very difficult ethical and moral questions to be answered as issues surrounding the productions came up. He would often struggle between his various hats and somehow come up with the best compromise without losing theatrical clarity.

My work on these productions has been a great complement to my "normal" theatre work.

This form of theatre is an amazing and very rewarding way to affect change in our society.

Preface

I grew up in the beautiful little New England college town of Amherst, Massachusetts. I went to kindergarten in a small white brick building next to an apple orchard. I can still smell the apple blossoms in springtime. Without a doubt, I come from a background of privilege.

Over the hill from our house on 86 Kellogg Avenue, about the distance of five football fields, was the house where Emily Dickinson grew up in the mid-1800s. I have always felt a close spiritual kinship with my neighbor over the hill in Amherst. When I was a high school student I raked the leaves by her grave site. I, too, am a bit of a rebel against the stony Calvinist Yankee heritage of white Anglo-Saxon Protestantism.

Emily Dickinson has written many wonderfully enigmatical poems. Perhaps one of the most strange and arcane of these is her poem, "Trust in the Unexpected." You can look it up on Google, as I recently did, and find dozens of people trying to explain its meaning. "Trust in the Unexpected." What was Emily really trying to say, here? What did that mean to her own life?

Somehow, looking back at my own life, I see it has been filled with the unexpected. I did not expect to be a father at 23. I did not expect to drive a taxi cab at night for seven years in New York City. I expected to become a professional actor when I graduated from Emerson College in 1968 and won the Carol Burnett Performing Arts Award. I expected to become a professor of performance theory when I graduated with a Ph.D. in Performance Studies from NYU. None of this happened. Instead, the unexpected kept on moving me in different directions. I certainly did not expect that a part-time job in a nursing home's recreation department, while I was writing my dissertation on a fellowship, would become my career. I certainly did not expect to end up living in Montreal for 28 years, teaching drama therapy at a Canadian university. Nor did I expect to write a book that brought all my trainings – in theatre, performance ethnography and drama therapy – together, in one method. But these things have all happened and I am grateful for them.

Trust in the unexpected. Life has its way of taking us up and moving us where it wants to go. Maybe trusting in the unexpected is a way to accept the mystery and miracle of life, no matter what one's conditions are. Maybe this is what my ghostly Amherst neighbor meant by these words in her poem. She certainly was able to capture so much of the profound beauty and mystery of life in her poetry.

My hope for this book is that it will be a service to the whole community of drama therapists, theatre practitioners and scholars who use theatre to effect individual and social change. It carries a message of hope – Emily's "the thing with feathers" – for effecting real change in society and emancipatory healing experiences for individuals. I trust it will move out into the world in many unexpected ways, as well.

Stephen Snow
Easter Sunday, April 4, 2021,
Dorval, Québec, Canada

Acknowledgments

As this book is an integration of many aspects of my life and an integrative reflection of a long professional career, I have many people to thank and acknowledge.

First of all, I want to thank my mother and father, Bernice Frances Eddy Snow and Ernest Augustus Snow, Jr., and my brother, Ronald Edwin Snow, for their deep support of my theatre dream. I owe a special debt of gratitude to my parents for paying for my theatre education at Emerson College in Boston. I would also like to express my appreciation for my theatre professors at Emerson: Leonidas Nickole, Harry Morgan, Richard Arnold, Alfred Sensenbach and Thomas Haas. When I went on to get a Ph.D. in Performance Studies at New York University, I had the privilege of being mentored and guided by two formidable scholars: Richard Schechner and Barbara Kishenblatt-Gmblett. I thank them both.

I began my career in drama therapy at Wartburg Lutheran Home for the Aging in Brooklyn. I am very grateful to have had that opportunity. I especially want to thank Eileen Gerard, formerly Director of Recreation, for her support and faith in me. At my 5-year "apprenticeship" at Bronx Psychiatric Center, I was supervised by Dance Movement Therapist Miriam Berger and Music Therapist Gillian Stephens. I wish to express my gratitude for their great support at the beginning of my career. It helped me to get a real grasp of the creative arts therapies.

For supporting my first job in teaching drama therapy, I wish to thank Dean Sondra Farganis of the New School for Social Research (now the New School University) in New York City. For hiring me to teach at Concordia University, in Montreal, I am extremely grateful to Barbara MacKay, with whom I collaborated to establish the graduate Drama Therapy Program in 1997. Barbara was a wonderful friend and colleague over many years. I would also like to thank Professor Gene Gibbons for being so supportive of me and the field of drama therapy while he was Chair of Theatre. He helped to get the M.A. program pushed through the faculty senate. My heartfelt gratitude goes to Theatre Professor Eric Mongerson, my friend and creative collaborator in producing theatre for over two decades. Partnership with you has helped me to grow dynamically as a theatre practitioner.

To all of my colleagues in the Department of Creative Arts Therapies at Concordia I send my warmth and gratitude. It has been 25 years of creative and scholarly collegiality. Thank you. I especially want to acknowledge my three close colleagues in the Drama Therapy program, Bonnie Harnden, Jessica Bleuer and Simon Driver. Now, being just retired, I have great confidence in a bright future for the program under your leadership.

At Concordia, I also want to thank two Deans of the Faculty of Fine Arts: Rebecca Duclos for granting me a six-month sabbatical that allowed me to begin work on this book, and Annie Gérin, for releasing me from teaching for the Fall 2020, which allowed me to further advance the writing of this book. Merci beaucoup. I also want to acknowledge the substantial funding that I have received from the Office of the Vice-President of Research and Graduate Studies, in terms of several Start-up and Accelerator grants for my research projects.

In regard to other financial support for my research, I owe a great debt of gratitude to the Social Science and Humanities Research Council of Canada, as well as to the Raschkowan Family Foundation, the Ellen Foundation, the Mills Foundation, the Seagram's Fund for Academic Innovation and the Centre for the Arts in Human Development.

In 1996, Social Worker Lenore Vosberg, Educational Psychologist Miranda D'Amico and I founded the Centre for the Arts in Human Development (CAHD) at Concordia University. I want to thank them both for their friendship and support through the years. Lenore is a powerful advocate for the field of development disability and has provided great leadership to CAHD for 25 years. Dr. D'Amico has been a wonderful research colleague, especially supporting the quantitative aspect of our research. In that light, I also wish to thank my friend and colleague Dr. Norman Segalowitz of the Psychology Department for his invaluable assistance on statistical analyses and quantitative research for our ethnodramatherapy projects since 2014.

I wish to express my great gratitude for their friendship to my close international colleagues in the field of drama therapy: David Read Johnson, Saphira Linden, Susana Pendzik, Daniel Wiener, Armand Volkas, Phil Jones, Robert

Landy and Renée Emunah. I have learned so much from you all! I especially want to thank Robert for his mentorship of me, back in the late 1980s and early 1990s, when I was first getting my sea legs as a drama therapist. To Renée, I express a deep gratitude for the gift of her Foreword to this volume. Over the years, I have found your personal approach to drama therapy a genuine inspiration. Thank you. In terms of international colleagues from other disciplines, I want to express my appreciation for the support and kindness of two psychiatrists, Dr. Shavindra Dias of the University of Peradeniya, Sri Lanka, and Dr. Mona Rakhawy of the University of Cairo and the Rakhawy Institute, in Egypt, as well as psychologist Dr. Li Weixiao, Founder of Apollo School Education China.

To my two colleagues from the disciplines ethnodrama and theatre, Jim Mienczakowski and Eric Mongerson, thank you, so much, for your thoughtful and supportive Forewords. They mean a great deal to me.

I have been very fortunate to have had master teachers in the disciplines of psychodrama and playback theatre. From the former I wish to express my gratitude to Peter Pitzele, James Sacks, Tobi Klein, Heidi Landis, Dale Richard Buchanan and Nina Garcia. From the latter, I express my great appreciation to Jonathan Fox and Jo Salas.

At Routledge, I want to thank Senior Editor Stacey Walker for seeing the value of my unique project, Editorial Assistant Lucia Accorsi who has offered steadfast guidance throughout the writing process and my Production Editor, Lauren Ellis, for bringing the ship safely into harbor. My gratitude to you all.

I also wish to especially thank my friend and long-time collaborator, Phil Herbison, for shooting, editing and narrating three documentaries we co-created based on theatre productions at The Center for the Arts in Human Development (2000–2022).

In my nearly three decades at Concordia University, I have had many wonderful research assistants. I thank them all for their hard work and support of my many research projects. Here, I want to specifically recognize Rosy Kuftedjian who has been an outstanding research assistant for this book project, helping me to locate scholarly materials and drafting designs for line drawings, among many other tasks. Thank you, Rosy.

Last, but definitely not least, I want to thank my wife, Shelley Huffaker Snow, and my daughter, Robin Snow, for their constant love and support.

Part I
Background and Development

1

The Concept of Ethnodramatherapy and Its Origin

Despite Victor Turner's (1986) initial call for research that also participated in performance, the worlds of theatre and research at that time were too far apart for a viable elision between the aesthetic assumptions of performance and the methodological and theoretical ambitions of research to truly take place.

(Jim Mienczakowski, 2001)

Big Word, Big Concept

Ethnodramatherapy. It is a big word. It is made up of seventeen letters. Some might say it is an overwrought, fancy-dancy neologism. As the inventor of this term, I feel a big responsibility to clarify its meaning and to answer the central question: is it an authentic concept? This is the essential purpose of this book.

Ethnodramatherapy is a big concept. There are several different ways to review the word as it relates to the overall construct. The first of these derives from the tripartite construction of the word. It could be called the triangulated perspective (see Figure 1.1).

The term is made up of three separate words derived from Greek: ethno, drama and therapy. To begin with *ethno* is not just used as a prefix, as in *ethno*botany or *ethno*musicology or *ethno*psychiatry. *Ethno* is derived from the Greek word *ethnos*, which means a nation, a people (*Oxford Dictionary of English*, 2005, p. 595). It implies a group with a common language and shared traditions. In this way, it relates specifically to disciplines like *ethno*logy or *ethno*graphy – the study or portrait of a people – the latter being a method of research, quintessentially relevant to the concept and practice of ethnodramatherapy. The second noun, drama, is derived from the Greek verb *dram*, indicating "to do," or "to act" (*Oxford Dictionary*, p. 527). It reflects Aristotle's succinct definition of tragic drama as "an imitation of an action that is serious, complete, and of a certain magnitude" (Aristotle, 1961, p. 7).

DOI: 10.4324/9781003083818-2

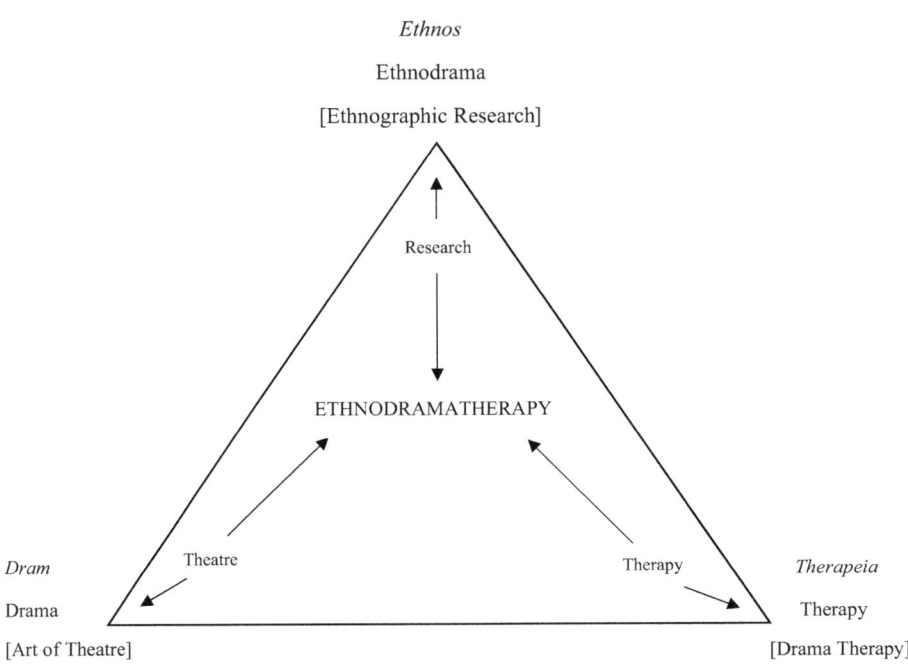

Figure 1.1   The Triangulated Perspective

It refers precisely to the performance of a such dramatic action. The third component, therapy, is also derived from a Greek word, *therapeia*, fundamentally meaning a "healing" process (*Oxford Dictionary*, p. 1830). Although outside the scope of this study, the alignment of healing and the Greek Theatre has been well established (Hartigan, 2009).

Putting all these words, together, what do we get? Ethnodramatherapy is "the preparation and performance of a play based on the study of the actions and thoughts of a group of people, with deeply shared common experience, which aims to have a therapeutic effect on the individuals in the group." This is a pretty good summation of the ethnodramatherapy process from the triangulated view. It is also a good umbrella formula for the chapters that follow in the **Applications** section of this book.

The second point of view could be called the "binary perspective." It defines ethnodramatherapy as the integration of two things: ethnodrama and drama therapy. It constitutes, therefore, the synthesis of a performance-based research process, ethnodrama, and a theatre or drama-based therapy process, drama therapy. In terms of a scholarly conceptualization of ethnodramatherapy, this way of looking at the intellectual invention of the method is probably the most accurate. It immediately recognizes the immense significance of Dr. Jim Mienczakowski's ethnodrama approach (Mienczakowski, 1995a, 1995b, 1997, 2001) and my great debt to him. Mienczakowski is the creator of the performance-based method of ethnographic research, known as ethnodrama. He formulated this approach in Australia, in the 1990s, as a participant in the emerging discipline of **performance ethnography**, or what Denzin (2003) describes as a new movement towards "a performance-centered pedagogy [that] uses performance as a method of investigation, as a way of doing ethnography, and as a method of understanding, a way of collaboratively engaging the meanings of experience" (p. 31). Mienczakowski was very much part of this movement, as is witnessed in his statement in the epigraph at the beginning of this chapter. So, it completely makes sense that he would advocate that his own method of "the ethnographic construction of dramatic scripts, validated by contributors, peers, and informed others, is potentially able to achieve vraisemblance and cultural ingress as effectively, if not more effectively, than some traditional means of research reporting" (1995b, pp. 365–366). Much more about this, later.

Drama therapy has been my professional discipline for 35 years. I will describe some of my work in this domain, in the third section of this chapter. One of the most commonly used and succinct definitions of drama therapy is "the intentional and systematic use of drama/theatre processes to achieve psychological growth and change. The tools are derived from theatre, the goals are rooted in psychotherapy" (Emunah, 1994, p. 3). Drama therapy is, itself, a synthesis, combining the many media of dramatic art with the principles and practices of psychotherapy.

It falls under the wider rubric of **creative arts therapies**, sometimes, in Europe, especially, designated as expressive arts therapies, or simply as the arts therapies (Jones, 2005). Whereas ethnodrama was developed by one person (although, in Chapter 9, we will look at how Moreno first coined the term in the 1950s), drama therapy was created collectively, over many years by many separate individuals (Jennings, 1992; Jennings et al., 1994; Jones, 1996, 2007, 2010; Johnson & Emunah, 2009, 2020; Landy, 1986, 1993, 2008; Lewis & Johnson, 2000). It is practiced, today, worldwide, in North America, Europe, the Middle East, Africa, Asia and Australia. There are graduate training programs in many countries.

Ethnodramatherapy (henceforth to be abbreviated as EDT) is, then, the dynamic fusion of the performance ethnography method, known as ethnodrama, with the praxis of drama therapy. It is the substantial merger of two disciplines. Although, as will be shown, it also represents a synthesis of research, therapy, theatre and social activism.

My First Encounter with Ethnodrama

In 2002, my Drama Therapy graduate student, Ron Scott, handed in a research proposal, "The Place of Performance in Qualitative Research." It was largely based on Mienczakowski's ethnodrama. I had never even heard of the term before. My eyes opened wide as I read through my student's text. The method seemed extraordinarily familiar to me. Mienczakowski was talking about the "performance of ethnography." In my doctoral program in **performance studies** at New York University, I had studied with the famous anthropologist Victor Turner who had devised his own approach called "**performing ethnography**." As he and his wife Edith had written in *The Drama Review* (1982): "For several years, as teachers of anthropology, we have been experimenting with the performance of ethnography to aid students' understanding of how people in other cultures experience the richness of their social existence" (p. 33). Saldana (2011) mentions how Turner coined the term, "Ethnodramatics" and goes on to explain how valuable this approach has been to his own work in ethnodrama (pp. 47–61). For myself, I was fascinated with Turner's approach and was fortunate to have several lectures and workshops with him during my studies at NYU. I especially remember Turner's phrase, "to put experiential flesh on these cognitive bones" (1982, p. 41) as a justification for the performance of ethnography. Mienczakowski, in his own writing, cites "Victor Turner's (1986) initial call for research that also participated in performance" (2001, p. 468) (see the rest of the quote in the epigraph at beginning of this chapter). Saldana quotes Turner from Turner's book, *From Ritual to Theatre: The Human Seriousness of Play*, honing in on this harbinger of ethnodrama: "I've long thought that teaching and learning anthropology should be more fun than they often are. Perhaps we should not merely read and comment on ethnographies, but actually perform them" (1982, p. 89). Turner's ideas and perspective were a major part of my training in performance studies.

I am very grateful to my former student for "introducing" me to Mienczakowski and ethnodrama. From that point on, I plunged into the world of ethnodrama, reading all of Mienczakowski's work, including his doctoral dissertation, as well as the work of Canadian sociologist Ross Gray and his collaborators (Gray and Sinding, 2002; Gray et al., 2003). Later, the writings of Johnny Saldana (1998, 2005, 2011), the major American interpreter of Mienczakowski, became very valuable for my grounding in ethnodrama.

As the development of ethnodramatherapy is profoundly intertwined with my own personal life journey, I hope the reader will allow me to indulge in a little more autobiographical framing, here, in order to elucidate the origins of my method.

Two Formats for Living History Performance

Two other factors enhanced my immediate grasp of this performance ethnography approach. In 1984 and 1985, I had done field work for my doctoral dissertation on the performance of "Living History" at the **"Living Museum"** of Plimoth Plantation. The embodied approach to first-person interpretation where costumed enactors speak in a 17th-century English accent, saying "I did this or that," was used at this site, also, as a way of putting "experiential flesh on cognitive bones." In this case, the bones of ethnohistory. I utilized the Turners' perspective to analyze the performance of ethnohistory that was taking place at Plimoth. Eventually, I published my thesis as a book, *Performing the Pilgrims: A Study of Ethnohistorical Role-Playing at Plimoth Plantation* (Snow, 1993). This whole experience, from field work to analysis, gave me a great familiarity with the concept and practice of performing ethnography (see Figure 1.3).

There was one other significant factor which made the ethnodrama approach, so easily accessible to my understanding and use. *It was actually a major turning point in my life.* During the year 1985, when I was writing my dissertation on a fellowship, I took a part-time job at Wartburg Lutheran Home for the Aging, a nursing home in Brooklyn, New York, in their recreation department. I began doing plays with a unique method of therapeutic theatre, called **"Living History Theatre."** It was an amalgamation of **oral history**, ethnography and the psychological process of life review (Charnow et al., 1988). I got trained in the method by its creators. I had studied a little drama therapy as part of my performance studies coursework at NYU. I was combining that with what I knew of performance ethnography and, at the same time, studying the well-known gerontological therapy technique, the **"Life Review"** process (Butler, 1963). My first piece was actually entitled "The Life Revue." It re-created scenes from the actual life stories of the seniors' own developmental process. As I wrote about it, "life stories of residents of a nursing home are evoked, sensitively processed in a small group therapy context, and finally transformed into theatrical scenes. These scenes are, then, constructed into 'Living History' plays which are taken on tour and shared with audiences" (Snow, 1986, p. 1).

If anything laid the groundwork for my development of EDT, it was this early work in living history theatre. I interviewed the residents at Wartburg about their personal experiences of growing up; I processed these experiences through drama therapy and psychodrama; I directed the plays; and I drove the bus that took them on the "tour" of the plays to schools, colleges, psychiatric hospitals, senior centers and other nursing homes. An example of the creation of one scene that embodies this whole process is the personal story of a West Indian woman who had an extremely strict mother who refused to let her go to a dance party as a teenager. So, this 13-year-old girl (at the time, actually a 70-year-old woman), snuck out of the house and went anyway. The 80-year old resident who played her intransigent mother, naturally had some of the mother's rigid and demanding characteristics and seemed to really enjoy playing that role. The argument between them was dynamically portrayed. The audience cheered when the young woman did the Charleston to represent her freedom at the dance party. Combining oral history and ethnodrama with life review and drama therapy was the vital precedent to my work in EDT.

In another instance, I collected the memories of the Wartburg residents around their experiences of WWI and WWII. Oral history was catalyzed by questions like: "Do you remember where you were on December 7, 1941?" We would locate the time, the room, the people there, the smells, the sounds, etc. This would initiate all kinds of intimate memories and out of these kinds of interview questions, we constructed a play called "War Stories." It was presented at the Living History Theatre Festival, sponsored by Elders Share the Arts, on Friday, May 13, 1988 (see Figure 1.2).

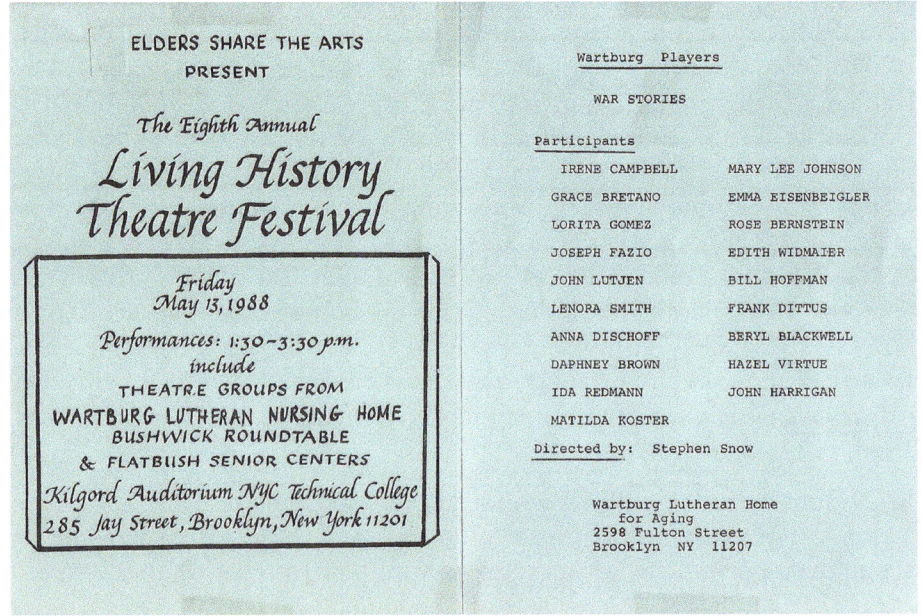

Figure 1.2   Programme from Living History Theatre Production, 1988

I created several of these "Living History" plays at the Nursing Home. These were some 20 years before my first ethnodrama project in 2006. They were also the beginning of my career as a drama therapist. The use of theatrical process and performance as therapy, known as "Therapeutic Theatre," became my major mode of working throughout my career in drama therapy (Snow in Gersie, 1996; Snow, D'Amico & Tanguay, 2003; Snow in Johnson & Emunah, 2009; Snow & Bleuer in Johnson & Emunah, 2020).

After my first readings of ethnodrama in 2002, I began to envision a plan for creating a large-scale ethnodrama. At that point, I had been a professor of drama therapy at Concordia University in Montreal for ten years. It took a few more years for this plan to come to fruition. I had co-founded a special center for research and practice in the creative arts therapies – the Centre for the Arts in Human Development (to be described in detail in the next chapter). We needed a dynamic research project, so I began to formulate a project around our central clientele, adults with developmental disabilities. In 2005, my grant application to the Canadian Social Science and Humanities Research Council was entitled: "Visually Performed Research: Creating Theatre with Adults with Developmental Disabilities through *Ethnodrama.*" In April 2006, we received major funding for a three-year research project. The central goal of the project was to:

> utilize the methodology of *ethnodrama* to create a theatre production with a new cohort of participants (20) at *The Centre for the Arts in Human Development* in order to explore, reveal and communicate their unique vision of the world, and, in this way, to empower them and, subsequently, to enlighten health providers, health educators and the public-at-large to the special needs and special ways of perceiving reality of our clients.
> (Snow et al., 2005, p. 3–4)

After three years of studying Mienczakowski's writing, I was very strictly following his design of using ethnodrama to "reflexively inform health educators and health service providers of health consumer needs; by voicing informant agendas in their own words and by presenting performances within informant habituses" (1995a, p. iv). The word *habitus* is very relevant, here, as the 20 participants from CAHD had just completed two years of our program in creative arts therapies, meeting twice a week from October to April, at the house on 7079 rue Terrebonne, in Montreal. Although a day program, it can be said that this group *lived together* for a good portion of time. The job of ethnodrama was now to capture the culture and psychology of this lived experience. In Fall 2006, we set out to do just that, and, as will be described in Chapter 2. This first ethnodrama production became "The Seedbed of EDT."

The Three Trainings in My Background that Supported the Creation of EDT

From the triangulated perspective (Figure 1.1), there are three essential components to EDT: the art of theatre, ethnographic research and drama therapy. Fortunately, and perhaps, fatefully, I had serious trainings in all of these areas *before* I began to conceive of the EDT method. My personal journey in life laid the groundwork for the creation of this approach.

Training and Practice as a Theatre Artist

In 1963, I entered the Theatre Arts B.A. program at Emerson College in Boston. I studied Acting, Directing and Speech. After graduation, I went to New York City and furthered my training with two acting coaches: Julie Bovasso at La Mama and Pierreno Mascarino from the John Lehne Studio. Also, during my time in New York, I participated in theatre workshops with many theatre artists such as Peter Brook, Eugenio Barbra, Augusto Boal and Richard Schechner. The meeting with Schechner in a workshop with the Performance Group in 1970 (Sainer, 1975, p. 214) was indeed fateful, as in 1979, I entered what was to shortly become the performance studies graduate program at NYU, and Richard Schechner became my mentor for the next seven years.

All of this is to say that I have had extensive experience in theatre. I have been a member of fifteen theatre companies in New York, New England and Montreal. I have been a member of Actors' Equity Association since 1980. I have performed in over 100 theatre productions on all levels. I have created two solo pieces, *Seething Brains: Madness in Shakespeare and Myself* (1994) and *Nightride in the City* (2003). The former dealt with mental illness in my family, my experience working in a psychiatric hospital and the many images of madness in Shakespeare's plays. The latter focused on my experiences of driving a taxicab at night for seven years, in New York City, during the 1970s. This **Self-Revelatory Performance** is cited in Saldana's book, *Ethnodrama* (2005, p. 11).

Over these many years, I have also directed over 30 theatre productions. Although, most of my productions have been in the vein of therapeutic theatre and ethnodrama (14 in all), I have also directed plays for experimental and traditional theatre, at Stage 1 Drama Workshop in Boston, Off-Off Broadway in NYC and Place des Arts in Montreal.

I believe with the background of all this artistic and creative experience, I have substantially lived in the role of "Theatre Artist." But, does one have to be a "Theatre Artist" to do EDT? This is perhaps a more difficult question for the field of drama therapy, where a clinical framework is predominant (Pendzik et al., 2016). However, for ethnodrama, where the major frame is performance-based research, the place and function of the *art* of theatre is clear. Saldana would have practitioners in this field aspire to the artistry of plays like *The Laramie Project* and the works of Anna Deavere Smith, which demonstrate how "gathering the voices of real people and transferring them on the stage in aesthetically sound ways can become riveting theatre" (2005, p. 9). So, my answer to the question is "Yes": one of the main functions of the ethnodramatherapist is that of "Theatre Artist." At a very significant level, the practitioner must have sufficient training to use the *art* of theatre as both a process for healing in the group and a vehicle of communication for the research report. Or, she or he must collaborate with individuals that have these skills.

Training as a Performance Ethnographer

I entered the MA in Graduate Drama at NYU in 1979. In 1980, it was re-named the Department of Performance Studies. It was the first full program in performance studies ever given at a university (Harding & Rosenthal, 2011). This was a discipline that brought together the theories and prac-tices of theatre and anthropology (Schechner, 1985). It was the brainchild of Richard Schechner, a renowned experimental theatre director (1973) and a brilliant performance theorist (1977).

Immediately, we were asked to study the work of Clifford Geertz, a formida-ble anthropologist, who defined his concept of culture as "a semiotic one" and describes his view of ethnography as "Thick Description." He writes:

> Believing, with Max Weber, that man is an animal suspended in webs of significance that he himself has spun, I take culture to be those webs, and the analysis of it to be therefore not an experimental science in search of law, but an interpretive one in search of meaning.
>
> (1973, p. 5)

And so, our assignment was to explore performances in this way, looking at the multiple "webs" of significance that are the meaningful substructures of any given performance in any given culture. This is exactly what led me to study the performance at Plimoth Plantation (Snow, 1993). I followed the lead of ethnographers like Geertz, who in his famous essay, delineating the performance of the Balinese Cockfight, worked with "describing and analyz-ing the meaningful structure of experience (here, the experience of persons) as it is apprehended by representative members of a particular society at a particular point in time – in a word, a scientific *phenomenology* of culture" (italics mine, 1973, p. 364). As students of performance studies, we were learning to be dynamic writers of the description and analysis of cultural performances. I italicize the word "phenomenology," here, as the phenomenological approach would eventually become an important aspect of EDT, especially in regard to its use in ethnography (see Chapters 5 and 9).

One of the visiting professors in performance studies who made a lasting impression on me was Barbara Myerhoff, an anthropologist who taught a course on "Self-Narrative." She was accompanied by theatre artist Arthur Strimling who helped us embody the narrative expositions we developed. In this course, we were also being taught how to do *ethnographic interviews*; how to really listen and hear the story behind the story; how to uncover the deep structures. I will never forget Barbara telling the class how difficult it can be to really get to know someone. She described a wealthy young man in her class on the same topic as ours at the University of Southern California who decided to choose the family maid as the subject for his interview. As he interviewed her, he learned all kinds of new things about her life, but the biggest was that she sent all her earnings to her son who was in medical school. He was flabbergasted. He had had no idea. His interview completely changed his concept of this family employee. I had a similar experience. I chose an older man who lived in my building in the East Village, who always walked around in a white leather jacket and a black beret. A piece was missing from the top of one ear. He walked with a limp. In telling his story, I came to know that he had been a U.S. Army combat soldier, incarcerated in a German prisoner of war camp, in WWII. Also, he was an artist who made his living for over 30 years as a night guard at the Metropolitan Museum of Art. He described his passion and delight for one particular painting, he would walk by on his security tour, each night. *It was from this experience that I learned the tremendous value of the interview in research* that I applied both in Living History Theatre and in EDT.

As Victor Turner wrote, in his Introduction of Myerhoff's book, *Number Our Days*, based on her interviews with elderly Jewish people at a Senior Centre in Venice, California: "While her work is always informed by her anthropological training, it goes beyond the usual reports from the field. It can perhaps best be described as compassionate objectivity or better yet, a realistic humankindness" (1978, p. xvii). Myerhoff's work truly inspired me. As noted, her class turned me on to the great value of interviews. This significantly influenced me when I began my own work in Living History Theatre, at Wartburg Nursing Home, in 1985. It also foreshadowed for me the place that interviews would play in my future EDT work. As Denzin wrote on this topic in 2001, "The present moment is defined by a performative sensibility, by a willingness to experiment in different ways of presenting an interview text. The performative sensibility turns interviews into performance texts, into poetic monologues" (p. 24).

Richard Schechner, the founder of performance studies, had courageously plunged into the studies of ritual and theatre performances in Papua New Guinea and India and was developing models for theories of performance that correlated ancient dramatic ritual forms with the experimental theatre in the West (1977). I was very inspired by this work and these new models of performance. I had planned to go and study dramatic rituals in Bali, Sri Lanka and the Himalayan countries. But, as they say, "life intervened." I was impressed by the way Schechner, like Geertz, could develop multi-leveled analyses and penetrate structures under structures in performances. Nowhere is this more observable than in Schechner's essay on "Restored Behavior." I utilized this concept for my own analysis of the ethnohistorical "Living History" performance at Plimoth Plantation. As he writes:

> In fact, restored behavior is the main characteristic of performance. The practitioners of all these arts, rites, and healings assume that some behaviors – organized sequences of events, scripted actions, known texts, scored movements – exist separate from the performers who "do" these behaviors. Because the behavior is separate from those who are behaving, the behavior can be stored, transmitted, manipulated, transformed.
>
> (1985, p. 36)

This model became a way for Schechner to analyze multiple types of cultural performances that are kept alive as traditions and sometime even "invented traditions"! It was from Schechner that I came to see Plimoth Plantation as a great potential site for the exploration of performed ethnohistory via a participant/observation approach. As he stated, the "'first-person' interpretation technique used at Plimoth is very effective theatre." As part of my participant–observation research, I performed several of the historical characters at Plimoth over two seasons, including Governor William Bradford (Figure 1.3). I got a good deal of firsthand experience of "performing ethnography." It prepared me for later, when I began to practice the performance ethnography method of ethnodrama.

Training as a Drama Therapist

In 1986, in my second year of working as a "Drama Therapist" at Wartburg Lutheran Home for the Aging, I began to realize that I was going to

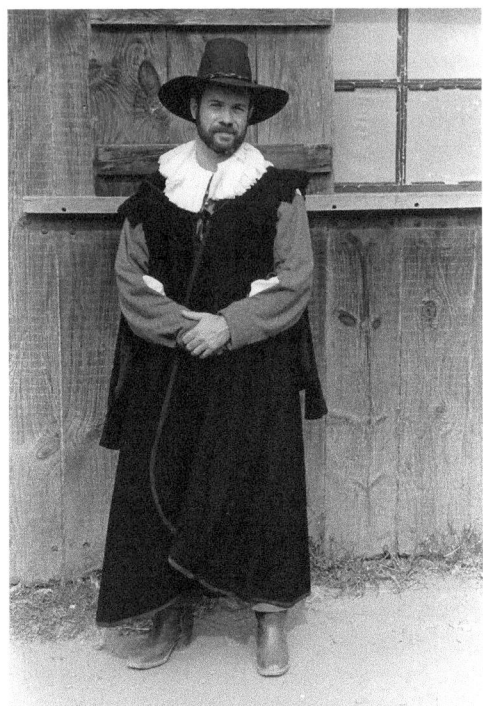

Figure 1.3   Participant/Observation of Ethnohistory at Plimoth Plantation, 1986 (photo courtesy of Plimoth Patuxet Museums)

need more training to justify the use of the title, "Drama Therapist." I had only taken two courses at NYU: "Introduction to Drama Therapy" with Gertrud Schattner and "Psychodrama" with Peter Pitzele. From my study of healing ritual performances and shamanism in my performance studies courses, I had become very interested in the idea of the "Healing Function" of drama and theatre. So, it felt very natural to ask Dr. Robert Landy, the founder and director of the Drama Therapy MA program at NYU, if I could take some drama therapy courses in his program. Fortunately, he agreed.

To get more training, I began to formally study the **psychodrama** method with James Sacks at the Psychodrama Center of New York. I put them to use in my living history theatre groups to help participants process remembered experiences that were painful or traumatic for them. By 1990, I was an "Assistant Director-in-Training." I had also continued my drama therapy training, doing a year of supervision with Dr. Robert Landy. In order to gain my professional registration in drama therapy, I applied to the NADT Registry

Committee and submitted my training and experience in drama therapy.[1] In 1991, I received my RDT (Registered Drama Therapist). Also, to increase my knowledge of psychotherapy process, I completed two and a half years of training in Psychoanalytic Psychotherapy Training at Institute for Expressive Analysis, New York City, 1988–1991. This was an institute specifically created for creative arts therapists.

It may also be important to note that during this entire transition period in my life, from theatre to performance studies to drama therapy, I had been in a long-term Jungian analysis. I don't believe I could have become a therapist without this personal therapy.

A Deep Exploration of Mienczakowski's Method as the Necessary Foundation for Creating EDT

In 2002, after reading my student's research proposal on Mienczakowski, I began to immerse myself in all his writings on the topic of ethnodrama as a *research method*. Somewhere, around 2005, someone handed me a copy of Mienczakowski's dissertation (1995a). I made a copy of it. It became one of my central "go-to" resources for interpreting Mienczakowski's theory and practice of ethnodrama. I think perhaps the person who lent me that copy was Dr. Nisha Sajnani, who, at that time, was my Ph.D.-level research assistant for the first ethnodrama project. She analyzed this first ethnodrama production in her own dissertation, *Permeable Boundaries: Towards a Critical Collaborative Performance Pedagogy* (2010). Through a deep reading of all of these materials, I believe I established a firm foundation in what Mienczakowski's intentions were for his own creation – ethnodrama.

Mienczakowski's Definition for Ethnodrama as a Method of Research

From the beginning, Mienczakowski was concerned with the "theoretical and methodological ambitions of research." At the end of his doctoral dissertation, he writes: "The reconstruction of ethnographic research into consensually validated and open-ended forum health theatre represents an original, practical and viable methodology for bringing about individuated

---

1 In 1996, this would become the Alternate Training program at NADT for persons with an M.A. or Ph.D. in Theatre or Performance, or a graduate degree in a mental health professions. For information, see www.nadta.org/education-and-credentialing/become-a-bct.html.

emancipation through the conditions prescribed in this study" (1995a, p. 276). This statement underscores the major themes of his method. First of all, it is an ethnographic form of research that uses theatre to make the research report. Secondly, it is "consensually validated," meaning that the informants in the project must give their consent that the data is true and valid. This particular strategy is one of Mienczakowski's most significant and original contributions. I will review it in more detail, shortly. Finally, the purpose of the method is to catalyze an experience of "enlightenment" or "*emancipation.*" This latter may be the most important construct to understand, in terms of the ultimate value of Mienczakowski's method. In his dissertation, he goes to great lengths to describe and define what this means. Although he has written many articles, and many articles have been written about his work, I highly recommend the reading of his dissertation by anyone who wishes to understand the full scope of the ethnodrama method.

Between 2002 and 2004, as I dug into Mienczakowski's writings, I discovered one definition of his method that really resonated with me. In his chapter in the *Handbook of Ethnography*, (2001) he states:

> ethnodrama is explicitly concerned with decoding and rendering accessible the culturally specific signs, symbols, aesthetics, behaviours, language and experiences of health informants using accepted theatrical practice. It seeks to perform research findings in a language and code accessible to its wide audiences.
>
> (p. 468)

This definitely brought me back to my study of Geertz and his semiotic approach to culture (1973). I felt very close to the ideas of looking at "specific signs, symbols, aesthetics, behaviours, language and experiences" of a group. Hadn't I done that with the performance of ethnohistory at Plimoth Plantation? And, I could really understand how Mienczakowski had looked at these elements in persons with **schizophrenia** in his very first ethnodrama called "*Syncing Out Loud.*" It was between 1987 and 1992 that I had spent five years as a drama therapist and participant/observer at Bronx Psychiatric Center. I really related to the exploration of the "nitty-gritty" elements that constitute the "cultural" realities of a specific group that shares a great deal of common experience. In the Bronx, I had done several therapeutic theatre pieces on the cultural life of my patients. One in particular was about their personal experience with many years of psychopharmacological treatment and its effects on them. There were many specific codes connected to these shared experiences that we presented in the form of a play. So, I agree with Mienczakowski's assertion that the "reconstruction of ethnography into a validated research report in play form, which is appropriate to both academic and informant needs, is a new interpretation of *research practice*" (italics mine, 1995a, p. 278).

The data of the lived experiences of informants is collected through ethnographic interviews and focus groups. It is important to note that this is all done in a participatory action research framework. Everyone involved in the process of exploring the theme of the play is an equal partner in the research endeavor (Chevalier & Buckles, 2019). As he confirms, Mienczakowski's goal in the creation of his method was "to construct a new form of action research which utilizes participatory and 'interactional' theatre to negotiate and construct understanding and meanings with participants and audiences" (Mienczakowski & Morgan, 2001, p. 219). It is this very democratic approach to process and communication that establishes his method as a new form of ethnography. In this period, anthropology was under the gun for its colonialist heritage. An expert comes in from outside the given culture and writes an expert report, a monograph, on that specific culture, without giving anything back. This point of view and practice was being harshly criticized at the time Mienczakowski was studying ethnography (Trouillot, 1991). He found a solution to the problem through putting the control of the data and its presentation back into the hands of the informant.

The Powerful Innovation of Informant Validation

In focusing on health systems, where patients are often highly marginalized and disempowered, Mienczakowski found a way in his research to create a more even playing field. In his dissertation, he delineates this approach in detail:

> In order to overcome this lack of interpretive neutrality, a multi-voiced narrative and processes of *extensive validation are used to guarantee reliability and authenticity of meaning in the plays*. The guarantees are that the ethno-drama plays faithfully construct a reality in the language of and recognizable by its respondents; the plays reflect the agendas of concern and values of the respondents and that the artifice of literary construction and fictional penetration, inferred in all report construction process, is limited to *only that which is agreed upon by the respondents*.
> (italics mine, 1995a, p. 123)

He uses the term "respondents" and "informants," interchangeably. These are the participants who are consensually giving all the information on their lived experience; in the two ethnodramas that are the basis of his dissertation, these were persons with schizophrenia or those who experienced addiction to alcohol and drugs.

This technique of giving the informants the opportunity to review and finally approve of the material to be presented is called "Informant Validation." It plays a crucial role in the process of ethnodrama. As Mienczakowski relates, "The public performance of ethnography in the argot of its informants may be argued to de-academize the report construction process. Significantly, ethnodrama also returns *the ownership*, and, therefore, the power of the report to its informants" (2001, p. 471). This happens at two major junctions of the process: first of all, when the draft of the script is completed, the informants are asked to review, correct, edit and add to it; secondly, at the time when the performance is fully prepared, again, the informants are asked to review it and to critique it; it can only go forward to public performance when it is validated by them. This is a wonderful ethical way to confirm the authenticity of the performed report. As one might imagine, it can also be very challenging when there is a production schedule to adhere to. It was also developed more for the type of ethnodrama where the informants and performers are different people. I have done much more of what Mienczakowski calls the "confrontational" format for ethnodrama (Mienczakowski, Smith & Sinclair, 1996, p. 441), where the informants *are also the performers*. I will describe the challenges with this approach in the next chapter.

The Concept of Emancipation

One of the most exciting, dynamic and complex concepts in Mienczakowski's method is that of "Emancipation." All in all, it may be *the* most important concept. In developing his own theory of emancipation, he draws heavily on the works of Habermas (1992), Foucault (1972), Alberoni (1984) and Freire (1978). In a 1997 article in *Research in Drama Education*, he discusses taking a workshop with Augusto Boal in order to better understand the "emancipatory pedagogy" of the great Brazilian director/teacher who wrote *Theatre of the Oppressed* (1979). He was investigating Boal's use of theatre to confront political and systematic forms of oppression. It was very much in alignment with his own construct for relieving systematic oppression from healthcare systems. As he writes:

> Our performances come under the umbrella of a postmodern critical pedagogy which seeks to overcome the oppressive identifications and circumstances in health understandings. If we are very lucky, and we have been at times, the audiences of our ethno-dramas leave the auditorium changed in some way. In some cases, they have even claimed to have changed or modified their professional behaviours because of the staged interactions in which they have participated.
>
> (1997, p. 166)

Like Brecht and Boal, Mienczakowski's is an instructive theatre. He wants to see the audience changed after the curtain goes down on the play. He builds his theory of emancipation in his dissertation, by exploring the thought of many writers who address critical emancipatory concepts, especially Habermas and Alberoni. Again, this dissertation is the major text revealing Mienczakowski's full development of his conceptualization of emancipation, "examining in detail the relationship between critical ethnography and its dramatic presentation and emancipatory potential" (1995a, p. 7). This concept is at the very core of ethnodrama and must be fully grasped to appreciate and apply the ethnodramatic method. It also leads to a vision of ethnodrama that has an investment in social activism, as one of its essential purposes is to change and eliminate oppressive systems in society. In terms of ethnodrama-therapy, this has led me to formulate a "Quadrated Model" that includes a fourth function for EDT, that of the social activist (See Figure 1.4). Change *is* the essential purpose of the ethnodrama/research report.

In regard to the conceptualizing in his dissertation, Mienczakowski states that one of the "central tenets of the thesis problem is the question of ascertaining

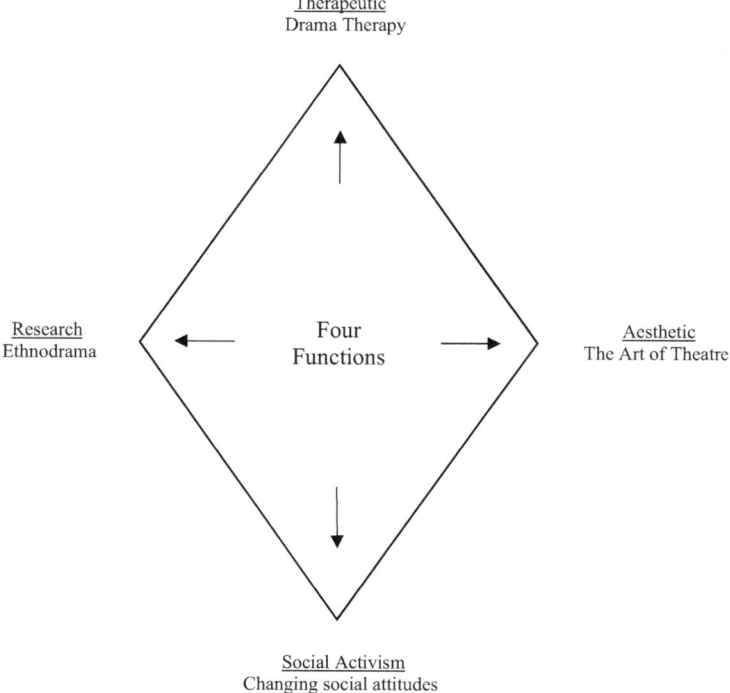

Figure 1.4   The Quadrated Model for EDT

emancipation as a recognizable outcome or product of ethno-drama" (1995a, p. 250). He frames this question with many theories of how to change systems but measures the effectiveness of producing an emancipatory experience in his informants and the audience through post-performance questionnaires and discussions. For his production of *Syncing Out Loud*, about the lived experience of schizophrenia, he documented through post-performance questionnaires how the health consumer informants felt that the play was "'insightful', 'therapeutic' and 'enlightening'," and how "Other comments described the performance as giving 'a great deal of insight into how other schizophrenics feel', and as 'relieving the stigma attached to mental illness'" (1995a, p. 261). Mienczakowski concludes: "I interpret this data as reflecting symbolic achievement (Alberoni, 1984) of emancipatory acts and insights as a direct result of the critical ethno-drama process" (1995a, p. 261). The questionnaire responses confirmed the effectiveness of the play.

A major focus for the emancipatory potential of ethnodrama is changing ideas, attitudes and perspectives of audience members. I have worked in a similar way as Mienczakowski, providing pre-and post-performance questionnaires to audience members. For instance, in *Through the Eyes of Caregivers* (see Chapter 5), we used questionnaires to see if the performance changed audience attitudes about mental illness. If we want to change and challenge deficits in our health systems, then everyone involved in them, administrators, government agencies, medical professionals and patients have to be in the audience and use the post-performance forums to strategize how to implement change.

Mienczakowski also focuses on change in the informants and in the actors, as well. This really caught my attention. Here is where his writing became very significant to me, as a therapist who wants to utilize the processes of theatre for *psychological* change. Mienczakowski writes: "Typically, critical ethno-dramas have been used in the training of nursing students and as health education and *therapeutic vehicles* for detoxing alcoholics and persons with schizophrenia" (italics mine, Mienczakowski, Smith & Sinclair, 1996, p. 457 n4). In this last phrase, I found a nugget that I wanted to unearth: how ethnodrama could also be used as a therapeutic experience for the participants. In fact, this is what led me to develop ethnodramatherapy.

References

Alberoni, F. (1984). *Movement and institution* (Trans. P. Arden Delmoro). Columbia University Press.

Aristotle. (1961). *Aristotle's poetics: With an introductory essay by Francis Fergusson* (Trans. S.H. Butcher). Hill & Wang (Original work published ca. 350 B.C.E.).

Boal, A. (1979). *Theatre of the Oppressed.* Urizen Books.

Butler, R. (1963). The life review: An interpretation of reminiscence in the aged. *Psychiatry, 26*(1), 6–76.

Charnow, S., Nash, E., & Perlstein, S. (1988). *Life review training manual.* Elders Share the Arts, Brooklyn, NY.

Chevalier, J.M., & Buckles, D. J. (Eds.) (2019). *Participatory action research: Theory and methods for engaged inquiry* (2nd ed.). Routledge.

Denzin, N. (2001). The reflexive interview and a performative social science. *Qualitative Research, 1*(1), 23–46.

Denzin, N. K. (2003). *Performance ethnography: Critical pedagogy and the politics of culture.* Sage Publications.

Emunah, R. (1994). *Acting for real: Drama therapy process, technique and performance.* Brunner/Mazel Publishers.

Foucault, M. (1972). *The archaeology of knowledge* (trans. A. Sheridan Smith). Tavistock Publications.

Freire, P. (1978). *Education for critical consciousness.* Seabury Press.

Geertz, C. (1973). *The interpretation of cultures.* Basic Books.

Gray, R., & Sinding, C. (2002). *Standing ovation: Performing social science research about cancer.* Altamira Press.

Gray, R., Fitch, M., Labrecque., M., & Greenberg, M. (2003). Reactions of health professionals to a research-based theatre production, *Journal of Cancer Education, 18*, 223–229.

Habermas, J. (1992). *Postmetaphysical thinking: Philosophical essays* (trans. W. M. Hohengarten). MIT Press.

Harding, J.M., & Rosenthal, C. (Eds.) (2011). *The rise of performance studies: Rethinking Richard Schechner's broad spectrum.* Palgrave Macmillan.

Hartigan, K.V. (2009). *Performance and cure: Drama and healing in ancient Greece and contemporary America.* Duckworth.

Jennings, S. (Ed.) (1992). *Dramatherapy: Theory and practice 2.* Routledge.

Jennings, S., Cattanach, A., Mitchell, S., Chesner, A., & Meldrum, B. (1994). *The handbook of dramatherapy.* Routledge.

Johnson, D.R., & Emunah, R. (Eds). (2009). *Current approaches in drama therapy* (2nd ed). C.C. Thomas Publisher.

_____. (2020). *Current approaches in drama therapy* (3rd ed.). C.C. Thomas Publisher.

Jones, P. (1996). *Drama as therapy, theatre as living*. Routledge.

_____. (2005). *The arts therapies: A revolution in healthcare*. Brunner-Routledge.

_____. (2007). *Drama as therapy: Theory, practice and research* (2nd ed., Vol. 1). Routledge.

_____. (2010). *Drama as therapy: Clinical work and research into practice* (Vol.2). Routledge.

Landy, R. (1986). *Drama therapy: Concepts and practices*. C.C. Thomas Publisher.

_____. (1993). *Persona and performance: The meaning of role in drama, therapy, and everyday life*. The Guilford Press.

_____. (2008). *The couch and the stage: Integrating words and action in psychotherapy*. Jason Aronson.

Lewis, P., & Johnson, D. R. (Eds.). (2000). *Current approaches in drama therapy*. C. C. Thomas Publisher.

Mienczakowski, J. (1995a). *The application of critical ethno-drama to health settings* [Unpublished doctoral dissertation]. Griffith University, Australia.

_____. (1995b). The theatre of ethnography: The reconstruction of ethnography with emancipatory potential. *Qualitative Inquiry, 1*(3), 360–375.

_____. (1997). Theatre of change. *Research in Drama Education, 2*(2), 159–172.

_____. (2001). Ethnodrama: Performed research – limitations and potential. In P. Atkinson, A. Coffey, S. Delamont, J. Lofland & L. Lofland (Eds.), *Handbook of Ethnography* (pp. 468–476). Sage Publications.

Mienczakowski, J., Smith, R., & Sinclair, M. (1996). On the road to catharsis: A theoretical framework for change. *Qualitative Inquiry, 2*(4), 439–462.

Mienczakowski, J., & Morgan, S. (2001). Ethnodrama: constructing participatory experiential and compelling action research through performance. In P. Reasons & H. Bradbury (Eds.), *Handbook of action research: concise paperback* (pp. 219–227). Sage Publications.

Oxford Dictionary of English. (2005). (2nd ed. Revised). Oxford University Press.

Pendzik, S., Emunah, R., & Johnson, D.R. (2016). *The self in performance: Autobiographical, self-revelatory, and autoethnographic forms of therapeutic theatre*. Palgrave Macmillan.

Sainer, A. (1975). *The radical theatre notebook*. Discus Books.

Sajnani, N. (2010). *Permeable boundaries: Toward a critical collaborative performance pedagogy* [Unpublished doctoral dissertation]. Concordia University, Montreal, Quebec, Canada.

Saldana, J. (1998). Ethical issues in an ethnographic performance text: the 'dramatic impact' of 'juicy stuff', *Research in Drama Education, 3* (2), 181–196.

_____. (Ed.). (2005). *Ethnodrama: An anthology of reality theatre.* Altamira Press.

_____. (2011). *Ethnotheatre: Research from page to stage.* Left Coast Press.

Schechner, R. (1973). *Environmental theatre.* Hawthorn.

_____. (1977). *Essays on performance theory, 1970–1976.* Drama Book Specialists.

_____. (1985). *Between theater & anthropology.* University of Pennsylvania Press.

Snow, S. (1986). *Theatrical outreach by the elderly: The value of sharing life stories through living history theatre* [Unpublished manuscript]. Wartburg Lutheran Home for the Aging, Brooklyn, New York.

_____. (1993). *Performing the Pilgrims: A study of ethnohistorical role-playing at Plimoth Plantation.* University Press of Mississippi.

_____. (1996). Focusing on mythic imagery in brief drama therapy with psychotic individual. In A. Gersie (Ed.). *Dramatic approaches to brief therapy* (pp. 213–235). Jessica Kingsley.

_____. (2009). Ritual/Theatre/Therapy. In D.R. Johnson & R. Emunah (Eds.), *Current approaches in drama therapy* (2nd ed., pp. 117–143). C.C. Thomas Publisher.

Snow, S., & Bleuer, J. (2020). Ethnodramatherapy. In D. R. Johnson & R. Emunah (Eds.), *Current approaches in drama therapy* (3rd ed., pp. 250–283). C. C. Thomas Publisher.

Snow, S., D'Amico, M., Tanguay, D., & Mongerson, E. (2005). Visually performed research: Creating theatre with adults with developmental disabilities through *ethnodrama.* Grant application to the Social Science and Humanities Research Council of Canada.

Snow, S., D'Amico, M., & Tanguay, D. (2003). Therapeutic theatre and well-being. *The Arts in Psychotherapy, 30,* 73–82.

Trouillot, M.R. (1991). Anthropology and the savage plot: The poetics and politics of others. In *Recapturing Anthropology: Working in the Present* (pp. 17–44). School of American Research Press.

Turner, V. (1978). Foreword. In B. Myerhoff, *Number our days: A triumph of continuity and culture among Jewish old people in an urban ghetto* (pp. xiii–xvii). Simon & Schuster.

_____. (1982). *From ritual to theatre: The human seriousness of play.* Performing Arts Journal Publications.

Turner, V., & Turner, E. (1982). Performing ethnography. *The Drama Review, 26*(2), 33–50.

2

The Seedbed of the New Method

The catharsis we are seeking is not only emotionally experienced but can be logically related to therapeutic strategies leading to individual change.

(Mienczakowski, Smith & Sinclair, 1996)

A Special Context

This chapter will describe how ethnodramatherapy was first conceived and formulated in the context of developing the first ethnodrama at The Centre for the Arts in Human Development (CAHD) at Concordia University in Montreal. One of the main game-changing discoveries was that Mienczakowski had already envisioned a therapeutic function for ethnodrama (see epigraph, above) and, in the context of CAHD, we were able to enhance and further develop this function, integrating our arts-based therapy process into the performance-based research framework. This began to define a new method: ethnodramatherapy. As this project was the "seedbed," where EDT was, in fact, conceived, I will delineate the process in full detail, so that those readers who might like to practice EDT in the future can get a complete grasp of the multiple steps involved in this synthesized method.

The Centre for the Arts in Human Development

The Centre for the Arts in Human Development, established in 1996, at Concordia University, is a research, clinical and educational center serving adults with intellectual and developmental disabilities, as well as other special needs populations. CAHD is presently a Research Unit within the Faculty of Fine Arts. The Centre has had an active partnership with this faculty since its founding through its research initiatives and graduate student education. Implementing both clinical practice, clinical training and dynamic

DOI: 10.4324/9781003083818-3

public outreach, along with multiple research projects, makes CAHD a unique Research Unit. This uniqueness is also grounded in its clinical approach which is based on a creative arts therapies' paradigm. **Art therapy, drama therapy, music therapy** and **dance movement therapy** are all utilized at CAHD, which has a close association with the Department of Creative Arts Therapies at Concordia. Many students fulfill part of their first-year practicum requirement working at CAHD. Students in creative arts therapies also participate in the research projects.[1]

The founders of CAHD are Lenore Vosberg, MSW, a social worker, Miranda D'Amico, Ph.D., an educational psychologist, and, myself, a drama therapist. We three presently serve as Director of Clinical Services and Public Outreach and the two Co-Directors of Research, respectively. CAHD has a long history of doing research in the creative arts therapies (Lister et al., 2009), especially performance-based research (Snow in Lewis & Johnson, 2000; Snow in Johnson & Emunah, 2009; D'Amico et al., 2014).

In 2003 (November) and in 2005 (both in January and October), we submitted research proposals to the Social Science and Humanities Research Council of Canada (SSHRC), to create a theatre production with our cohort of 20 adults with developmental disabilities, based on the ethnodrama method. The first two applications failed, but the third was successful. So, in April 2006, we received major funding for a three-year project, "Performance-based Research: Changing Perspectives on Developmental Disabilities through *Ethnodrama*." This was a project, similar to, but also different from, the performance-based research we had been implementing since 1994 (Snow & D'Amico in Johnson, Pendzik & Snow, 2012). In fact, the Centre was founded after our first therapeutic theatre piece, *Oh! That Aladdin …* in 1994. The productions in the first decade were all based on famous fairy tales. In 2006, we began to create theatre based on the actual life stories of our participants at CAHD.

The Tradition of Therapeutic Theatre at CAHD

This foundation of previously producing **therapeutic theatre** at CAHD was an excellent seedbed for adding a dynamic therapeutic component to our new work with ethnodrama.

So, what is "therapeutic theatre," then? And what was our "tradition" of this at CAHD?

---

1 For a complete profile of CAHD, visit its website at www.concordia.ca/finearts/research/cahd.html.

The concept of therapeutic theatre has been developed in the field of drama therapy for many years, now. As Emunah stated in 1994:

> Performance transforms notions about theatre and about therapy. The setting of the therapy scene changes from the closed room to public stage; the cast changes from client and therapist to client/*actor*, therapist/*director*, and outside *audience*. The therapeutic impact of performance is different from and often greater than process-oriented drama therapy.
>
> (p. 251)

In their recent co-edited book, *The Self in Performance* (2016), Pendzik, Emunah and Johnson make a simple differentiation between theatre that has a therapeutic purpose and that which does not: "*nontherapeutic* forms (where the aim in primarily artistic, educational and advocacy) and *therapeutic* forms (where the aim is personal growth)" (p. 2). When cursorily reviewing the ethnodrama literature, I would have said it fundamentally fits into the first form. However, when taking a much deeper look, I saw that it had the potential to fit into the latter. And, I began to realize that our unique context at CAHD could substantially actualize the therapeutic function, already present in ethnodrama (Mienczakowski et al., 1996).

After more than a decade of producing therapeutic theatre and thinking about it, I felt a real need to define it. In 2003, I set out to do just that. In "Therapeutic Theatre & Well-Being," my colleagues at CAHD and I state:

> To properly belong to its domain [therapeutic theatre], a play *must be developed with therapeutic intentions and goal-setting; be facilitated by a therapist skilled in drama or a drama therapist; and be brought to culmination in a performance for a community beyond the social sphere of the therapeutic group, itself* … And, finally, there [must] be *post-production processing by the group to deal with all the issues that have been provoked and evoked by the performance experience.*
>
> (Snow et al., 2003, pp. 75–76, emphasis in original)

Over the previous decade we developed a complex system of integrating the therapeutic work into the theatre productions. This always began with establishing therapeutic goals for each of the participants. We would follow the progress with these goals over the period of the play production, just as we would over the clinical year. The participants had already had two years of drama and art therapy, and one of music therapy and dance movement therapy, before we began devising and rehearsing the play. So, they were ready and, for the most part skillful, in various forms of creative expression. Transitioning from the clinical year (September to April), our professional consultants would shift their focus: the music therapist would become the composer and musical director; the dance movement therapist, the choreographer; the art therapist, the related art exhibition coordinator (and consultant with the scene and lighting designers); and the drama therapist would become the script writer and director. Each would bring their clinical training to this theatrical work, as well as their artistic training. For instance, in our 1994 production of *Oh! That Aladdin …* the young man in the starring role of Aladdin had been physically abused as a child in various foster homes that he lived in. He carried these emotional scars, and it was hard for him to open up. The music therapist, as his vocal coach, used certain music therapy techniques to help open him up, emotionally. He sang his major solo, a song called "I am Someone," with such authenticity that an audience of 400 people, instantaneously stood and gave him a standing ovation – a powerful validation of his personhood and a powerful moment of theatre (Snow in Lewis & Johnson, 2000).

Over this period (1994 to 2004), we worked with fairy tales like *The Wizard of Oz*, *Alice in Wonderland* and *Pinocchio*, not because they are classics of children's literature, but, as Bruno Bettelheim points out (1975), because they often reflect the initiatory journey of a hero or heroine. From my own point of view, the archetypal symbols in the story and the ritual process of creating a drama can have a therapeutic effect. During this period, I was using a kind of Jungian approach to activate the symbolic values of healing in these powerful stories and have them embodied in theatrical art (Snow in Lewis & Johnson, 2000). I had established this approach, earlier, in my work with psychiatric patients (Snow in Gersie, 1996).

We had established a pattern at CAHD that, at the end of the second year of a cohort, we would produce a large-scale therapeutic theatre production. It became a definite ritual expectation of the cohort, each spring of the second year in their program. There were two other components that also enhanced therapeutic potential. By *Pinocchio* (2002), we began to realize, a *therapeutic community* was being established during the two clinical years. Working on their therapeutic goals in groups, eating together, attending community meetings, waiting in a common room for transportation to and from the Centre, all these experiences created coherency and trust in the group. Not that its was without problems and challenging issues of group dynamics, but it did seem to provide "a milieu that will maximize therapeutic effort" in Sharp's definition of *therapeutic community* (1975, p. 24). The two clinical years led into the ensemble play creation; then, participants were offered a third year to process their experience at CAHD.

Secondly, from 1998, we had been developing a method of **assessment** through an improvisational enactment, "The Drama Therapy Role-Play Interview," created by myself and two student assistants, with the advisement of Dr. Miranda D'Amico (Snow, Maeng-Cleveland & Steinfort in Snow & D'Amico, 2009). This assessment tool became more and more valuable, as we developed it, as a way to discern speech skills, performance skills, empathy, and concentration and focusing ability. Towards the end, knowing we would be using it as a kind of audition method for the therapeutic theatre productions, we even put in a testing category, called "Ability to Follow Directions." This became an invaluable resource for casting participants in the most potentially therapeutic role for them. Case examples of this are described in detail in our chapter, "Casting the Healing Role: Assessment in Therapeutic Theatre" (Snow & D'Amico in Johnson, Pendzik & Snow, 2012).

It is interesting to note in regard to the therapeutic potential of our play productions: past research had shown that the greatest therapeutic gain for our participants was not in the clinical year, but actually during the time of creating the therapeutic theatre productions (D'Amico et al., 1998).

Measurement in the Research Process at CAHD

The transition from fairy tales to autobiographical stories of participants was an enormous shift, but it was very clear that the therapeutic procedure that we had developed for the former therapeutic theatre projects would be equally effective with ethnodrama, and we used our research to evidence this phenomenon.

Ethnodrama is primarily a performance-based research method with an expectation for evaluation and measurement of its effects on audiences. This is clearly articulated in Mienczakowski's dissertation: "Data were recorded indicating the effectiveness of the critical ethno-drama process to produce both insight and explanation. Data were also gathered on the methodology's potential to generate discussion and to alter paradigmatic understanding" (1995a, p. 267). Our model of therapeutic theatre at CAHD also had a frame for evaluating the effects of the play experience on the therapeutic goals set for the participants: "Pre- and post-interviews ... were conducted to measure the therapeutic benefits of a public performance in a play production for individuals with diverse intellectual and developmental disabilities" (Snow et al., 2003, p. 77). Our focus was the "growth" of the informants; the value of the experience to their enhanced psychological well-being. In the end, we considered that: "From the qualitative evaluation of 'running records' and the comparison of pre- and post-performance interviews, it would seem that the therapeutic goals for participants in the *Legend of Pinocchio* were accomplished" (Snow et al., 2003, p. 81). These accomplishments included reduced sense of stigmatization, enhanced interpersonal skills, improved self-confidence, increased capacity for spontaneity and freedom of expression and a more positive sense of self (Snow et al., 2003, p. 81).

CAHD was well set up to take on the research protocol required by ethnodrama. The major difference was that the ethnodrama research focuses mainly on the effects on the audience, whereas the therapeutic theatre evaluations are aimed at measuring emotional and psychological effects on the participants/actors. In the beginning, to merge these two perspectives in our first ethnodrama research project at CAHD (2006–2008), we looked to the potential to gather data on measurements for both the audience response and the informant/actors' therapeutic experience. This was to become a major frame of the research as we developed ethnodramatherapy over the next 15 years: *how to evidence both the therapeutic and educational value of the whole process from workshop to performance to post-performance forum?* As shall be seen, there were many challenges to this research goal.

The Game Plan

Having finally received funding for our ethnodrama research project in spring 2006, we went to work further developing our research design, which would be implemented in fall 2006. Because it took three times to acquire the grant funding from SSHRC, we had a long opportunity to review Mienczakowski's method, *very thoroughly*. It was in this period that I came to realize that his method already suggested a potential therapeutic framework. For this reason, one of the goals for our project was stated, thusly:

> as the Centre operates specifically under a Creative Arts Therapies paradigm, with the goal of using the arts as instruments of healing, rehabilitation and development, the theatrical production created through the *ethnodramatic* approach may help the participants experience *catharsis* that "is not only emotionally experienced but can be logically related to therapeutic strategies leading to individual change" (Mienzakowski, Smith & Sinclair, 1996, p. 445). So, in this way, the methodology of *ethnodrama* aligns itself perfectly with the mandate of The Centre for the Arts in Human Development.
>
> (Snow, 2005–2008)

In spring and summer of 2005 we were refining a game plan to utilize the ethnodrama method with our cohort of 20 adults with developmental disabilities. We would use this method as a way of "relating postmodern critical theory to health settings" (Mienczakowski et al., 1996, p. 439) in order to enlighten our audiences about their special needs and special ways of perceiving reality, with the ultimate goal of improving health services for this population. At least, this was our plan as we started out. And this was strictly aligned with Mienczakowski's earlier work with individuals with schizophrenia and persons in drug detox (1995a), with the exception that, in these two ethnodrama projects, *actors performed the stories of the informants.*

The Model in Mienczakowski's "Confrontational Theatre"

We were planning on having our cohort of 20 informants *also be the performers*, as this was the tradition at CAHD. Performance in our therapeutic theatre productions was part of their therapeutic process. We found a model for this in Mienczakowski's case study of what he designated as "Confrontational Theatre" (Mienczakowski et al., 1996). His team, in 1995, created an ethnodrama project called "A Good Smack in the Head," focused on the lived experience of informant/performers with brain damage. In a footnote in their article on this project, they define "Confrontational Theatre," as "a form of research-based theater that operates through intentional emotional confrontations with its audiences" (1996, p. 457 n1). What "confrontation" seems to mean here is the goal of waking the audience up to problematic practices in health service for this population. They give an example which I found inspiring. I will describe it in detail, here, as it epitomizes the emancipatory potential of this form of theatre. In this moment, an informant/actor had just completed a scene about the routine questioning of a brain-injured patient by doctors in which they talked about him as if he wasn't present. The performer/patient was playing himself, so this was an authentic incident. He tells this story with the anger he felt being trapped in a body that could not respond and articulate his feelings and sense of humiliation in a powerful way (Mienczakowski et al., 1996). After the performance a doctor in the audience shared her own reaction to this scene:

> The doctor was sort of excited and shaky, emotional. She didn't know where to begin. "That was me!" she said. You know. Really surprised. "I've been doing that, doing that for years." She was devastated. She described it as a sort of realization, like she knew she was talking to a person, but because they'd had a bash on the head or a tumor and couldn't reply to her, she assumed they were veggies even though she was working in the hospital to prove just the opposite.
>
> (Personal conversation as quoted in Mienczakowski et al., 1996, p. 443)

This is a dynamic example of how ethnodrama can produce enlightenment in health providers and, therefore, have the capacity to change a health system. As Mienczakowski states: "the critical ethno-drama process precipitates reflexive emancipatory insights amongst health service providers and the health community at large" (1995a, p. 276). This was our goal for our project. I must have quoted this anecdote to our research team, as a model for our work, a dozen times! We also intended our research-based theatre to effect changes in the health system related to developmental disabilities.

There were many similarities of our project to Mienczakowski's ethno-drama research about the lived experience of persons with brain damage. As the director and coauthor of this production wrote: "our performances end with everybody doing a 'therapy thing' and hugging the cast members" (Mienczakowski et al., 1996, p. 442). This would often happen at the end of our own performances when we played Bob Marley's "One Love," in a final moment of communal sharing, as part of the curtain call. Audience members would come directly onto the stage to emotionally embrace the actors (Snow & Herbison, 2012).

There were some big differences, as well. Our production was not so harshly confrontational. It was ultimately titled by the informant/actors, themselves, "It's A Wonderful World" and they chose Louis Armstrong's singing the song of the same name for the opening entrance of the performers. However, the dark and light of their personal experiences were shared with the audiences. In this way our central goal was the same as Mienczakowski's team: "to produce active emotional responses from health audiences and evolve critical and intellectual and emotional awareness that (potentially) will become the foundations for constructing political and social action" (Mienczakowski et al., 1996, p. 454).

A Challenging Ethics Review

For students and professionals who might wish to practice EDT, this section provides a good profile of the "facts of life" in regard to requirements of **ethics review**s for this kind of research. As with all research projects that include work with human subjects, our university ethics board, the Human Research Ethics Committee (HREC), requires a Summary Protocol Form, a complete outline of the project, to be completed, reviewed and passed by the committee, *before* any research can begin. So, in order to get a little "ahead of the game," we submitted a **Summary Protocol Form (SPF)** for our ethnodrama project in September 2005, with the hope that we would receive the grant. The main reason for this was the big topic asked in section 4 of the

SPF: "Assessment of Risks to Subjects' Physical Wellbeing, Psychological Welfare, and/or Reputation" (Concordia University SPF Form, 2003, p. 7). We knew we were dealing with an "at-Risk" situation by unearthing personal stories of individuals that were already potentially in the "fragile" category.

Who were these participants to be? These were 18 individuals between the ages of 19 and mid-forties, all with some kind of developmental disability. They were the fifth cohort to go through the CAHD program since 1996. The rubric, "developmental disability," covers many diagnoses and syndromes. All of the participants had some degree of intellectual challenge, mostly in the moderate range. Actual diagnoses in the group included **Down's syndrome**, **Autism**, **Tourette's syndrome**, **Asperger's syndrome** and **ADHD**. We had two individuals who did not speak (one a **selective mute**) and four with **epilepsy**. One individual had **cerebral palsy** and was in a wheelchair.

With all the potential physical and psychological hazards involved, it was not surprising that the HREC rejected our first SPF and asked for more information. As they wrote on October 13, 2005: "As your protocol requires more than minimal levels of risk (participants with an impaired ability to consent), you must establish adequate peer review" (Reid, 2005), p. 1). We immediately reached out to two psychiatrists, who taught at McGill University and were familiar with our work at CAHD. They supplied the necessary "Peer Review." One by one we answered the HREC queries. We were asked to write our information letter and consent forms in a lower than grade 7 reading format. One of the normal HREC questions is about discovering "problematic situations," such as suspected abuse or inadequate care of one of our participants. We were asked to be sure there were adequate resources in case of a "heinous discovery, or if participation should in anyway cause emotional harm for those involved" (Reid, 2005, p. 2). As we were planning to deeply explore the personal stories of our participants, we made sure to answer these questions, carefully and sensitively. By November 7, we answered all queries and shortly after this received our **Ethics Certificate** to move ahead with our project. This turned out to be good practice, *as every research protocol we would develop in the next 15 years* would require this kind of scrutiny and careful articulation, usually more than once, by an HREC. In the end, we must have done a good job for this one, as Adela Reid, the Research Compliance Officer at Concordia, eventually used our project as a model for an article she published with a colleague, "Ethics Review for Qualitative Inquiry: Adopting a Values-based Facilitative Approach (Connolly & Reid, 2007).

By September 2006, we had all the funds necessary to support our three-year research project in the performance-based method of ethnodrama. We also had some extra funding made available through a foundation that supported CAHD. That fall, our cohort was entering their second year as participants in the CAHD program. Our research design was in place; we had reviewed their backgrounds, very carefully. We had earned our Certificate for Ethics Approval. We were ready to go.

The Process

It Began with Playback Theatre

Playback theatre was to play a very big part in our process. One year before, on October 28, 2005, we began a special form of meeting with Group 5. We were looking for a way to gently introduce the group to self-revelatory storytelling. Knowing that personal story and experience would be at the very heart of our ethnodrama project, we looked for a highly sensitive tool to evoke and capture self-narrative. We found it in the drama therapy technique of playback theatre (Salas in Johnson & Emunah, 2009).

Playback theatre is a wonderful technique used by drama therapists all across the world. It was created by Jonathan Fox, in 1975, as a way to serve the community by finding "effective dramatic forms for the enactment of any and all personal stories" (Fox, 1994, p. 3). As he says in the Foreword to his wife and creative partner Jo Salas's book, *Improvising Real Life: Personal Story in Playback Theatre*, "I envisioned citizen actors in towns and cities everywhere acting out stories of their people" (Fox in Salas, 1993, p. i). A group of my drama therapy MA students volunteered to come to the Centre at noon on Fridays and present an improvised performance of playback theatre, so our participants could tell their stories and see them performed on the spot. This was inoculating them with the sensibility of sharing stories and, at the same time, creating what Armand Volkas calls a "culture of empathy" (Volkas in Johnson and Emunah, 2009, p. 148). We did this from October 2005 to March 2006, even before we received the SSHRC grant in April!

In September 2006, we sent out a letter of information, along with a consent form, to all the prospective research subjects in Group 5. We wanted to explain what our ethnodrama process would be and that playback theatre would still be a part of it:

> Last year after lunch on Fridays everybody did Playback Theatre together. Just to remind you, Playback Theatre was the special kind of theatre that helped you tell stories about your life to the group. It can help people let others know what their lives are like. It can help people let others know

how they feel. Then people can understand each other better … [*Please notice the simple language level used to explain the complex concepts. This had been a requirement of the HREC. This information letter was meant to assist the participants in understanding the whole research program, before they signed their consent forms*]

[the letter continues]

> Here is a reminder of how Playback Theatre happens. Somebody wants to tell a story, then the other people in the group show how they understand the story. They might use role-playing, movement and puppets. They might also use music, dance and song to do this. The person who told the story gets to say if what they did feels right or not. Sometimes the whole group can tell a story together in this way. Playback Theatre will be an important way stories for the play will be developed in this project.
>
> (Snow & Anthony, 2006)

Here, we are reminding the group that we will deeply share stories from their lives, and playback is the vehicle. Playback theatre is an improvisational form of theatre in which an audience member, ready to tell a personal story, voluntarily comes up to the Teller's Chair, just between the Conductor and the actors (usually four) who are seated towards the back of the playing area. To their left (stage left) is a musician with musical instruments, and further upstage, a step ladder with many colored materials (often scarves) on it. The Conductor is a kind of MC and facilitator for the story; he/she needs to be a profoundly empathic listener. The Conductor asks the Teller to tell their story. As the Teller begins to narrate their real-life experience (this is the one absolute requirement of playback: *it must be something that actually happened to you, personally*), the Conductor casts the actors in the roles, asking the Teller for a few words to describe the characters in their story. When all roles are cast, the Conductor succinctly recapitulates the story and, then, may ask the Teller to give their story a title as if it was a novel or a movie. At this point, the Conductor says, "Let's watch!" and the actors respectfully create an improvisational performance of the Teller's story. When they are done, they often make the gesture of a gift to the Teller. The Conductor asks the Teller if the performance was true to their story, and, if so, to thank the actors. In closing, the Conductor thanks the Teller for sharing his story. There is one other main possibility. If the Teller felt the portrayal of their story was way off, then the Conductor can offer to Correct or Transform it, but this is a fairly rare occurrence.

This is an extremely simplistic formulation of a nuanced and complex art form that is practiced all over the world (Fox & Dauber, 1999). I was fortunate in that I had been given the opportunity to fully train with Jonathan

Fox and Jo Salas, over several years, and, by the time we began this project, I was a certified playback theatre practitioner, having conducted or performed in hundreds of playback performances. I knew the techniques very well.

So, in fall 2005, we created the context for using playback, and, in fall 2006, we began to utilize it as a way to collect stories for our ethnodrama on what it is like to live the life of a person with a developmental disability. Let me give one example. We will call this individual "George." He was a 32-year-old client diagnosed with mild cerebral palsy, in the moderately intellectually handicapped range. Like many of the participants, he offered up a simple but very beautiful story for a Playback session. It was about his joy at becoming an uncle. He described the whole circumstance with his family and the celebration at their household and how he was allowed to hold the newborn infant. This sent him into a kind of rapture. It was acted out and someone else played himself and his family. The musician accompanied it with appropriate joyful music. It was a good playback of his life experience, and he got great pleasure from it.

Later on, when we developed the ethnodrama play script and had decided that "Small Pleasures" was an important theme, George performed a piece of this story, himself, with a prop baby (a wrapped up blue scarf) in his arms, as a monologue:

This is my story
I like to hold my little nephew

And this baby to me is very special.
When I hold him I feel him, I love him,

And I care about him.
And when I feel him I want him to know,
I like him a lot,
And I care about him,
And I was an uncle to him.

This is a good example of how the eventual ethnodrama performance was distilled from the two years of playback theatre workshops. In fact, our goal was to train the participants, so that eventually they could practice the playback method, themselves, as Conductors, Tellers, actors and musicians. This was part and parcel of the therapeutic goal of enhancing individual autonomy as part of our process. And by 2007, this goal was attained as can be seen in the first scene in our documentary, "In Their Own Voices" (Snow & Herbison, 2012).

Playback theatre has become a major part of the ethnodramatherapy tool kit. It blends in beautifully with the search for authentic narrative. It can also be, and is used, as a therapeutic method, especially in its workshop format (Salas in Johnson & Emunah, 2009). Although essentially an improvisational theatre form, it has an underlying purpose of healing. As Jo Salas writes: "Art and healing are both irreducibly part of this work" (1993, p. 130). And this correlates specifically with the therapeutic and aesthetic functions of EDT (Figure 1.1).

The Creative Arts Therapies Groups

As with the playback theatre process, we created workshops in all the creative art therapies, with the same purpose of locating powerful authentic narratives of personal experience.

In the same Information Letter of September 2006, we wrote to the participants:

> In the Ethnodrama Project you will also be in an art group, a music group and a dance/movement group, as well as the Playback group. In these groups you can explore ways to make pictures, make music, and move and dance to tell your stories. You will also have a chance to explore a true-life story by using a sand tray and figurines.
>
> (Snow & Anthony, 2006, p. 2)

All of these groups, led by either professionals or M.A. student interns guided by professionals in the field of creative arts therapies, were implemented in fall 2006. They were the nitty-gritty processes out of which we would evolve the script.

An art therapy intern came up with the idea of each participant creating a "life box" that would be a graphic portrayal of their life. This led to many powerful self-explorations that would be expressed through painting, drawing and sculpture. As with all the expressive workshops, we set up a system of recording, so that material could be reported to the whole research team, using codes for the real participant's name. These notes turned out to be extremely useful in developing the collective theme of the play. Here is an example of a note on a participant we will call "Perry."

> [Perry] made a box about "passion" which he may have confused with "compassion." He spoke about his box being like the collection box at church. He said that people fill the box with passion to help the poor and

the sick people. The main theme for him this week was altruism. He was very happy to be able to do something to help other people.

(Student Intern Notes from October 11, 2006)

Another art therapy intern led a group in **sandplay therapy**, a form of therapy in which the client creates a small world by placing figurines in a 22 inch by 29 inch by 3 inch tray filled with sand (Ammann, 1991). Here is a note on a "world" by participant, "Don," with description and notes by the intern:

[Don]:

The couple is dancing in the house. The dove is swimming in the river. The horse goes to see the couple. It's a sunny day. The boss is walking, he is a mean boss. The couple works for the boss. The couple is dancing, and they're happy. The horse is galloping and the dove is swimming. The couple gets married. They get married in Spring, in a church. Their family is there, but they don't invite the boss. After they all go to the house to party. Confetti is falling down on them.

[Don] seemed to really enjoy the sensorial aspect of the sand and played with it, pouring it on top of the figurines, especially the couple. He kept taking away the sand to make a lake for the dove, then would put the sand back and would then take it away again many times.

(Student Intern Notes from October 24, 2006)

Don was an individual with fragile x syndrome, with some autistic features. Not very verbal, sandplay was a great way to "enter his world" and get a full sense of him. This was true for many of this group with developmental disabilities. As Tanguay writes:

Individuals with developmental disabilities present the researcher with a challenge when it comes to psychological assessment … sandtray assessment deserves close attention. It uses the body without necessitating fine motor skills, and it appeals to a natural tendency in the human being, that of play.

(Tanguay in Snow & D'Amico, 2009, p. 219)

These "self-portraits" expressed in sand were often very powerful and sometimes we used them as scenographic backgrounds (projected slides) in the play (see Figure 2.1), because they felt like such an authentic portrait of the inner world of our participants. In fact, in one part of the play, Don played music on a small xylophone, as various art and sandplay images on the theme of "Longings" were projected.

Music therapy and dance movement therapy were used in a similar way: to address major issues in the lives of the participants and to help them tell *their* stories through music and dance.

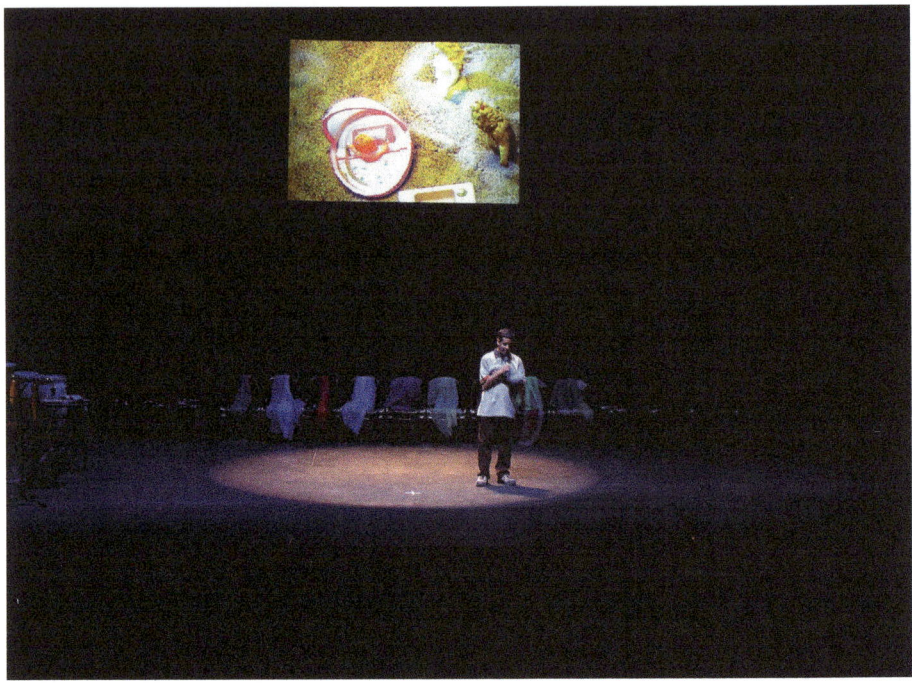

Figure 2.1   "George" Performing His Personal Story on Becoming an Uncle (photo courtesy of Eric Mongerson)

Dr. Shelley Snow, the Centre's music therapist, published an article on the project in the *Canadian Journal of Music Therapy* (Snow et al., 2008), in which she explains how she adapted a special form of "Community Music Therapy" for both group and individual work in the project. She writes:

> In group musical improvisations, much time was spent exploring how to give expression to different feelings. The group would choose four and five different feelings to play and then reflect on how successful the improvisations were in expressing a particular feeling.
>
> (2008, p. 40)

This process greatly sensitized them to musical expression and to each other; again, enhancing the "culture of empathy" we were generating for the project. Dr. Snow, a seasoned music therapist, was quite impressed with the impact on the group, over time. She states: "The joy and spirit expressed by the clients in these groups – of which they took complete charge –was unparalleled in my experience as a music therapist" (2008, p. 41).

She also carefully delineated a case vignette of in-depth individual work with one participant: Annette. She worked with Annette, intensely, over the nine months of preparation that preceded the preview performances. Annette expressed a deep desire, an almost desperate desire, to be in the spotlight. Her formal interview gave details from Annette's life for the background of this longing. In her private session with the music therapist, "She began by expressing how important the arts were to her: 'I want to act,' she said. 'I want to sing – I want to perform. This is my life'" (2008, p. 42). Steering the process away from a narcissistic self-indulgence, the therapist listened sensitively to the client's deep-seeded need and helped her to develop lyrics for the song, helping the client overcome her vulnerability and fears. Snow writes: "Thus, the focus of our work became the creation and performance of a song using Annette's own words and embodying her own feelings about things that had important meaning to her" (2008, pp. 42–43). The intimacy involved in the therapeutic process was later manifested in the power of the performance. Here is the song that Annette sang, as her contribution to the ethnodrama:

> I want to act
> I want to sing
> I want to sing like Celine Dion
> I want to see
> my family
> I want to see them be proud of me
>
> 'Cause I'm here
> on the stage
> like princess in a play
> (verse repeats)
>
> Feeling good
> Feeling free
> This is what I want to be
>
> I want to be something in my life!

Thunderous applause. This was one of the highlights of the show.

The Centre's dance movement therapist, Joanabbey Sack, oversaw the movement groups and the choreography, much of it implemented by her students Farah Fancy, Dana Kneeland and Sylwia Dyjak. Again, both group and individual work was done in this modality. Throughout the process, the team would receive notes from the movement specialists on the development and progress of movement and dance expressions in the piece. Although, in the beginning these were often in the Effort/Shape language of dance movement therapy (Bartenieff & Davis,1965), by the last month, these were put in precise terms of choreography. Here is an example from April 11, 2007, in regard to a number based on a karaoke version of Celene Dion's "I'm alive."

> **Choreographed by**: the group of 8 performers.
>
> **Beginning**: [William] plays the steep pan to act as a conductor of the group.
>
> **Progression**: the group dances only when the steel pan plays, pauses in place when no music.
>
> **Big Movements**: movements that take up the entire space according to individual tastes
>
> **Ending**: all end together in frozen pose.
>
> **Visual**: impression/interpretation: A dance that shows active listening and cooperation.
>
> (Student Intern Notes from April 11, 2007)

This was the biggest production number in the show (Figure 2.2), largely based on William's extraordinary talent with the steel pan. William was a

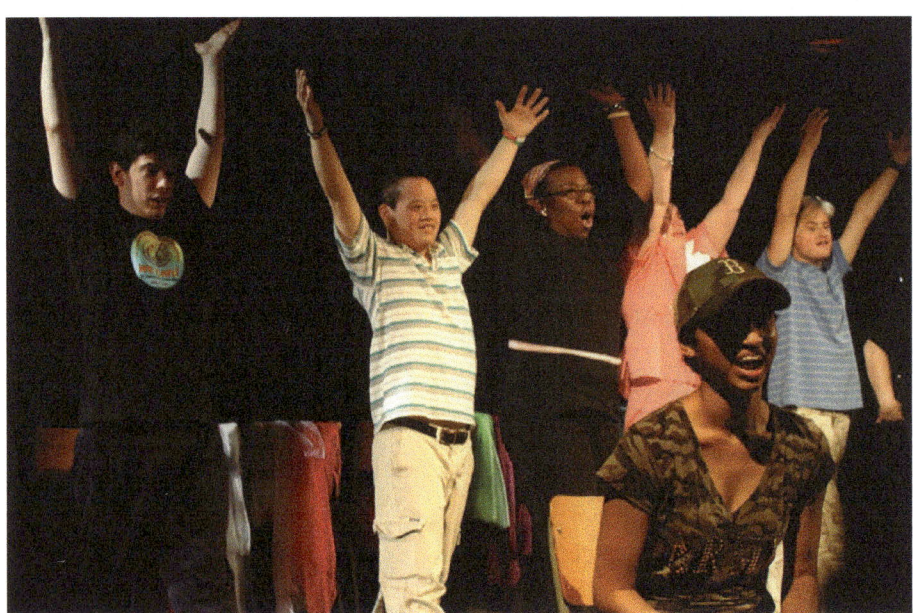

Figure 2.2   The Chorus Line for "I'm Alive!" (photo courtesy of CAHD)

29-year-old man with autism and epilepsy who was largely nonverbal. To some degree, this scene, which had various diagnoses of developmental disability simultaneously projected on the back screen, was meant to show the talent, creativity and humanity of this "population." Certainly, the movement work was another factor in creating the "culture of empathy" and the coherence of the ensemble.

The Weekly Drama Therapy Groups

We had also held two-hour workshops in drama therapy, every Wednesday, since September 13, 2006. These workshops followed **Emunah's Integrative Five Phase model** of drama therapy (1994, 2020). We utilized the first phase, "Dramatic Play," to build trust and confidence in the ensemble. To accomplish these goals, we employed basic sound and movement and trust exercises, many of these borrowed from Viola Spolin (1963) and experimental theatre, and adapted by Emunah for drama therapy. For example, we used "Group sounding the movement" in which one person in front creates a unique movement and the "…group makes sound or voices words that correspond to the person's motions" (Emunah, 1994, p. 155). We used dozens of exercises like this to catalyze a spirit of fun and play in the group; to get them warmed up to performing, especially in the frame of improvisation. Emunah's second phase, "Scenework" was most valuable in getting the group ready to perform scenes from their own lives. It should be remembered that most participants had already had two years of drama therapy groups by this point and were on very familiar territory, here. The main philosophy was to engage them in "drama reality" (Pendzik, 2012) in a safe and enjoyable way. In this case, "**dramatic reality**" meant the construction of a theatrical performance.

Each informant/performer was respected for their unique individuality; the drama therapy was focused on enhancing their individuality, autonomy and creative self-expression. Therapeutic goals were established for each participant. Many of these goals were around developing greater confidence in themselves and a positive **self-image**. As previously described, members of this group had many cognitive and physical challenges and these had to be taken into consideration in terms of staging and developing their performances. In the section on *Rehearsals*, I will delineate in detail a case example of one participant's therapeutic journey in the rehearsal process.

It was in exploring the third phase of Emunah's method that we developed the material for the play and simultaneously provided a therapy experience for the informant/performers. This stage, known as "Role Play," is where actual life experiences are rendered as dramatic scenes. As Emunah states:

> The stage becomes a laboratory setting in which real life can be explored and experimented with in safety … Through dramatization and ensuing discussion, clients gain a clearer view of the roles they play in life and the patterns that emerge in their interactions.
>
> (1996, p. 34)

Stories that spoke of their fears, their passions, their longings and their hopes were presented and explored through dramatic improvisation. These became scenes directed by a drama therapist, either myself or one of the research assistants. This was in the context of Emunah's major perspective that: "One of the primary means of intervention in drama therapy is through the direction of improvisational scenes" (1994, p. 111).

We also used improvisation to further explore scenes that had been established in the Friday playback theatre meetings. In fact, we used improvisation to explore everything. In this way, stories and ideas could be tried out several times, in several ways, before they were congealed, or set down for good. This is a principle practice in ethnodramatherapy. Also, in this way, other people could play the parts in someone else's story, to see what was most comfortable for the performers and, in this exchange, we also nurtured the desired "culture of empathy."

Drama therapy was the essential modus operandi in this endeavor to create a therapeutic performance based on autobiographical experience. Our approach was very much in agreement with Bailey's conception of the value of performance in drama therapy:

> Performing plays is a dynamic drama therapy approach which allows clients to expand and practice their role repertoire; gain confidence; be witnessed for their creativity, expressiveness and strengths; share their stories and ideas; and learn how to work more effectively with other people toward an end product that makes a difference.
>
> (Bailey in Johnson & Emunah, 2009, p. 387)

Interviews and Focus Groups

As Mienczakowski writes in his chapter in the *Handbook of Ethnography* (2001): "The development of ethnographic narratives into a full-scale performance vehicle is clearly an elaboration and enhancement of ongoing, world-wide interest in evolving ethnographic construction and practices" (p. 470). One of the main practices of ethnography is the use of interviews. As ethnographer Julian M. Murchison writes: "talking and *listening to* informants are key parts of the ethnographic process" (2010, p. 43). Along with all the modalities of creative arts therapies used to collect information, we also utilized the traditional practice of interviews with individual participants.

Here are the basic questions:

1. What story would you like to share today from your life or about yourself? (Whatever story you want to tell, we want it to have really happened in *your* life.)
2. Is there something you're proud of having done or accomplished in your life? Can you tell me about that?
3. What do you enjoy doing in your life?
4. How much fun do you get out of life? Little? Some? A lot?
5. How much control do you have over things you do every day, like going to bed, eating? Little? Some? Complete?
6. What do you want someone to know about your life so they could understand you better?
7. Is there anything you would like to do that you feel you can't?
8. If there's something you could change about your life, what would that be?
9. How would you go about making that change? Who might be there to help do that?
10. What do you think about yourself and what you're doing now in your life? (Prompt: How do you feel about yourself?)
11. What do you see yourself doing in the future?

(D'Amico, 2007)

These questions catalyzed many intimate responses about personal lived experience. We were following, here, Mienczakowski's directive to "allow respondents to explain themselves in their 'unique ways of defining the world'" (1995a, p. 160). It was these unique and idiosyncratic moments of experience that we wanted to capture in monologues that would become part of the play. To do this, we would follow up with the participant and further explore what had been presented in the interview. For example, one research assistant wrote these comments about "Mitchell," a 43-year-old man with a diagnosis of fragile x, with whom she was working:

> During the rehearsal [Mitchell] and I went over his interview and talked about what we might want to include in his monologue. Some ideas he wanted to talk about were:
>
> - the story he tells of seeing his girlfriend on the bus
> - working with his girlfriend
> - taking his girlfriend out on a date
> - marriage and children
> - intimacy (kissing and he got a big smile on his face when he talked about his girlfriend tickling him)
> - pet names (she calls him "teddy bear"
>
> (Student Intern Notes from May 19, 2007)

In fact, almost all of this information did end up in the brief, poignant monologue that Mitchell performed in the play.

The interview is a vital tool in the ethnodrama process. As Denzin reflects, "The performative sensibility turns interviews into performative texts, into poetic monologues" (2001, p. 25). In the context of trust that is built up between the interviewer and interviewee, very authentic moments can be captured. We will go much deeper into the dynamic role that the "reflexive interview" plays in the ethnodramatherapy method in Chapters 3, 4 and 5.

In searching for the most essential themes related to our research question, "What is it really like to live the life of a person with developmental disability?" we also implemented group discussions or focus groups. In one group, a lot of anger was evoked around the issue of being stigmatized and made fun of. Here is the description of that group by the research assistant who led the discussion:

> Main feelings were anger at people who make fun of people with disabilities; feeling vulnerable, desire to be recognized as strong and able to defend self. When participants expressed fear of being judged or made fun of by being in the play, we discussed how educating people can be a more effective way to change attitudes than physical violence ("Dora" and "Andrea" both wished to physically hurt people who had insulted or mistreated them). The courage and strength of the group members was emphasized. We talked about how this is a special group of people who can help prevent other people from being treated badly because of their differences, by making a play to teach others about what it is like to live with disabilities.
>
> (Student Intern Notes from November 20, 2006)

This group discussion identified a major theme that would eventually be represented in the play by a scene of people being arrested for proclaiming derogatory words about others. The idea came from one of the participants that "people should be arrested and put in jail for making fun of or denigrating others." And, a very positive expression of hope and advocacy came from one member of this group who designed an image for the flyer for the play (see Figure 2.3).

Scripting

After seven months of work, with all the various means we had for collecting information on the lives of our "research subjects" – "our informants" – we had an enormous amount of information. In my research office, I had kept a very large piece of paper on one of the walls, maybe 5 ft x 5ft. On this,

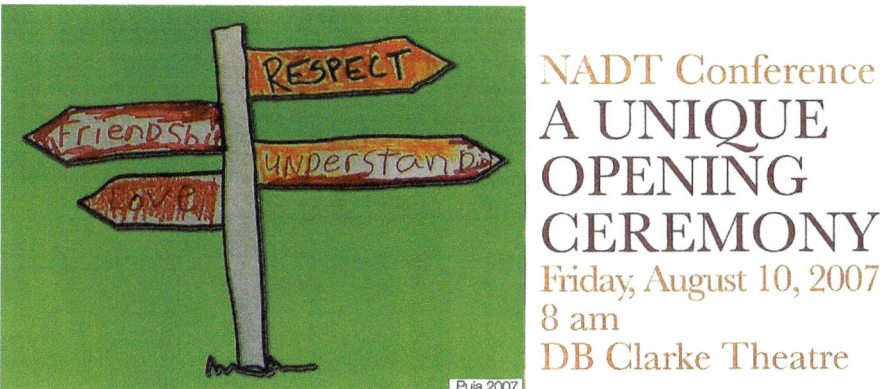

Figure 2.3   Poster for the NADTA Performance at 8am

I put all the major ideas that had arisen from the various groups, meetings and individual interviews that might be considered as the central themes for the ethnodrama play production. I would write thematic ideas in large colored letters, color-coding themes, and under these in black magic marker I wrote down scenes, songs, monologues and dances that would fit under each theme. I would highly recommend this to future practitioners of EDT as a great means for initial *mapping* of themes prior to script creation.

By March 2007, I had put a scenario together that organized all the material into seven sections by themes. The seven themes were: "Sources of Pride," "Small Pleasures," "Family and Friends," Vulnerabilities," "Romance, Love and Marriage," Stigma and Name-Calling" and "Desire for Independence and Dreams." This was the first step towards a full script that would contain everything to be said or done on stage. We would need this for cues to be called by the stage manager, and the lighting and sound technicians. A special stage was being designed by our long-time designer Eric Mongerson that would provide a very intimate atmosphere in a three-quarter format, with audience on raised platforms, in front and on each side.

At this point the scenario just had the theme heading and then, under it, an outline of the actions to take place on stage. For example:

SECTION 5: [SLIDE: "ROMANCE, LOVE AND MARRIAGE"]

Mitchell's Rhapsody on his girlfriend

Amy's PBT scene of "Fake Love"

Lucinda's PBT scene on meeting boyfriend on bus in Israel

Dora's monologue: "Being married is the most important thing …"

[**Statement of participants** about their desire for marriage within slides of their Sandtray and Art images. **Don** plays music underneath.]

By mid-March 2007, the script was completely articulated – everything to be done or said on stage was in it – and we had to go into the next important phase of the ethnodrama process: Informant Validation.

Informant Validation of the Script

As will be recalled, "Informant Validation" is one of the key strategies in Mienczakowksi's method, as it "returns the *ownership*, and, therefore the power, of the report to its informants" (Mienczakowski, 2001, p. 471). It should also be remembered that the script, at this point, actually represents a full research report on "What is it like to live the life of a person with a developmental disability?" All the material of the script had been constructed to create such a portrait of our group, literally embodying the essential meaning of *ethnography* (*graph*, a picture or portrait; *ethnos*, a group with deep common experience). Now, it was up to our informant/actors to tell us if the script represented a truthful portrayal. As Mienczakowski writes, the play/report must "reflect the agendas of concern and values of the respondents" and "the artifice of literary construction and fictional penetration, inferred in all construction process, is limited to only that which is agreed as real by all respondents" (1995a, p. 123).

In mid-March, we held a meeting with all 18 participants. The detailed draft script was read aloud, so all could hear it, clearly. Also, realizing some participants had very minimal reading skills, a clearly spoken version was the best option. Everything was discussed, some small changes were made, and the group agreed that the script was "real" in regard to authentically portraying their life experiences. At this time, they were also given the option to give the play a title. They choose "It's A Wonderful World." I don't remember exactly why, but it seemed to capture the essence of the life-affirming content in the script.

Rehearsals

Now, we were ready to go into full theatrical rehearsal mode. We had hired a professional stage manager, who had worked very effectively on a previous production with us. She had the "right" sensibility for working with our population and was very organized.

The value of improvisation in this kind of therapeutic theatre work is that you can discover contents of scenes that are aesthetically and dramatically effective and, then, frame and repeat those moments until they are memorized as words and actions. So, as we had spent months in the drama therapy workshops building these dramatic moments, it was not so difficult to bring them together for two months of rehearsal in April and May, 2007.

At this point, rehearsing an ethnodrama is like rehearsing any other kind of theatre production. As a director, I am looking for flow and an honest and skillful enactment of all the units. The main challenge was that this was a pretty big production with 18 actors, a "performance support team" of 17, and a production team of designers, choreographer, musicians, a wardrobe coordinator, etc. of more than a dozen. Our SSHRC grant allowed us to give the script a full artistic, theatrical embodiment, and we used every minute of rehearsal time left to us to be ready for the opening on June 7.

The major strategy we used to accomplish this was multiple rehearsals in multiple spaces, and the use of several assistant directors. We could break a rehearsal day down to some in music rehearsals, some in dance, group rehearsals of scenes and private rehearsals for monologues. Many of our team were used to the special contingencies of doing theatre with individuals with developmental disabilities (four participants with epilepsy!). The essential modus operandi is "safety first." We accomplished this through excellent stage management and having logistic coordinators, along with volunteers, whose goal it was to keep things safe. Finally, everyone on the production was made aware of the therapeutic goals of this project and therefore treated the participants with great sensitivity and care. A very strong feeling of trust had evolved in the group.

An Example of Adapting Drama Therapy for the Unique Requirements of One Informant/Performer

Truth be told, almost every informant/performer in this project had a physical or cognitive challenge that required special adaptation of drama therapy techniques to prepare them for their performances. One obvious case was Charlene who had minimal capacity for speech. We helped her create an onstage performance to express herself through hand-painting on a large fiberglass panel. She also did sign language for the "I'm Alive" production number (see Figure 2.2).

Here, I want to focus on the adaptations made for "Eliza." Twenty-four years old, at the time, she was diagnosed with epilepsy that manifested as petit-mal seizures on a regular basis. She also had a moderate intellectual disability. The goals set for her from her entry into the CAHD program in fall 2004 were: "to improve her social skills (encourage positive interactions with others and encourage awareness of and consideration of others) and to work on listening skills" (Notes from CAHD clinical files, 2006). She could be quite dominant in groups and, sometimes, very attention-seeking, even to the point of faking seizures. On the positive side, she took initiative, could express her feelings and really enjoyed music and drama. She had participated in a production of *Grease* a few years before she came to CAHD.

It was in the process of her individual interview for the EDT project that we discovered an issue that seemed very important to her. The question was: "If there was something you could change about your life, what would that be?" Her response was:

> Maybe moving out of my house … I would take my dog, take Pikachu with me, and we'd move to maybe another street … so I would move there, and I'd take Pikachu, put my stuff there and make my own meals, be independent like do my own medication for the week (sometimes I forget to take it!) … but I would definitely like to move out someday when I'm older. That's what I would like to do.
> (Interview at CAHD on March 7, 2007)

Like so many of our participants, her longing for autonomy was very strong. We looked at this as a healthy and age-appropriate desire. So, the team worked with Eliza on this in the frame of **surplus reality**, i.e. as a "dimension of alternative past, present and future events which are a 'reality' in our imagination, if not in the outside world" (Blatner, 1973, p. 73). The art therapist helped her create a beautiful painting of the house which in her imagination was turquoise and which, later, served as a projected background for her performance. The dance therapist assisted her in developing her movement skills for a performance on stage.

She was paired with a second-year drama therapy M.A. student who was trained in how to work with epileptic seizures and had a very good repertoire of drama therapy techniques that could be adapted to this situation. This student was also assigned the duty as "Performance Coach" for Eliza. The first step was to create a sense of safety through trust exercises like "Partner Blind Walks" (Emunah, 1994, p. 173), in order for the participant to feel safe in the rehearsal space and to build trust with her therapist. They worked together on developing her future projection of a house of her own into a monologue. These individual drama therapy and coaching sessions were designed so that Eliza could feel very confident in delivering her monologue. As I had previously written in a chapter on my earlier approach to therapeutic theatre, "The role of the drama therapist in this performative frame is multifocal and multivocal. The single most important function is integrating the therapeutic and the aesthetic, sacrificing neither for the other" (Snow in Johnson & Emunah, 2009, p. 131). That was equally true, here. I went on to describe how the role of the therapist is to pay "exquisite attention to the person," a phrase I had learned from drama therapist Remi Barclay (Snow in Johnson & Emunah, 2009, footnote on p. 131). The drama therapist/performance coach did exactly that. Through drama therapy exercises in voice, sound and movement, and concentration exercises (Emunah, 1994), she thoroughly prepared Eliza to feel confident in her own self-expression and to give a very strong performance of her monologue:

> There is a house in the neighborhood.
> I would like to move there some day,
> When I am older.
>
> I would like to be independent,
> Put my stuff there,
> And do my own medication for the week.
>
> I can see my house there all turquoise outside and inside.
> My bedroom will be blue,
> And my bed will be pokeman.
>
> There I will learn how to read, write and do math.
> I will take Pikachu with me,
> Because she is beautiful.

As far as I can recall, Eliza never had a seizure during her performance. But, we were ready if she did. She mastered the skill of the monologue and presented her unique individuality to the public. She learned to listen, very carefully. She developed better interpersonal skills through the collaborative process of creating a play. Without a doubt, her self-confidence grew. One of my most satisfying moments as a drama therapist/director was at the end of one show, when Eliza's father came up to me and said how proud he was of his daughter's performance and how he had seen her develop a new self-confidence.

The Performance

We opened the play production for three previews on June 7, 8 and 9, 2007. As an ethnodrama performance, it was "performed research" – again, the production, itself, was the "research report." It was also the culmination of two years of creative arts therapies at CAHD, coordinated now under the drama therapy paradigm of therapeutic theatre. As an ethnodrama, it was aiming "to use research and the public performance of research reports as a means to give insight into the lives of those who have become marginalized and disempowered through their relationships with health" (Mienczakowski, 1997, p. 163), i.e., what is it like to live with a developmental disability.

Tip of the Iceberg

As with any theatrical production, the performance represents just the "tip of the iceberg," founded on many months of building strong human bonds of trust and mutual respect; hours of developing moments to be performed, finally accepting what works the best and rejecting others; and, in our case, the coordination of a community of nearly 50 people, including informant/performers, performance coaches and the production team. As our performance was a pastiche of moments, collected from playback theatre, interviews, art, music, dance and drama workshops, it had a kaleidoscopic feel. One moment quickly flowed into another, making it difficult to capture in a written description as it was a *living performance*.

The set could not have been simpler: a black dance-type matted floor, semicircular, with the audience on three sides, seated on raised platforms. Wooden chairs and colored scarves were moved about and turned into everything. For example, in one informant's memory of a campfire sing-a-long, three chairs were piled up with red scarves on them. Our lighting designer placed a red light under the pile of chairs. Our sound designer created the crackling sound of fire. The performers set around it and warmed their hands.

Each of the main thematic units was introduced by a slide on the screen that filled the back of the performing space. One after another, scenes that represented simple moments of their own experiences were portrayed. One actor expressed how in real life he gets great pleasure from shopping and doing the laundry. Another told of the joy they get from walking their dog. Another moment of a Christmas eve church service had been turned into a playback theatre scene. Dora came out and did a monologue of going to a wedding in the country of her cultural origin.

For instance, the unit marked as "Vulnerabilities" began with the playback enactment of an epileptic seizure, with a performer who did not have epilepsy performing the role of the original Teller. Another scene was the enactment of falling in the shower, with one actor actually performing the role of the shower, using a white scarf. This was followed by a very brief monologue of what it feels like when one gets depressed. These were all shared moments of authentic experience translated into theatrical expression. It was very moving for the audience, at times, being given the privilege of entering the lives of these actors.

One of the most powerful units was entitled "Stigma & Name-calling." As mentioned, this theme had come, very dynamically, out of a focus group. Once the slide was shown, Dora stated how angry it made her when people made fun of herself or others. This monologue was wrought with strong emotion and set up the scene where the company all mingled about to music. Then, a very hurtful epithet would be called out, a whistle blown, and a policeman would take the villain away and put him or her in jail. It ended with one name-caller shouting out "Retard!" The music stopped. All froze for a minute. Then the whistle and the policeman took the culprit off to prison. Then, one of the performers, also a performance coach and a graduate of the Centre, with a developmental disability, himself, proclaimed: "Where do labels belong? Slap them on jars. That's where they go. C'est une bonne question, tout le gang!"

Artistic Images

It should not be forgotten that making an ethnodrama is creating theatrical art. As Saldana puts it: "Ethnotheatre employs traditional craft and artistic techniques of theatre production to mount for an audience a live performance event of research participant's experiences and/or the researcher's interpretation of data" (2005, p. 1).

All of the content of this production was shaped by artistic techniques of theatre, including lighting, sound, staging, music and dance. I believe the positive tone of the piece – "It's A Wonderful World" – came from the informant/actors, themselves, but I used my skill as a theatre director to shape the content in the most pleasing aesthetic forms I could conjure. For instance, the very climax of the performance was the steel pan version of "I'm Alive!" It was meant to be a joyful confirmation of life by the participants, manifesting their own joy in being alive. One of the performance coaches, a student in the drama therapy M.A. program, had an exceptional singing talent. She sang, "I'm Alive," the song made famous by Celine Dion. Partly for legal reasons, we used a Karaoke version. The research assistant brought her

vibrant skill to the singing of it. There was a back-up group of eight participants dancing to the music and William, our non-verbal autistic participant,
played his heart out on the steel pan. It was a rousing production number and
brought the house down, every night (see Figure 2.2).

The Social Message

We began to discover as we brought the play from rehearsal into performance
that a central theme of *fighting the stigmatization placed on persons with developmental disabilities* had emerged. The group in the developing of the play
had shown that they really wanted to advocate for themselves. Our original
primary goal, "to enlighten health providers … In order to advance knowledge of how to best serve such individuals" (Snow (Principal Investigator),
2005–2008, pp. 1–2), began to seem less necessary. Indeed, there were many
health professionals, such as therapists, social workers, managers and educators, who work with the population, in the audience at the June previews. It
did not seem to change their views a great deal. It was more like a "coals to
Newcastle" type of experience. However, we began to realize that our "real"
audience were very young people who had not yet formed prejudices that
would lead them to stigmatize this group. This will be explained in greater
detail in the section on "Post-Performance" outcomes. One of the values of
the performance process is that is shows you how the research report, and the
research itself, may need to be revised.

Our aim had been to use the theatre as a powerful tool to capture the authentic lived experience of our participants. We used ethnodrama as a method to
"influence change among providers and audiences, while retaining the potential to construct new understandings" (Mienczakowski & Morgan, 2001, pp.
219–220). In this vein, we were developing a kind of quasi-participation action research (PAR) approach in which our informants also had a stake in the
research, especially in the truthfulness of the research report. We were utilizing what I would call a "qualified" PAR approach (Snow et al., 2017, p. 244).
This also meant being self-advocates against discrimination, stigmatization
and inequity. Our social message was one of social acceptance and integration.
The play itself was an advocacy piece for correcting these social phenomena.

Therapeutic Theatre Perspective

Beside the social activist goals, this ethnodrama also had therapeutic intentions. We were watching the progress of the participants' therapeutic goals,

from the beginning. The frame of performance is part of the clinical process in our therapeutic theatre mode. We will discuss measurement of the therapeutic success in the "Post-Performance" Section. For now, let it suffice to say we were looking carefully at the therapeutic value of the performance for our actor/informants. As one audience member wrote: "The experience of creating theatre from authentic experience is a journey of discovery shared by both the participants and the therapists working with them. It also creates a bond that is therapeutic, in its own right, for everyone involved" (Kristine Berey, *La Scena*, 2008).[2]

Post-Performance

As Mienczakowski states: "It is this reconstructive and reflective post-performance debate that separates ethnodrama from other health theatre and versions of verbatim theatre which perform to, rather than discuss with their audiences" (Mienczakowski & Morgan, 2001, p. 221). The importance of the post-performance frame has been articulated, very clearly, by Nisha Sajnani in her doctoral dissertation, *Permeable Boundaries: Towards a Critical Collaborative Performance Pedagogy* (2010). While a Ph.D. student, I had hired Nisha as a research assistant for our project and one of her major responsibilities was to organize and facilitate the post-performance forum. This fitted in beautifully with her doctoral research which aimed to "examine approaches to audience engagement within three applied theatre projects towards defining the necessary elements of a critical, collaborative performance pedagogy" 2010, p. 7). One of her case examples was "It's A Wonderful World."

Post-Performance Forum

The three previews were focused on three separate audiences: June 7 was for family and friends; June 8 for health providers, educators and social service professionals; June 9 was for the general public. For each evening, Dr. Sajnani provided an assortment of post-performance events. The first of these was the *Audience Feedback Questionnaire*.

1. One word describing your response to the play:_____.
2. What in this play is most meaningful to you?

---

2 For any readers who would like to view a documentary that shows many parts of this performance, just go to psychotherapy.net and write in Snow in the search space. Also see Snow & Herbison (2012).

3. The scenes were presented under the following themes [All themes listed]:
   A) Which themes were covered well?
   B) Which them were not addressed that you feel need to be?
4. Who do you think should see the play AND why?
5. What questions/comments do you still have about the play?

(Sajnani, 2010, Appendix: "It's A Wonderful World," 4. Questionnaire)

Many powerful and useful responses came from each audience cohort: Family & Friends (22 responded); Healthcare Professionals (47 responded); General Public (73 responded). This type of feedback gathered in these questionnaires was invaluable to revising the research protocol and reshaping the performance. The use of post-performance questionnaires became a standard practice as we further developed EDT (for an example of a full quantitative analysis of questionnaire responses, see Chapter 5).[3]

Sajnani also developed several other post-performances activities for the audiences: *Direct Questions*, immediate verbal responses to Sajnani as MC; an *Actor Talkback* (basically Q&A with the actors); an *Art Corner*, where audience members could make an art response to the performance; a *Video Response*, in which audience members could make a reflection on camera; and a **playback theatre** period, through which the audience could process their experience of the play. This latter was to be done by our staff playback theatre team, but it was cancelled as the research team felt this could possibly "overshadow the accomplishments of the Centre's participants" (Sajnani, 2010, p. 68). All of these activities demonstrate the creative potential in developing the post-performance forum which "seek[s] debate and to inform further our data, which is continually under construction. Each performance is considered an opportunity to add further data to the report" (Mienczakowski & Morgan, 2001, p. 221).

Sajnani also presents a sound critique of "It's A Wonderful World" in her dissertation. Some of this is quite nuanced, but it deals with the central issue of who holds the power and is it equitably distributed? As we were aiming to work in a participatory action research style, I think this was a fair and thought-provoking criticism.

the absence of any representation of the relationship between caregivers, service providers and the participants causes the audience to temporarily "suspend their disbelief" about the capacities of their relatives, peers and

3 The actual responses can be read in Sajnani's dissertation, *Permeable Boundaries: Toward a Critical Collaborative Performance Pedagogy*, 2010 (pp. 65–67), open to all researchers on Concordia University's *Spectrum Research Repository* at https://spectrum.library.concordia.ca/

clients on stage. The near invisibility of those who hold the power to *permit* and *shape* the conditions in which participants' expression could be heard is what preserves the rigid binary of the rescuer and the rescued in the long term and prevents sustainable alliance between these centres and margins of power. Thus, though the *overt* message celebrated through such performances is one of the empowerment of the marginalized group, the *covert* message (i.e., that they are not capable) is held in the shadows, as a conversation that cannot be held simultaneously, and that therefore goes unexamined or challenged.

(2010, pp. 70–71)

We took this significant commentary into consideration, later on, when we developed other PAR-oriented ethnodramas at CAHD (see Chapters 4 and 6). The point is always to extend the validity of the research approach.

Closure

Closure is important in any drama therapy process. As Emunah writes: "The closure is in itself an important developmental process, facilitating the integration and assimilation of the therapeutic progress made in the preceding phases" (1994, p. 43). Closure encompasses this integration of new attitudes and perspectives, acknowledges the growth and accomplishment of the group, celebrates the uniqueness of the group and also looks towards the future. As Emunah and Johnson say about their therapeutic theatre work with psychiatric patients: "the gradual construction of the Play, which is developed from scratch, and the gradual formation of the Group, which had developed out of separate individuals, serve as a model to the patients for the creation of an identity" (1983, p. 235). It might be emphasized, here, the outcome can be the creation of a *new* identity. As Amorim and Cavalcante say about their performance work with individuals who have developmental disabilities, performance provides "opportunities to deconstruct the current disabling constructions and to reconstruct new and more powerful identities" (1992, p. 154). Many of the staff of CAHD and family members observed positive changes in the ethnodrama participants, but their comments are only subjective. Here, is where a better system for measuring these changes would be invaluable, but this was not developed for this research program. However, the transformative power of therapeutic theatre obliges the provision of careful and sensitive closure.

On June 11 and 13, the Monday and Wednesday after the preview performances in 2007, we provided a substantial closure process of the group. We had been working together for ten months. They had just completed the "culminating" experience of performing a play about their own life experiences. They needed a calm, more distanced way to process this experience. For this reason, we only used a modicum of Emunah's excellent drama therapy closure exercises (1994, pp. 228–247) and focused rather on an art therapy process, guided by Elizabeth Anthony, the Centre's Art Therapy Supervisor. This procedure took place on two mornings and was fully documented by Anthony. There were three questions for individuals to respond to by creating images via drawing and pasting photographs onto paper.

> **MURAL #1:** Participants were asked to make images of positive aspects of their experience of the play, or of parts of the play that they liked.
>
> One example was Don who identified friendship and love as two of the most important positive aspects of his experience, along with singing, dancing, music, his family saying "You were great!" as well as his speech into the microphone. He drew a picture of himself and Gilbert as best friends, and included the titles of three songs: "I'm Alive," "This [Little] Light of Mine" and "Amen."
>
> **MURAL #2:** Participants were asked to make images of aspects of their experience of the play that were difficult or challenging, or that that they did not like.
>
> Amy stated that it was challenging to deal with feeling nervous about performing. In addition to the nervousness, she stated that she did not like going to jail in the name-calling scene. She said it made her feel like she had done something bad.
>
> **MURAL #3:** Participants were asked to make images of what they had learned from their experience in the play, or what they could take with them from the experience.
>
> Perry contributed written thoughts suggesting that friendship and the opportunity to develop and have his own creative material (dreams and music) valued by others in this public way was what he will take with him from the experience.
> (Anthony, 2007, Notes from art therapy closure)

So, these are examples of responses to the art therapy process. Exercises from drama therapy, music therapy and dance/movement therapy were also implemented in the closure on June 11 and 13. The closure process embodied the same values of the whole ethnodrama process: to allow the participants to "tell the truth as they see it, so as to give them voice" (Mienczakowski, 1995b, p. 367).

Informant Validation of the Play

In the afternoons of these two days, we also gave the participants an opportunity to validate their performance that had been documented on video. They observed and made comments. Some of these led to changes in the script or the production. For instance, some of the participants really liked the idea of using masks for the "Name-Calling" scene so they would not feel exposed as being mean people who cast derogatory epithets at others. This suggestion about "integrating some sign to the self and the audience, such as masks, that would indicate 'this is not me speaking,' was greatly appreciated by Amy, Ronald and others" (Anthony, 2007, Notes from the art therapy closure). It also reflected some confusion about responsibility for words when one is acting. As we began to plan for the next phase of the project, these issues and ideas arising in the "Informant Validation" of the performance we incorporated.

After the closure, we were breaking until August when we would begin to plan Phase II of the project. As stated in the 2005 SSHRC application:

> The second phase will consist of a planned "tour." This could mean either going to conferences of "specialists," such as neurologists, social workers or educators, or bringing such groups to a performance space in Montreal. Four of these 'tours' would be set up over the course of the academic year.
> (Snow (Principal Investigator), 2005–2008, p. 6)

The Tour

The "tour" began on August 10, 2007. We adapted the performance to fit into an "Opening Ceremony" of the Annual Conference of the National Association for Drama Therapy. We performed "It's A Wonderful World" on the main stage of Concordia's major theatre venue, the D.B. Clarke Theatre. It was an 8am performance!

As one young Drama Therapy student in the audience reported:

> I wasn't sure what to expect at the 8am opening ceremony on the first day of the conference. My eyes were still adjusting to the light of day as I settled inconspicuously into the theatre chair … I pretended to read the program that had been handed to me at the entrance although nothing significant was actually entering my brain at that hour. So, when the performance began I was shocked to see twelve developmentally disabled adults dance onto the stage waving colorful scarves. As the song played and the actors danced it seemed as though they were asking us for something that would make them feel comfortable enough to proceed

with their show. Indeed, they were requesting a "return to innocence," a washing away of disillusionment, disappointment and tainted views of the world we live in. What they needed from the audience was genuine attention and an open heart …

When the lights came up at 9am there was not a dry eye in the theatre. Many of us found ourselves onstage hugging the performers and no one knew what to say to each other. As I made my way to the first session of the day, I asked myself why I could not stop the flow of tears that had run onto the theatre floor. Was it pity? Was it embarrassment? Was it joy? Was it fear?

We witnessed the beauty and the struggles, the needs and the desires of a person who lives with a developmental disability. We heard stories of love and courage as well as stories of vulnerabilities and rage. Each story was written, staged, and performed by a person who had lived it.

(Shatzkes, 2007, p. 22)

This review certainly captures the power of theatre based on personal lived experience and authentically performed by the informant/actors.

Over the next two years, we took the show on tour to high schools and colleges, finally ending up with a large-scale public performance in the D. B. Clarke Theatre on May 15, 2008. As the play was being revised, constantly, we had to seek new consents from the performers.

We took great care to be certain no ethical boundaries were violated, as in this kind of work great attention must be paid to every aspect of the ethics involved (see Chapter 8).

As mentioned, even after the first performance, we began to realize our "research audience" was elementary school children. We brought some groups of these to the Centre at Concordia University, so they could witness and respond to the play. There is documentation of a really interesting set of questions asked by these students, after a performance (see Snow & Herbison, 2012). Because of the success we were having reaching this population, we toured several elementary schools. Out of these experiences, our logistical coordinator, Poppy Baktis, and the Co-Director of Research at CAHD, Dr. Miranda D'Amico, developed an educational toolkit, entitled "The DisAbility Awareness and Empathy Building Kit" (Baktis & D'Amico, 2009). It contained our DVD, "In Their Own Voices" (Snow & Herbison, 2012), as well as instructions and resources on how to work with elementary school children on these issues. It was an important outcome of our research.

Mienczakowski's concept of "Critical Ethno-drama" embraces an agenda for bringing the research to wide audiences, i.e. "touring." He says,

Ethno-drama seeks explanation and expression in a public form which opens its meaning to its informants as well as to wide audiences including the academy. In so doing it "de-academises" its research reporting format by translating data into scripted performances.

(1997, p. 170)

In developing the ethnodramatherapy method since this first production in June 2007, "touring" had been a regular part of our procedure, to get our performances/research reports out to "wide audiences."

A New Method Defined

All of the material and processes developed in this project served as the seedbed for the emergence of ethnodramatherapy. From the first failed research proposal in 2003, "Creating Theatre with Persons with Developmental Disabilities through Ethnodrama," through the final performance in May 2008, each step along the way added to the evolution of a dynamic synthesis of ethnodrama, drama therapy, theatre and social activism (see Figure 1.4).

What's New?

The main new ingredient added to Mienczakowski's well-established formula for ethnodrama is the actualization of an intentional and systematic use of a therapy process integrated with the ethnographic research procedures. In carefully reviewing his writings on ethnodrama, I had discovered a latent ambition to implement therapeutic strategies (see the epigraph for this chapter). In his scholarly writings, this therapeutic concern is often implied under the rubric of "Emancipation," which he defines as "a democratically founded process in which oppression is not defined for health consumers but by them" (1995a, p. 107) The lifting of this oppression is also conceived as therapeutic action. As Mienczakowski writes elsewhere: "constructive action implies a desired (limited emancipatory) potential and an embracing terminology describing the therapeutic effects of ethno-drama on participating informants" (Mienczakowski et al., 1996, p. 455).

Bringing the ethnodrama method into the context of a therapeutic Centre, based on the therapeutic use of the arts, created a new alchemy for this approach, by synthesizing what was essentially a performance ethnography research framework with arts-based clinical practices.

CAHD had already established a model for therapeutic theatre. Extending its practices of this model into the use of ethnodrama as a research activity established a new method.

As it was the drama therapy domain of therapeutic theatre that most essentially characterized the new perspective, the emerging practice was defined as a combining of ethnodrama and drama therapy. *Mienczakowski's method was a theatre-based approach to research. Therapeutic theatre is a theatre-based approach to therapy.* It felt like a natural fit. As the principal investigator of the project, I oversaw all aspects, including research and arts-based clinical practices. As director of the play production, I supervised the theatrical creation and its **social justice** message about stigmatization and marginalization of persons with developmental disabilities. In bringing together these four elements (see Figure 1.4), I began to conceive of ethnodramatherapy as a complete methodology, in itself.

The New Formulation of Steps

The ethnodramatherapy procedure, adapted from the original formulation of ethnodrama, is applied to any "health consumer group" in the following way. Here are the basic stages:

Stage 1: The group of "health informants" is brought together. Many techniques of spontaneous play and trust-building from drama therapy are utilized to build trust and coherence in the group. Focus groups and ethnographic interviews with individuals are established and transcribed. They will be used to develop an authentic portrait of the lived experience of the group. We also use many creative arts therapies methods to evoke this material. These, in turn, provide music, dance, art images, scenes and monologues, to help develop the "authentic portrait" to be realized in the ethnodramatic theatre production. Drama therapy is the coordinating modality as all is created in the framework of *therapeutic theatre*.

Stage 2: Out of the focus groups, interviews and creative arts therapies workshops, coordinated with the drama therapy process, essential themes for the playscript are developed. A script is created through constant consultation with the informants. When ready, a process of *informant validation* of the script is implemented in which the participants correct, edit and verify what they want in the script in order to best tell *their* stories.

Stage 3: Rehearsal is instituted for the preparation of the performance of the script. Usually, in the ethnodramatherapy process, the informants are the actors. However, there are instances when outside actors, either professionals or students or community volunteers may be the actors (as in the case of the Mienczakowski's first study with persons with schizophrenia, where theatre students and nursing students performed the play. Also, see Chapter 5 on the "Caregiver" project). Rehearsal time is organized strategically to genuinely accomplish the therapeutic *and* the aesthetic goals of the play production.

Stage 4: A process of *informant validation* of the performance of the play, *before* it is presented to any audience, is completed by participants. The group makes certain that the performance of the play, as it stands, truthfully represents their life experiences. They have the final voice on this. They dictate the changes required.

Stage 5: Performance of the ethnodrama for an audience (typically of healthcare providers and audiences relevant to the issues presented in the play). When the play goes on "tour," the multiple performances often engender necessary changes in the script and/or performance. This may require further *informant validation*.

Stage 6: Post-performance forums with healthcare providers and health consumers are established to identify problems in the healthcare system and ways to correct them. These forums can take multiple forms, but their purpose is to allow for debate of the issues and strategizing to create ways to make changes in oppressive systems.

Stage 7: Because the therapeutic purpose of a project is now emphasized, proper closure is needed after the performances, including at the end of a "tour." This will give participants the opportunity to review and process their experience. It will also allow the clinical staff to evaluate the therapeutic value for each participant.

Stage 8: As any project in ethnodramatherapy has both research and therapeutic outcomes, final analyses of the effectiveness in both these domains must take place. The former is usually based on data from pre- and post-questionnaires that will evidence the educational efficacy for audiences. The latter, which still needs development, is aimed at demonstrating the value of the therapeutic experience for the informant/actors. The detailed analyses of this data will lead to future dissemination of the research.

This is the basic formula for the design, implementation and evaluation of an ethnodramatherapy project. Over the next 12 years, we were to create five more projects and implement several workshops in different countries.

What Was to Follow

I have spent some pains to delineate this first project in great detail, as I truly see it as the seedbed of what was to follow. The formulation of the EDT

Table 2.1   EDT Projects from 2006 to 2018

Year	Production	Organized by	Themes
2006–2008	It's A Wonderful World: A Musical Ethnodrama	CAHD	Self image, stigma, living the life of a person with a developmental disability
2011–2012	Inside the System: An Ethnodrama in One Act with Two Songs	w/the Youth Protection Centre	Self image, stigma, living the life of a 14- 18-year old girl under Youth Protection
2012	Our World: A Musical Ethnodrama	CAHD	The place of culture in the lives of adults with developmental disabilities
2014	The Amazing Adventure of Relationships: A Musical Ethnodrama	CAHD	The place of relationships, romance and sexuality in the lives of adults with developmental disabilities
2015–2017	Through the Eyes of Caregivers: An Ethnodrama on Mental Illness in the Family	w/AMI-Québec	The experience of being a caregiver for a loved one with a serious mental illness
2017–2018	Nobody's Perfect: A Theatrical Exploration of Mental Health	w/AMI-Québec	Two questions for the whole community: What is Mental Health? What is Mental Illness?

method, although it was to be developed more in future projects, was fundamentally established with the three-year process of "It's A Wonderful World" (2006–2008). Table 2.1 is a chart showing the EDT productions that were created over the next decade.

In the following chapters, I will delineate how the formulation was further developed and describe how it was applied and actualized in four other productions in Montreal and a series of workshops in China.

References

Ammann, R. (1991). *Healing and transformation in sandplay: Creative processes become visible*. Open Court.

Amorim, A. C., & Cavalcante, F. G. (1992). Narrations of the self: Video production in a marginalized subculture. In S. McNamee & K. J. Gergen (Eds.), *Therapy as social construction* (pp. 149–165). Sage Publications.

Anthony, E. (2007). *Notes on closure process for It's A Wonderful World, June 2007*. The Centre for the Arts in Human Development, Concordia University.

Bailey, S. (2009). Performance in drama therapy. In D. R. Johnson & R. Emunah (Eds., 2nd ed.), *Current approached in drama therapy* (pp. 374–389). C. C. Thomas Publisher.

Baktis, P., & D'Amico, M. (Eds.). (2009). *The disability awareness and empathy building tool kit.* The Centre for the Arts in Human Development, Concordia University.

Bartenieff, I. & Davis, M. (1965). *Effort-shape analysis of movement: The unity of expression and function.* Albert Einstein College of Medicine, Yeshiva University.

Berey, K. (2008). Gained in translation. *La Scena, 1*(2), 10.

Bettelheim, B. (1975). *The uses of enchantment: The meaning and importance of fairy tales.* Vintage Books.

Blatner, A. (1973). *Acting-in: Practical applications of psychodramatic methods.* Springer Publishing.

Concordia University Summary Protocol Form, Rev. 10 (December 2003). Concordia University.

Connolly, K., & Reid, A. (2007). Ethics review for qualitative inquiry: Adopting a value-based, facilitative approach. *Qualitative Inquiry, 13*(7), 1031–1047.

D'Amico. M. (2007). *Questions for participants in first Ethnodrama project.* The Centre for the Arts in Human Development, Concordia University.

D'Amico, M., Barafato, A., & Vargas, S. (1998). *The Centre for the Arts in Human Development: A progress report, 1996–1998.* Concordia University.

D'Amico, M., Lalonde C. & Snow, S. (2014). Evaluating the efficacy of drama therapy in teaching social skills to children with Autism Spectrum Disorders. *Drama Therapy Review, 1*(1), 21–39.

Denzin, N. (2001). The reflexive interview and a performative social science. *Qualitative Research, 1*(1), 23–46.

Emunah, R. (1994*). Acting for real: Drama therapy process, technique, and performance.* Brunner/Mazel Publishers.

_____. (1996). Five progressive phases in dramatherapy and their implications for brief dramatherapy. In A. Gersie (Ed.), *Dramatic approaches to brief therapy* (pp. 29–44). C. C. Thomas Publisher.

Emunah, R., & Johnson, D.R. (1983). The impact of theatrical performance on the self-images of psychiatric patients. *The Arts in Psychotherapy, 10,* 233–239.

Fox. J. (1993). Foreword. In J. Salas, *Improvising real life: Personal story in Playback Theatre,* (p. i). Kendall/Hunt Publishing.

Fox, J. (1994). *Acts of service: Spontaneity, commitment, tradition in the nonscripted theatre.* Tusitala Publishing.

Fox, J., & Dauber, H. (1999). *Gathering voices: Essays on playback theatre.* Tusitala Publishing.

Lister, S., Tanguay, D., Snow, S., & D'Amico, M. (2009). Development of a creative arts therapies center for people with developmental disabilities. *Journal of the American Art Therapy Association, 26*(1), 34–37.

Mienczakowski, J. (1995a). *The application of critical ethno-drama to health settings* [Unpublished doctoral dissertation]. Griffith University, Australia.

_____. (1995b). The theatre of ethnography: The reconstruction of ethnography with emancipatory potential. *Qualitative Inquiry, 1*(3), 360–375.

_____. (1997). Theatre of change. *Research in Drama Education, 2*(2), 159–172.

_____. (2001). Ethnodrama: Performed research – Limitations and potential. In P. Atkinson, A. Coffey, S. Delamont, J. Lofland & L. Lofland (Eds.), *Handbook of Ethnography* (pp. 468–476). Sage Publications.

Mienczakowski, J., Smith, R., & Sinclair, M. (1996). On the road to catharsis: A theoretical framework for change. *Qualitative Inquiry, 2*(4), 439–462.

Mienczakowski, J. & Morgan, S. (2001). Ethnodrama: constructing participatory experiential and compelling action research through performance. In P. Reasons & H. Bradbury (Eds.), *Handbook of action research: Concise paperback*. Sage Publications.

Murchison, J. M. (2010). *Ethnography essentials: Designing, conducting, and presenting your research*. Jossey-Bass.

Pendzik, S. (2012). The 6-key model – An integrative assessment approach. In D. R. Johnson, S. Pendzik & S. Snow (Eds.) *Assessment in drama therapy* (pp. 197–222). C. C. Thomas Publisher.

Pendzik, S., Emunah, R., & Johnson, D. R. (Eds.) (2016). *The self in performance: Autobiographical, self-revelatory, and autoethnographic forms of theatre*. Palgrave Macmillan.

Reid, A. (2005). *Results of your human research ethics application: Queries*. Human Research Ethics Committee, Concordia University.

Sajnani, N. (2010). *Permeable boundaries: Toward a critical collaborative performance pedagogy* [Unpublished doctoral dissertation]. Concordia University, Montreal, Quebec, Canada.

Salas, J. (1993). *Improvising real life: Personal history in Playback Theatre*. Kendall/Hunt Publishing.

Salas, J. (2009). Playback theatre: A frame for healing. In D. R. Johnson & R. Emunah (Eds.), *Current approaches in drama therapy* (2nd ed., pp. 445–460). C. C. Thomas Publisher.

Saldana, J. (Ed.). (2005). *Ethnodrama: An anthology of reality theatre*. Altamira Press.

Sharp, V. (1975). *Social control in the therapeutic community*. Saxon House.

Shatzkes, S. (2007). An open heart. *Dramascope, 28*(3), 22.

Snow. S. (1996). Focusing on mythic imagery in brief drama therapy with psychotic individuals. In A. Gersie (Ed.). *Dramatic approaches to brief therapy* (pp. 213–235). Jessica Kingsley.

_____. (2000). Ritual/Theatre/Therapy. In P. Lewis & D. R. Johnson (Eds.), *Current approaches in drama therapy* (pp. 218–240). C. C. Thomas Publisher.

_____. (Principal Investigator). (2005–2008). *Visually performed research: Creating theatre with adults with developmental disabilities through Ethnodrama* (File No: 410–2006-1212) [Grant]. Social Science and Humanities Research Council of Canada.

_____. (2009). Ritual/Theatre/Therapy. In D. R. Johnson & R. Emunah (Eds.), *Current approaches in drama therapy* (2nd ed., pp. 117–143). C. C. Thomas Publisher.

Snow, S., D'Amico, M., & Tanguay, D. (2003). Therapeutic theatre and well-being. *The Arts in Psychotherapy, 30*, 73–82.

Snow, S., & Anthony, E. (2006). *Letter to participants explaining the first Ethnodrama project, September 2006–June 2007*. The Centre for the Arts in Human Development, Concordia University.

Snow, S., Maeng-Cleveland, J., & Steinfort, T. (2009). The development of the Drama Therapy Role-Play Interview. In S. Snow & M. D'Amico (Eds.), *Assessment in the creative arts therapies: Designing and adapting assessment tools for adults with developmental disabilities* (pp. 99–162). C. C. Thomas Publisher.

Snow, S., & D'Amico, M. (2012). Casting the healing role. In D. R. Johnson, S. Pendzik & S. Snow (Eds.), *Assessment in drama therapy* (pp. 91–117). C. C. Thomas Publisher.

Snow, S., & Herbison, P. (2012). *Ethnodramatherapy: A New Methodology as Applied to Diversity Training* (originally distributed by Mental Health Resources. Since 2014, distributed by psychotherapy.net, as *Empowering adults with developmental disabilities: A creative arts therapies approach*).

Snow, S., D'Amico, M., Mongerson, M., Anthony, E., Rozenberg, M., Opolko, C., & Anandampillai, S. (2017). Ethnodramatherapy applied in a project focusing on relationships in the lives of adults with developmental disabilities, especially romance, intimacy and sexuality. *Drama Therapy Review, 3*(2), 241–260.

Snow, S. H., Snow, S., & D'Amico, M. (2008). Interdisciplinary research through community music therapy and performance ethnography. *Canadian Journal of Music Therapy, XIV* (1), 30–46.

Spolin, V. (1963). *Improvisation for the theatre*. Northwestern University Press.

Tanguay, D. (2009). Adapting sandtray assessment for adults with developmental disabilities. In S. Snow & M. D'Amico (Eds.), *Assessment in the creative arts therapies: Designing and adapting assessment tools for adults with developmental disabilities* (pp. 219–256). C. C. Thomas Publisher.

Volkas, A. (2009). Healing the wounds of history: Drama therapy in collective trauma and intercultural conflict resolution. In D. R. Johnson & R. Emunah, *Current approaches in drama therapy* (pp. 145–171). C. C. Thomas Publisher.

Part II
Applications

3
EDT with Female Adolescents in Youth Protection

The adolescents' anger towards their parents (which is frequently generalized to all authority figures) and sense of helplessness about their situation is compounded by this involuntary placement, and they enter the institutional setting ready to fight all aspects of treatment.

(R. Emunah, 1985)

Focusing on the Unique Voices of the Informants

Each project in EDT is shaped by *who* the group (the *ethnos*) is and *where* the process takes place. This is absolutely true for the present case. Our group was made up of 14–18-year-old female adolescents in a **Youth Protection** facility where they lived under residential care. These special circumstances helped to define the central focus of this project: to assist these informants to express their unique voices as they experienced life in this particular situation. This was the overarching goal of this project. Our phenomenological approach to ethnographic research was well matched to this task. As van Manen writes in *Researching Lived Experience*:

In phenomenological research the emphasis is always on the meaning of lived experience. The point of phenomenological research is to "borrow" other people's experiences and their reflections on their experiences in order to better be able to come to an understanding of the deeper meaning of significance of an aspect of human experience, in the context of the whole of human experience.

(2016, p. 62)

As with the first EDT project, delineated in Chapter 1, we wanted to come to understand, and we wanted the audience to learn, *what it is like to live the life of a person in this circumstance*. Our belief was, if we could capture the authentic voices of the informants, we could change perceptions about their lives, maybe even change the system of care in which they were forced to

DOI: 10.4324/9781003083818-5

live. So, there were other goals for this project, as will be described, shortly. However, the essential undertaking was to use our methodology to locate genuine expressions of these young women about their life experience. In this chapter, we will review our successes and failures with this endeavor.

How the Four Roles of the Ethnodramatherapist were Divided in this Project

As there are four major functions in the EDT process (see Figure1.4), there are four major roles for the ethnodramatherapist. These roles are: Drama Therapist, Theatre Artist, Researcher and Social Activist (Figure 3.1).

As has been stated, ethnodramatherapy is fundamentally a dynamic integration of ethnodrama and dramatherapy. So, the EDT practitioner must be both a drama therapist and an ethnodramatist, or find a partner who has the set of skills that she or he does not. The practitioner must also have skill as a theatre artist and drive and capacity as a social activist, or assign other team members to these specific roles. In terms of the social activist role, it should be noted by students and future practitioners of EDT, the approach *always* holds an intention to change systems through the mirroring the effects of theatre and genuine dialogue in post-performance forums.

In Chapter 2, I described how I mostly carried these four roles, myself, with the support and guidance of other researchers, clinicians and theatre artists. In the present case, the four roles were more divided, especially in regard to the therapeutic function. The frontline therapists were the art therapy and drama therapy interns, supervised by myself and an art therapy faculty member from Concordia University. I oversaw the producing of the theatre performance. I also coordinated all of the research, with the aid of my colleague Dr. Miranda D'Amico (Snow & D'Amico, 2015). The whole team

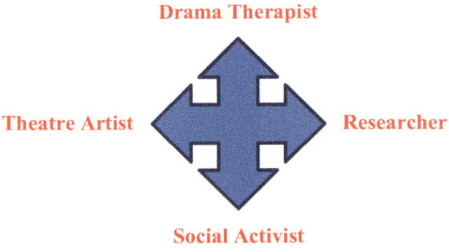

Figure 3.1   Four Roles of the Ethnodramatherapist

was dedicated to the social activism function of de-stigmatizing the inform-ants and improving the Youth Protection system that cares for them.

Setting up a New Project

The Preliminaries

As with every EDT project, certain basic preliminaries are required to get everything prepared to move ahead with the process. Students and profes-sionals who might like to do this type of work need to be very aware of these first steps.

First of all, a group must be located and gathered. In this case, our group was young women under Youth Protection who have been placed "in foster care, group homes or residential units with the goal of returning them to their families as soon as the situation permits" (Batshaw Youth and Family Centres, 2011–2012, p. 6). The *ethnos*, the group to be studied, needs to have certain common experiences that bind them, together, emotionally, psycho-logically and socially. Here, it was the common experience of living "inside the system" of Youth Protection. That is what was to be researched in the *ethno*-dramatherapy process.

Again, for this project, a very challenging ethics approval had to be accom-plished *before* we could begin. This included both an application to Con-cordia University's Human Research Ethics Committee and, because we were going to work under the auspices of a government agency, a second application had to be approved by the Centre Jeunesse de Montreal-Institut Universitaire. It is very important for students or professionals who wish to utilize the EDT method that they learn to effectively write these kinds of ethics applications. It is very detailed and time-consuming work.

Our project was entitled, "Diversity Training Outreach Program: Pilot Pro-ject with Batshaw Youth and Family Services." It was based on a concept of further developing ethnodramatherapy as a tool for emancipation and edu-cation with marginalized groups. It was a "pilot project," as this was the first time we had focused on this population. We planned to complete the project within a year. I began planning meetings with the Batshaw staff in May 2011 and submitted the ethics application to HREC by the end of that May. We had established goals in our application. The two main goals were:

(1) The primary goal was to utilize the synthesized ethnodrama method de-veloped at The Centre for the Arts in Human Development at Concordia

University to empower the youth-in-care at Batshaw by providing them with the opportunity to express their personal voices and narratives and to, thereby, reduce their sense of self-stigmatization, i.e., change their self-perception.

(2) The secondary goal was to measure if witnessing the ethnodrama created by the youth-in-care could change the perceptions towards these adolescents in an audience, made up of staff, family members and caregivers. It should be noted, here, that because of the extreme measures for confidentiality required by Youth Protection there could be no public performance of the ethnodrama (as there had been with Mienczakowski's work) nor could the video of the performance be shown outside the circle of the research team and Batshaw staff.[1]

(Snow & D'Amico, Batshaw Report, 2012, p. 5)

Another major preliminary task, of course, is securing funding. Our team applied for and received funds from Concordia's "Seed Funding (Team) Program." This gave us enough to hire four MA students as research assistants, two in art therapy and two in drama therapy, and a small amount of funding for professional consultants, such as a lighting designer, a stage manager and a music and dance teacher, and funding for the transcription of interviews.

From Spring 2011 on, we began strategizing on how to most effectively implement the full EDT process to accomplish our goals. However, the rubber did not hit the road until October 4, 2011, when our team first met the prospective participants at the "audition" held for all interested Batshaw residents. This was the beginning of an amazing, sometimes very challenging, sometimes inspiring, educational process for us and for our informants.

Stage 1: Gathering the Group and Exploring Who They Are

In order to help students and professionals interested in learning the EDT methodology, I am framing the description of our process in the **Formula of the 8 Stages**, outlined in Chapter 2. This provides a real map on how to do the work. Under each stage, the required actions are delineated through the way they were realized in this specific project.

---

1 Due to the strict ethics regulations, no photography or videotaping was allowed to have public exposure. Therefore, there is no visual documentation for this chapter, as there is for other chapters in this book.

Recruitment

To begin with, we developed a specialized flyer that staff on various Batshaw units could disperse to their adolescent residents (Figure 3.2). It succinctly outlined what the project would be about.

The flyer aimed to attract and inform the candidates for our program. It was advertised as a "Therapeutic Drama Program":

- What the Program is: "Drama therapy allows teens to tell their story to an audience."
- Why participate: "Be part of a research team and share your experience of being part of Batshaw."
- What you need: "An openness to new and exciting experiences."
- Fill in the Form (an attached form also asked questions): "Why do you want to join the Therapeutic Drama Program?" "Name 3 positive qualities about yourself."

We interviewed 22 candidates for this program. We used a rating scale of 1 to 10 (10 being the "best" potential participant). By the end of this process we had selected ten participants from three different units at one of Batshaw's residential centers. They were all female adolescents between the ages of 14 and 18. Now, we had to explore who they were and "what made them tick."

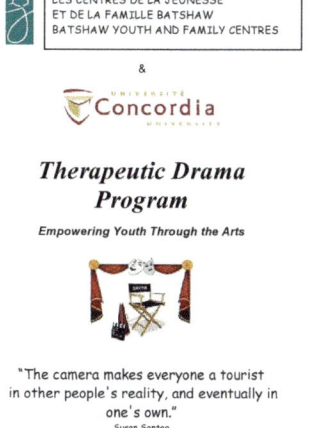

LES CENTRES DE LA JEUNESSE
ET DE LA FAMILLE BATSHAW
BATSHAW YOUTH AND FAMILY CENTRES

&

Concordia
UNIVERSITÉ

Therapeutic Drama Program

Empowering Youth Through the Arts

"The camera makes everyone a tourist in other people's reality, and eventually in one's own."
Susan Sontag

6 Weredale Park
Westmount, Quebec
H3Z 1Y6
(514) 932-7161 local 1183

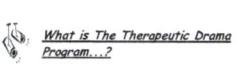

What is The Therapeutic Drama Program...?

Therapeutic Drama Program combines drama and therapy methods to offer teens new ways to express what they are thinking or feeling. This is a research project that will help others understand your experience of being part of Batshaw.

- Drama therapy allows teens to tell their story to an audience
- The story details and ending can be changed
- Looking at problems from a different perspective
- Combines drama, information, humor, and life experiences into several short sketches
- Foster a genuine love of the performing arts

Why participate...?

- Explore and expand your speaking, acting and auditioning skills.
- Receive skilled training and hands on experience with production elements, as you design, build and create the set, lighting, sound, props and costumes.
- Performers will develop and work on creating a show as their final performance.
- Be part of a research team and share your experience of being part of Batshaw.

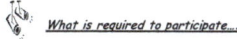

What is required to participate...?

- An openness to new and exciting experiences
- No acting experience necessary, just a willingness to try new things
- Youths between the ages of 14 and 18
- Open to all youth in Residential and Foster Care programs in the Montréal area at Batshaw.
- Be available to meet every Tuesday night from 6pm to 8pm, from September to February, at 6 Weredale Park.
- Be willing to present the piece before an audience composed of family members, Batshaw staff and researchers.
- You can participate even if no guardians or family members will attend the final presentation

How to apply...?

Fill in the following application form in the back of this flyer and send it to 6 Weredale: Attention Sam Barile

Then

We will contact you.
An interview process will occur, as places are limited.

If you have any questions please contact
Sam Barile at local 1183

Figure 3.2   Recruitment Flyer for the Batshaw Project

Who Are These Girls, Really?

Over the next few months we utilized several methods to investigate the background and present psychological status of each participant. These included individual interviews, discussion groups and drama therapy and art therapy processes, as well as one special music group for songwriting.

Demographically the group was diverse, with various cultural backgrounds, including Greek, Iranian, Moroccan, Afro-Canadian, Caucasian Canadian, etc. Many of them had very damaged self-images. Underneath their tough defensive front, they are often very vulnerable. As one 14-year-old girl put it: "I grew up a fuck-up." This sense of negative **self-perception** is also expressed in the art work they created in the art therapy workshops (see Figure 3.3).

This kind of negative self-perception is very common in this population (Gil-Kashiwabara et al., 2007; Scannapieco et al., 2007). "To achieve substantial improvement in the transition success of marginalized youth, many of whom have very little hope or chance of success, will require everyone to recognize and discard stereotypes and biases in favor of attitudes, practices, and policies that provide genuine opportunity and support of youth to realize their dreams" (Gil-Kashiwabara et al., 2007, p. 90). Overall, this statement reflects the essential goals of our ethnodramatherapy project with the girls at the Batshaw residence: to see if we could improve their self-images and the way others think about them (stereotypes and biases), and to help them actualize their dreams.

Another aspect of the lives of these young women was the degree of trauma that they had experienced. They definitely fit into the category of "at-risk youth," with problems including "psychological distress, suicide and high-risk behaviors" (Batshaw Youth and Family Centres 2011–2012, p. 6). These are "adolescents who have been placed in group homes due to court recommendations for out-of-home placement" (Dunne, 2012, p. 287).

Our participants have had their lives disrupted on many levels; in terms of dysfunctional family and/foster family relations, their placement by the courts in Youth Protection due to some kind of "acting out," and being adolescents with all the psychological dilemmas of that stage of development (Corradetti, 2012).

The first step in our research, then, was the ethnographic work of getting to know these young women. Our task was, as Mienczakowski writes: "decoding and rendering accessible the culturally specific signs, symbols, aesthetics, behaviours, language and experience" (2001, p. 468). This is the ethnographic work that is necessary to accomplish an "authentic portrait" of the group. Without a doubt, the role of Researcher (see Figure 3.1) is that of *ethnographer*. As Murchison states: "The goal of ethnography is to gain insight into cultural and social behaviors as well as the cultural understandings and underlying thought processes that produce behavior" (2010, p. 15). In this light, we looked at our small group of young women in the Batshaw residence as a microcosmic subculture. We needed to enter their world in an honest and authentic way.

The One-on-One Interviews

One of the most powerful tools of ethnographic research is the interview. Individual interviews are a crucial vehicle for capturing the authentic experience of the participants (Denzin, 2001; Mienczakowski, 1995a, 1995b; Saldana, 2005, 2011). As Murchison writes, "Since one of the primary goals of ethnography is to assess insiders' perspectives, interviews and conversations that allow you to record the thoughts and words of informants are absolutely essential" (2010, p. 44). It is a vital way to find entry into the "culture" of a specific group. Nine in-depth interviews were done with participants and transcribed, before developing the script for the ethnodrama. They were all used to build the background of "what it is like to live inside a residential unit as an adolescent girl." Seven of the interviews were eventually used in constructing the playscript. One interview was done with Jennifer Dupuis, the Batshaw Youth Empowerment worker, to represent the point of view of an individual who had made it through the system and succeeded in her life.

The questions were devised by my co-investigator, Dr. D'Amico, and were meant to evoke the girls' self-perceptions in regard to their situations and their images of themselves at this point in their life. All the interviews were implemented by myself, either on the units where the girls lived or in the large dining room at the front of the Dorval Residence. There were seven questions, presented in an open and adaptive manner in one-on-one sessions with the nine girls:

1. How would you describe your current situation?
2. Why are you living in this Batshaw Residence?
3. What does it feel like to be living in a Batshaw Residence?
4. What types of attitudes do you think that people generally have towards adolescents living in such a place?

5. List some words that you would use to describe to someone about what it feels like living in a Batshaw Residence.
6. Thinking about your life at this moment; how much control do you feel you have in terms of what you want your life to be?
7. What traits or skills do you think that you have which will help you overcome the difficulties that led you to be in a Batshaw Residence?

It took from 30 to 50 minutes to complete the individual interview. A composite profile of the girls emerged from the responses to these questions. The transcribed interviews revealed rich information about who the girls were, at this stage of their lives, in this situation. They seemed very earnest in their responses to the questions asked. There were four major areas analyzed in terms of themes present: how the girls thought about themselves (self-concept); their general attitude towards life; their specific attitude towards Batshaw; and their hopes and dreams for themselves.

Self-Concept

In the first category, there were many indications of a negative self-concept. As one 14-year-old participant put it: "anyone who likes living here is just messed up in their head." Another 15-year-old said, point blank: "I'm ashamed of myself." Another girl stated that "My life was going down the drain." Another girl, a bit older said: "Before [Batshaw] I had randomness ... I love being random ... that's *who I am*." One very reflective 18-year-old stated: "I've made a lot of stupid decisions and choices in my life ... then, at the end of the day when I sit in my room ... I'm like, why would I do that, like it's getting me nowhere." Some were able to express a more positive perception of themselves: "I know how to be my own person, like I don't follow what other people do," "I'm a fun person to be around." They saw themselves as "determined," "persistent," "creative," and "good." However, a major theme, as one girl expressed it was: "I'm less of the person that I was before, and I feel like I'm slowly forgetting like what it's like to live my life and that's just so wrong on many levels."

Attitude towards Their Situation

Their perception of environment within their Batshaw residence was embodied in the single words they used to describe what it was like for them to live there. Here are few examples: "irritating," "frustrating," "aggravating," "misery," "tiresome," "stressful," "depressing," "addictive," "shitty," "sad," "annoying," "horrifying." Not a very pretty picture of their conception of their own quality of life.

How They Think Outsiders See Them

A couple of interesting repeated themes came up. When asked how people *on the outside* perceived them, a couple of the girls used the term: "useless delinquent." Most of the time, these images were very negative: "people probably think we're the worst kids ever"; "what people think about when they hear about someone being at Batshaw, they think about mothers and fathers doing drugs and being alcoholics." One thoughtful young participant had another perspective "they're looking at a book, we're like the books, and they're just reading us, and then they're trying to say that they understand, but ... *you don't exactly understand because you haven't lived through it.*" A beautifully articulated rationale for our ethnodrama.

Fake It 'Till You Make It

Another motif that came up a number of times was: "you gotta fake it till you make it." A number of girls held this as a survival strategy, especially when they knew their designated time at Batshaw would be *long*. However, one 15-year-old cited this as a very bad philosophy to live by. She said: "I ain't gonna fake anything 'cause faking isn't gonna get you anywhere in life ... basically your whole life is a lie." Interestingly, she was also one of the very few who stated that Batshaw had really helped her.

Their Dreams for the Future

The girls' dreams ranged from very simple, present matters – "I can't wait to sleep in my own bed, talk on the phone whenever I want and eat whatever I want" – to more grandiose fantasies of becoming a famous singer or a backup dancer for a pop musician. Some were very pragmatic: "I can't wait to be able to go out there and get my own groceries or you know, have the responsibility of paying my own rent, you know, like have a house that's mine." As one 14-year-old plainly said in regard to her future hopes and dreams: "I don't really know at this point."

Certainly, the overarching goal of Batshaw Youth and Family Centres is, in the words of Gil-Kashawabara et al. (2007), to "provide a genuine opportunity and support of youth to realize their dreams," (p. 90), and the goal of our project was to enhance this potential through the ethnodramatherapy process. Interestingly, the girls' composite profile of themselves was corroborated by Youth Empowerment worker Jennifer Dupuis. At 12 years old she had been placed within a Batshaw Group Home and remained in the "system" until she was 18. She sees herself as a "system's kid," although, presently she serves as a "success story" and a role model for kids presently in the system. I interviewed her using an adapted version of the questions asked to the nine adolescent girls. On many levels, her responses corroborated the highly negative aspects of both the girls' perceptions of themselves and the notions held by the girls of the general public's attitudes towards "system's kids." Dupuis states:

> I think that they [the general public] don't really think about the reason for a child being in placement as like anything related to their family, but like more like labeling the kid as being a troublemaker or being, even if they think the kid ... might have family problems ..., they think that that kid is just like ... troubled and like have negative behaviours, or like I don't think they would want their children to hang around with children that live in the system.
>
> (Interview with Jennifer Dupuis, January 23, 2012)

This echoes the exact sentiment expressed by one of the seven participants in the project.

With all her experience of the "system," from both the inside and the outside, Dupuis seems to hold a very realistic and grounded perspective toward the Batshaw system. She goes on to say how she wouldn't want her own son being with "system's kids":

> I wouldn't want my son around them or any of those kinds of behaviours ... yeah, a lot of them do have problems ... they have a lot of knowledge of things that kids don't normally know at that age ... and I mean who wants their kids to learn stuff like that, right?
>
> (Interview, January 23, 2012).

From her six years inside the system, Jennifer's one or two word descriptions of that experience seem to be congruent with those of the nine interviewees: "lonely," frustrating," "lack of privacy," "difficult relationships." However, she also used the word, "beneficial."

This potential for improving "the system" was the one of the central purposes of the EDT project.

Drama Therapy and Art Therapy

One of the major innovations of EDT is to evoke personal experience and personal stories though creative arts therapies methods. Two modalities were used in this project: drama therapy and art therapy. These provided another way of entry into the world of these young women. The playful games of

warm-ups and improvisational role-playing of drama therapy were used at the beginning to create trust, bonding and coherency in the group.

As the principal investigator and the ethnodrama director for the project, I organized and implemented the first session at the beginning of November.

The First Groups

November 1, the first meeting was held in the gym at the Dorval Residence. We decided to try out the gym as a workshop space. In fact, it was too big with very bad acoustics, but for the first evening the idea was to start the process, here, and then go to a smaller room to create the *contract* for the ethnodrama process with the girls. Nine girls showed up that evening, all having signed or having had their parent or guardian sign their consent form. At this point, there were ten adults present in supporting roles. We soon realized we had way too many adults in the "therapeutic space"!

I facilitated the process in the gym, including clarification of the project, warm-ups, ice-breakers, some introductory drama therapy "games." There was an atmosphere of nervousness, shyness and awkwardness, which was to be expected in a first meeting in this environment with teenage girls. Next, the two drama therapy intern/research assistants reviewed the *contract* in Room 52. They emphasized (1) an agreement for confidentiality; (2) respect for each other and the workshop space and, finally, (3) the commitment to building a script based on stories of the participants' experiences in Batshaw and a subsequent performance. Later, the art therapy interns/research assistants took over the contract building process, using some art media. At midpoint, there was a break for juice and cookies (this break was a required and necessary part of the process for all the following sessions). The drama therapy interns led the group in some final drama therapy exercises and, so, we seemed to be on our way in terms of building a group process.

A Big Fight Breaks Out in the Second Meeting

As trust is a huge issue for this population, we wanted to spend time to build trusting relationships and focus on creating group cohesion. This element was very necessary for both the therapeutic process of art therapy and drama therapy and the development of the ethnodrama. In this meeting, it was decided to begin with the art therapy process and to continue at the beginning of the group with the large mural paper that had been placed on the wall, last time, to concretize the *contract* with large-scale writing and arts media. The second part of the evening on the following Tuesday was devoted to drama therapy process, which was done on the other side of Room 52. As is normal with both the framework for drama therapy and ethnodrama, the group needs to be trained in fundamental improvisational acting skills, to build their confidence and also to set the pathway for better communication via improvisational role-playing. Both drama therapist Renée Emunah's Integrative Five Phase model (1994, 2020) and her perspective on using drama therapy with resistant adolescents (1985) were used in our work. As described in the epigraph at the beginning of this chapter, Emunah perceives resistance as a natural component in the treatment of adolescents (1985, p. 71). Although she was doing her work with adolescents in a psychiatric day treatment program, her words certainly rang true for us. I can vividly remember one young woman, subtly giving me the finger, all through one part of a workshop, pretending she was touching her face. She wanted the white male "authority figure" to know that she was very angry. Emunah's approach to getting beyond the anger and resistance was a major component of our creative arts therapies' framework.

This second group was run by the drama therapy interns under my guidance. We explored different formats for the leadership of the groups; eventually, the evenings were split between being led, one half by the drama therapy interns and one half by the art therapy interns, and this pattern was alternated from week to week, for the rest of the "data-gathering" phase.

This night an explosion erupted in the group: during the drama therapy role-plays, one of the girls felt that another had insulted her – "dissed her" – and suddenly a fight broke out. What had been play suddenly became real. And factions were immediately set in place. This was because the girls came from different units, and they were rivals. There was also an age difference factor. Within two minutes the group of eight girls became all split up, yelling and cursing at each other; taunting each other, and, later, on the way back to the unit, one girl took a swing at and hit her adversary. The ideal of trusting group cohesion was instantaneously destroyed, and the adult researchers, staff and interns were at a loss about what to do *in this moment*. The group ended early, and the team met to figure out how to repair this rupture. The group had a real split between two factions. One of the older girls had told her rival, "don't speak under your breath about them," meaning the derogatory remarks her adversary had aimed at the younger girls. The team was now looking for ways to reset the frame for "safety" in the group and create a respectful process of communication in the group.

This second group was a real harbinger of the challenges ahead of us, and of the fragility of the girls and the tendency of the group to fragment. In the months to come, we were witness to the depth of distrust and pronounced negative self-images of the girls, which made it very difficult to build the kind of *ensemble* we needed for the ethnodrama.

Re-Setting the Structure for the Weekly Groups

We realized from the "Fight Night" that there were just too many adults present in the room. Basically, we re-set it so that only the interns ran the groups, all other staff and researchers were seated outside the group. It was cut down so that only one or two staff and one researcher were present. That meant only two or three adults in the space, besides the interns. Fortunately, the room had an accordion divider, so it could be at least partially shut to give even more a sense of privacy for the art therapy and drama therapy groups. These two sessions alternated between the first half of the evening and the second, with a ten-minute break in between the two 40–45 minute sessions. It had also been worked out in the revised *contract* that there would be pizza there for the break, every third week. The girls always looked forward to this.

Eventually the group "topped off" at seven. A new girl came in and two girls left: one ran away and one decided to drop out. By mid-December, the group was pretty constant. The seven young women that remained were the seven who performed in the ethnodrama on March 28, 2012.

The Use of Art and Drama and Processes to Capture the Girl's Authentic Experiences of Being "Inside the System"

The essential purpose of the art therapy and drama therapy groups was twofold: to give the girls a supportive and therapeutic experience while they were living in the Dorval Residence and to collect the data of their *lived experience* in order to build the background for the ethnodramatic play production.

The art therapy interns from Concordia's MA in creative arts therapies led over a dozen sessions, using various art therapy methods to help the girls express their feelings and internalized experiences. In these sessions, the girls produced various art forms such as collages or pastel drawings. The content often expressed their anger and frustration at being placed in the system. Here is a description of one process implemented by the art therapy interns:

Life at Batshaw Collage

- Participants were asked to create a visual representation of their experience of living in residential care, using a variety of visual media, including drawing materials, paint, and collage.

- Fostered self-reflection.
- Facilitated control and encouraged self-expression: Participants were free to express themselves and their experience of their environment without judgment or punishment.
- Visual representation offered containment and contextualization for a variety of conflicting and difficult emotions; Some felt Batshaw offered them security and stability, while others expressed anger as a result of loss (of freedom, home, friendships, and identity).

(C. Corradetti, personal communication, September 2, 2013)

Some of this artwork was later used as projected scenery in the actual *Ethnodrama* performance. Figure 3.3 is an example that expresses Georgia's[2] rage at the system:

The drama therapy interns who ran one-half of each evening's workshops, in the same way, used many **drama therapy** techniques to help build trust in the group, confidence in their expressing themselves and improvisational skills for role-playing:

The clap: The group stands in a circle. The leader claps her hands to her right. When she does so, the participants next to her must try and clap

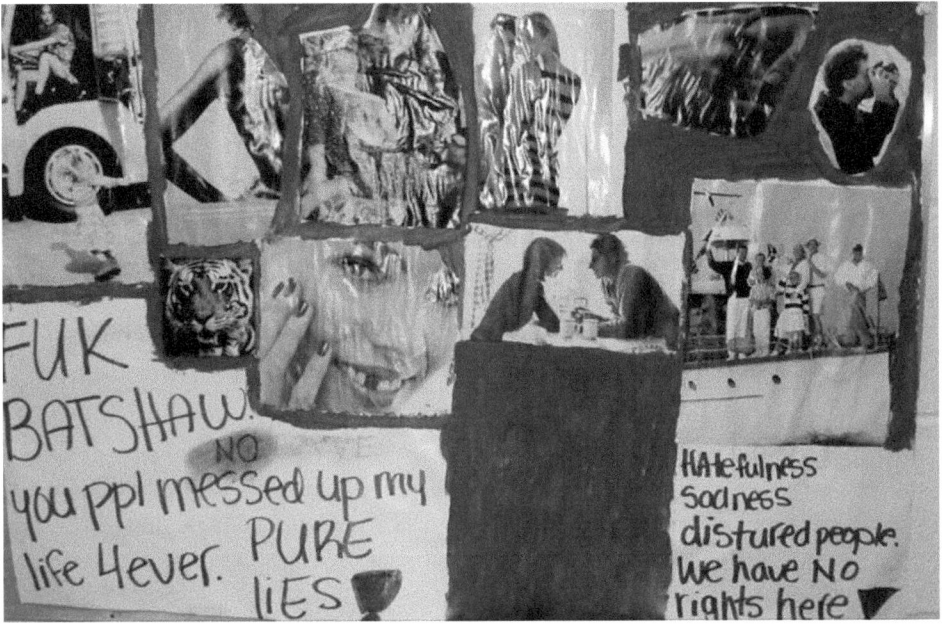

Figure 3.3   Georgia's Rage at the System (courtesy of *The Drama Therapy Review*)

2 All participants have been given pseudonyms to protect their identities per our ethics agreement.

at the same time facing her. This participant then turns to her right and claps with the next person trying to clap with her. The clap goes around the circle. The leader can play with intensity (speed, strength, etc.) Raise the group energy, concentration, and group work. Playful. Works well only if the whole group is in it together.

Numbers and shapes: The members walk in the room keeping to themselves. The leader calls out a number, and the participants team up in that number. The participants who were not quick enough to find a group are eliminated, which raises the stakes of the game. The leader can also call out shapes in which case the participants team up and create the shape with their bodies. Verify their capacity to listen to directives of group leaders. Figure out who the leaders in the group are (are they positive, creative). Raise the energy.

Three pictures: In small teams, the members choose a situation in which a specific action occurs. They create three embodied pictures of this situation: beginning, middle, end. Each person decides their character and position in the frescos. The members practice taking the pose without moving. They then present in front of the group without playing the actions between pictures. The group tries to guess the action. If the activity works well, after trying to guess, the presenters can act out the story going through the three images from beginning to end. This works on group cohesion, teamwork, decision-making, concentration, embodiment and performance. While onstage, the participants learn how to act in front of an audience (attitude, respect, presence, etc.).
        (M. Gendron-Langevin, personal communication, July 18, 2013)

As in all *therapeutic theatre* work, the participants must have some fundamental training in acting to be able to both evoke and perform their personal experiences. In Emunah's (1994, 2020) approach, the group moves from improvisational *play* exercises, which establish concentration and stage focus (as the first two exercises above) to *scenework*, in which they create fictional scenes to improve their improvisational role-playing capacity (like the third exercise above). This work then sets the platform for the *role-playing* phase in which real experiences are enacted. The final phase of each drama therapy session is a *closure* process, bringing the group back to its everyday reality; in this case, the girls' return to their units. The following are delineations of exercises for the last two phases mentioned:

Positive story told by someone else: Having created a timeline with positive highlights of their lives in art therapy, the participants now use this in drama therapy work. The participants are invited to pair-up with someone they've never worked with, that they don't talk to very often, or that they don't know very well. They share a positive story of their timeline. Two groups of two join. The member listening now tells the other members about her partner's positive story. **Embody the story**: Within the group of four, the members choose one story to embody they think could be fun (even if it's internal ex: different people playing different parts of the brain). They choose who plays whom, and direct the scene. They then come back as a big group and the teams play out their story to the rest of the girls.

The squeeze: Standing in a circle, the participants hold hands. The lights are dimmed and the group members are silent. The leader asks the participants to breath deeply three times and then starts a squeeze that will be passed around the circle. This exercise can be used as an opening and closure ritual. It invites the participants to calm down and concentrate as well as acknowledge the group they are working with.
(M. Gendron-Langevin, personal communication, July 18, 2013)

As can be seen in the description of the first exercise above, the art therapy and drama therapy interns worked in conjunction to evoke the personal experiences of the participants through the two media of art and drama. The art therapy interns had implemented a very powerful exercise called "Time Line" which intimately explored the girls' self-perception. Here is a description of it:

Time Line

- Participants were asked to create a timeline of significant events of their life using a variety of visual media, including drawing materials, paint, and collage.
- Emphasis was placed on creating a visual narrative of their past and present experiences, as well as helping to visualize goals and aspirations for the future.
- A variation of the self-portrait.
- Facilitates internal and external organization of what can often be a fragmented childhood due to incidences of severe and reoccurring trauma, abuse and/or neglect.
- Identity construction: addresses questions of who am I?, how did I get here?, and where do I go from here?
(C. Corradetti, personal communication, September 2, 2013)

The drama therapy interns then used the same framework to give the girls the opportunity to embody and enact their experiences. What was catalyzed by the **art therapy** process was then taken into embodied scenes, which the participants performed for each other, creating the pathway for the eventual performance of a playscript.

The Song-Writing Workshop: A Fiasco, or Nearly So

Music and song can always enhance the power of any theatre production, and this is also true with ethnodrama. We had planned to have a musical dimension in our project. I invited my Concordia colleague, Jeri Brown, a professor of music and an internationally known jazz singer, to do a song-writing workshop with the girls in February. Professor Brown prepared an evening-long workshop adapted to what she thought would be the girls' musical tastes. Everything Jeri Brown, in a highly skilled and open approach, offered that evening was rejected by the girls, saying, "this sucks!" They seemed to need to demonstrate their power to reject everything offered by "the adults." This was also true in the case of a professional choreographer that I had hired to help with the expected dance numbers that would be developed with the script. The psychology of the girls in this pilot project, in fact, beyond their defensive anger and sullenness, reflected their actual vulnerability and lack of self-confidence and seemed to predicate their unwillingness to "take direction." As the director, I felt that I was providing them with an incredible opportunity with this song-writing teacher and this choreographer, and they flatly rejected both. Their clear message was that they needed to be *in control* and not comply with some adult's agenda. This important issue will be discussed, shortly.

However, a day or so after the song-writing session, one of the angriest girls wrote down a song and sent it to me via one of the art therapy interns who had her internship at the Batshaw Residence during the day. This song, along with one written later by Teresa, was transcribed into musical notation and set down on a professional song sheet by Jeri Brown and her assistant Chris Tauchner. Both songs were used in the play performance.

From the drama therapy and art therapy processes, themes began to emerge from the artwork and the scenes created by these young women that represented their experiences within "the system." These included simple scenes like "doing chores," "a day in the life of a Batshaw resident." Later, some of the "obligatory scenes," like "going AWOL" or "my day in Court," were developed. The method of creating the playscript will be discussed next.

Stage 2: Building the Script and Validating It

Creating the Script

The script in an ethnodrama constitutes the "research report." As Mienczakowski states, ethnodrama is "a form of 'performed research' in an endeavor to motivate wider community analysis, discussion and dissemination of issues affecting and informing health informants' lives and healing potential" (Mienczakowski & Morgan, 2001, p. 219). In essence the script that is built represents a "research report," aimed at changing the system portrayed in the ethnodrama.

All the "data" collected in the art therapy, drama therapy and music workshops – the artwork, the scenes, the monologues, the songs – composed the content, ready to be shaped into a dramatic and authentic portrait of the girls' experience of being "inside the system." It represents a research process in Saldana's phrase, that moves "research from page to stage" (2011, frontispiece).

Validating the Script

After the series of workshops during November, December, January and early February, I began to collate the research data into a script. Having studied playwriting and having written many scripts over the past 20 years, it was a fairly simple task for me. The script was outlined in terms of essential themes and then material gathered from various workshops was inserted (see abbreviated script in the next session). The next crucial step was to get the girls to approve the script, as written. This is called *Informant Validation*.

A first reading was held with the girls on February 14. They seemed excited to hear their own voices embodied in the script. The script was based on verbatim extractions from the personal interviews that had been recorded and transcribed; themes and images that came out of the workshops; personal statements and scenes that had been explored in the drama therapy workshops; the two songs mentioned above; and a narration specifically developed for one of the girls.

At this juncture, the whole question of "Who is in control?" became even more accentuated. In every form of *therapeutic theatre*, a sense of ownership by the participants is quintessential. As the sense of control is a super vital issue with this population (see the interviews above), their ownership of the material, the script and the performance is a *sine qua non* for the success of the project. Mienczakowski's technique of *Informant Validation* is what allows the participants in an ethnodrama to have this sense of control and to develop ownership of the experience. This "technique" consists of all final approval of the script and its performance being left to the participants. Nothing moves forward unless they approve of it. This consequently "returns the *ownership*, and therefore the power, of the report to its informants" (Mienczakowski, 2001, p. 471). At least, this is the ideal. As the drama therapy interns led the script-reading sessions, they constantly checked in to see if the girls were satisfied with the script. Probably the fact that the girls did not outright rebel against the script, as they did in the song-writing session, was an indication that they recognized themselves in it. They recognized their own voices in the script. They "approved" it. Capturing their authentic voices was a goal from the start!

However, as then-art therapy intern Claudia Corradetti has pointed out in regard to our process:

> There were significant trust issues, in particular for youth who have experienced early developmental trauma – so more clarity was needed from the beginning about what the project entailed, and this would allow for us to maintain a sturdier frame. For such a group, consistency, predictability, and sturdiness is so essential; and would have allowed for a deeper process to unfold. We needed to listen better to the participants and have them be more in control of the process.
>
> (C. Corradetti, personal communication, May 2, 2020)

In retrospect, the more control these young women could have given in each stage of the process, the deeper their engagement might have been. In Chapter 8, we will discuss this as an ethical issue.

Script as 'Research Report'

The validated script consisted of an opening and a closing, with seven scenes in between. Each scene reflected a significant result of the previous phases of the research. The play was titled, "Inside the System: An Ethnodrama in One Act with Two Songs." It was expressly identified as "Co-created through a collaboration of the Concordia University Research Team and Eight Participants from Batshaw Youth and Family Centres." We said "eight," here, but one other girl dropped out before the performance.

Inside the System: an Ethnodrama in One Act with Two Songs

The Opening

Each of the girls entered and said a line of how they felt disrespected while in the Batshaw Centres residence. Here are a few examples:

GEORGIA: "I feel disrespected when they keep bringing up my past."

SAMANTHA: "I feel very disrespected when I am treated like an immature teenager."

HELEN: "I felt disrespected because I had absolutely no control over my own life when I was in Batshaw."

Then, they took a pose, representing their feeling about their statement and held it, thus creating a "tableaux vivant." This theme of "disrespect" emerged from the rehearsal process and the interviews. It vividly reflected their subjective experience.

Scene 1: "The Court Order for the First 30 Days"

This scene was set up by the Narrator, played by Sarah. As previously mentioned, pseudonyms are used here for all girls in the project. Sarah explained how the girls were to demonstrate what it was really like to live at the Batshaw Centre.

Then, each of the girls said a line expressing why they were in placement: "Ran away!," "Drugs!," "Family Issues!," "Robbery!." It is important to note that these lines, although developed by each individual, were not expressed by that individual. The Batshaw Centres Research Advisory Committee had asked for the script to be done this way for the sake of confidentiality, and the girls agreed to it. What followed next, was an amalgamated scene, based on the girls' collective experience of their appearances in court. This scene was inspired by the recurring stories of court appearances that occurred in the drama therapy group and the interviews.

Scene 2: "How We Got Here"

This consisted of two monologues, one of which was developed from Georgia's transcribed interview:

GEORGIA: I was fourteen years old. I was doing drugs, and I got abused. A lot of shit happened that you guys don't know. Batshaw doesn't know shit. I was out on the streets. I was hanging out with the wrong friends. They weren't my friends. These cocksuckers were traitors. I just wanted you to know ... they used me as a dog to get what they wanted ... Anyways, I was on AWOL and doing bad shit. I was at the hospital to make sure I was ok, and I was! Thank god there is a god. Then, the police came and asked me some questions. Then, Batshaw came to pick me up ... That's where I got my reputation for Batshaw!

Scene 3: "Once Inside the System"

This scene portrayed a typical day in a Batshaw Centres residence, with the themes selected by the girls – routine, boredom, loss of control, etc. – and expressed through mime and acting. The atmosphere came out of single-word descriptions the girls expressed in their interviews about their perceptions of the environment within their Batshaw residence: "irritating," "frustrating," "aggravating," "misery," etc.

Scene 4: "Going AWOL"

This was a re-enactment of one girl's experience of running away – going AWOL – her great sense of freedom, and then being picked up by the police. Theatrically, this was quite graphically portrayed, with sirens and flashing red lights, etc. This scene came directly from one individual's in-depth description of this experience during her interview:

PATTY: I used to love going AWOL. I felt free and that's the best part about it. The freedom! Me and whichever friends I met up with would have so much fun. I know that sounds bad, but I felt like I had a life outside of four walls whenever I got away.

Scene 5: "Stigma"

This scene consisted of two monologues adapted from the girls' interviews. One was almost verbatim:

MARCIE: I think that when someone realizes that you live in a place like this, they automatically see you as a negative influence, and they see you as someone who shouldn't be around their children if they're a parent and, then, children think, "Oh, I shouldn't be around this child because other people might get the impression that I'm involved in delinquent activities and so on." Yeah, there's a lot of negative associations with this place.

Scene 6: "Some Bad, Some Good"

This scene consisted of monologues expressing what the girls thought they did or did not get out of their residential center experience. It was accompanied by a backdrop of slides of their artwork:

JULIA: I don't think Batshaw can change my personality; they have the right to change me into a better person, but they don't have the right to change who I am. Like I'm still like the nice girl I used to be, I'm kind, I speak my mind, and stuff like that. They can't change me, but they changed the way I act.

Scene 7: "We're the Original, Not the Copy"

This came from an idea presented by Georgia. It was almost verbatim from her interview.

GEORGIA: Batshaw thinks like they bring you in and just because they have a bunch of papers and a bunch of books and all that stuff about you, it doesn't mean anything. There's a bunch of things that my unit doesn't know about me. They only know what they see, what they've heard of … they have the copy but they don't have the original.

This was a powerful theme about identity. Other girls picked up on this theme. One wrote a poem that closed the performance.

> The Closing
>
> You have hurt me
> You have scarred me
> For love I cannot truly feel
> Deep inside my soul, I wanna be love
> As much as I am loved.
> But because of all you've done to me
> I feel numb and hatred
> Tears I will not let fall
> For tears mean weakness and
> Pain
> Pain I wish to not feel again.

Stage 3: Rehearsing the Validated Script

As mentioned in the previous chapter, rehearsal time is organized strategically to genuinely accomplish the therapeutic and aesthetic goals of the ethnodrama production. By the end of February, 2012, a new two-day per week rehearsal schedule was initiated, and we eventually hired a professional stage manager to keep everything organized and flowing. However, the kind of resistance cited by Emunah (1985) was still activated during the rehearsal process, very likely, in this instance, due to the psychological stressors that she identifies: "The struggles of adolescents for a stable self-identity represent in part and to a degree on the depth of their psychopathology, struggles against the loss of boundaries, hence some authors conceptualize adolescence as a struggle against disintegration" (pp. 72–73). Due to these inner conflicts, it was very difficult for the participants to fully own this project. Even though they had validated the script, their commitment most often seemed half-hearted. This particularly showed up in the unwillingness to learn their lines and lyrics. It was for this reason, and because rehearsal time was so limited, we decided, together, that the performance would be a *Staged Reading* and would be advertised as such. This removed the anxiety about having to learn lines, which was already exacerbated by the fact that, due to confidentiality issues, the participants were *not allowed to take their scripts with them, back to their units, after rehearsals*.

With consideration of the specific context of the environment and population, rehearsals for an EDT project move ahead like any other theatre production: blocking is set, cues are learned, songs and movement are rehearsed, and lighting, props and costumes are brought in. As this was to be a *staged reading*, production values were kept minimal, with the exception of the projection of slides of the participant's artwork as backgrounds and a good sound system used to play music that the girls had either created or chosen for the beginning of scenes.

"Why Are You Trying to Turn Us into Great Actresses!?"

The stress of the final rehearsal process catalyzed some anger and frustration in the girls. This was likely the pressure of expectation, but, also, the questions came up again: Whose agenda is this? Who is in control? The drama therapy interns had been running the workshops for three months, but, now, in the final stage, I took over the rehearsal process. This has been the plan. I was, by far, the most experienced theatre director. However, the participants were used to young female facilitators, and I was an older white male, like many of the judges and school principals they had encountered. I think this fact precipitated some more rebelliousness on their part. I also wanted them to do their best and directed the rehearsal so they could have success. To them, I believe, in retrospect, this was experienced as more pressure. In one rehearsal, a young woman blurted out: "Why are you trying to turn us into great actresses!?" This gave me pause to reflect on the warning of Mitchell around the potential conflict within a therapeutic theatre director: "The dramatherapist is not there to theatrically realise their own vision and to use the 'company' to fulfill their own artistic ambitions, but to be a convenor, a resource person, to facilitate in the best traditions of dramatherapy practice" (Mitchell in Jennings et al.,1994, p. 52). This conflict, along with some struggles that began to emerge between myself and the art therapy and drama therapy interns, suggested the kinds of ethical issues which arise in the EDT process and will be addressed in Chapter 8.

Are We Ready?

This is the perennial question of all who create theatrical performances. Are things in place and well-organized enough to now bring in an audience? Two days before the scheduled performance we had installed a rented stage in the cafeteria of the Batshaw Residence. The lighting and slide projector were also set up. The readiness felt even more crucial as we would only do one performance for an invited audience, as specified by the Batshaw Advisory Committee. Only staff and family members were allowed to attend.[3] Surprisingly, as things got down to the final wire, the girls asked for an extra dress rehearsal, *one hour before the show*! This was an encouraging sign that they were, finally, perhaps, owning their performance.

Stage 4: Informant Validation of the Performance

This next step is crucial. The ideal is to have the group review the performance via video, or to have other members of the population witness a preview and provide formidable feedback on its veracity. This was easier in Mienczakowski's earlier work (1995a; 1995b): when the informants were not the performers, they could more objectively examine whether the performance was telling "their truth." In "It's A Wonderful World," as described in Chapter 2, the informants were also the actors, but they were able to view a *full videotaped performance* not long after the first previews, and in this way were able to give authentic feedback about the performance. This ended up in changes in the script and the performance, before we took the play on tour. As Mienczakowski writes: "ethnodrama, as an extension of forum theatre, renegotiates its meanings with every performance ... repeatedly seeking validation from those about whom it is written, and responding to a consensus of informed opinion by changing the research report/script accordingly" (1995b, p. 366). This is an incredibly valuable tool for the research and also for the authenticity of the performance.

---

3 Again, due to ethical restrictions, only one private performance was allowed for staff, family and the researchers. It was, in fact, videotaped, but this documentation could only be reviewed by Batshaw staff and the researchers.

How Did the Performance Validation Occur?

With each EDT project, the Informant Validation of the performance takes place in a different way. In the Batshaw project, we might say it took place through a constant osmosis as the female adolescents ingested the script (which they indirectly validated), the movement and blocking, the cues, and their lines and lyrics. Almost all of this material had come directly from their experience, so they were able to embrace it as "their truth." The one exception was the song, "Real Experience," which, although the lyrics were by one of the girls, had been professionally arranged and transcribed by Jeri Brown and Chris Tauchner. This was my idea but was accepted by the song's creator. In general, the participants accepted how the performance had been developed and staged. Otherwise, they would have refused to do it. As we have seen, they were not afraid to say "no"!

Stage 5: The Performance

In this case, it was the *one and only* performance. Sadly, there is no visual or audio record of this performance, that can be shown to the public or to other professionals in the field, because of the strict ethics regulations that were agreed to (see footnote on previous page). However, I do have my own research video of the performance that can only be screened for myself, the research team and the staff at Batshaw. I have reviewed it many times. From this, I will attempt to give some impressions of how the performance felt.

The performance was announced to the invited audience via a flyer. The improvised cafeteria/theatre was filled to capacity, about 50 persons in attendance. After the audience was seated at 7:15pm, Dr. D'Amico and her research assistant administered the pre-performance questionnaire to the audience (see presentation of this in next section). A few announcements were made, and the girls entered from the improvised "Green Room," around the corner. There was excitement in the air, but these young women were quite obviously nervous.

A Strange Beginning

Two things happened that got the performance off to a wonky start. First of all, the stage manager had put up the wrong slide. Because of a miscommunication from the director, this slide remained up all the time when the audience got seated and during the administration of the pre-performance questionnaire. This slide had large words in print: colored in purple were the words, FUCK THE SYSTEM; and in red and purple it stated, "NO modification ZONE – BITCHES." It certainly let the audience know, in "confrontational theatre" style, that the play was about the girl's anger and frustration. It was supposed to be a gentler slide with a special piece of music selected by the participants.

Secondly, after the girls introduced themselves with a line and a gesture about feeling disrespected, a song, "The Real Experience," was presented. Irene, who wrote the lyrics to the song, refused to perform them, but allowed the piece to be played over the sound system. The problem was the song was long and it left the girls on stage, seated in a line from right to left, with nothing to do. They looked very uncomfortable, as the audience looked at them and they looked back. It was a place for movement, but none had been prepared, after Irene decided not to actually perform her song.

A "Spontaneous" Moment

Thank goodness, this was followed by one of the funniest moments in the play, certainly a big surprise to the director who had never staged it, although probably pre-planned by the actress who "spontaneously" inserted it. It came in Scene 1, "The Courtroom Scene." One of the girls, who had been cast as a Court Security Officer, had to announce the entrance of the Judge (played by one of the girls in a real judge's robe). She proclaimed "All rise for the Right Honourable W. LaFonda!" That was her entire bit. What she did, also, then, was to look out toward the audience and very demandingly instruct: "*All rise!*" The entire audience of family members, staff, social workers, teachers, etc. stood up *as if they were really in court!* Some of the girls on stage, including the Right Honourable W. LaFonda, broke out laughing. The moment was so unexpected. They giggled and laughed, and could not contain themselves for a couple of minutes. It gave a delightful levity to a rather overly serious scene. It "broke the ice" for the rest of the performance.

According to the Script

The rest of the play moved along without any hitches, and the girls stuck to the validated script, previously described. Their performances were filled with all the emotions that they had infused in the scenes, songs and monologues. Teresa's song about an "imaginary friend," called "Down the Rabbit Hole," was an especially sensitive rendering and moved the audience with her vulnerability. The performance ended with individual lines about their unique personhood and their right to respect – "I am equal just like everyone else." I felt that this pastiche of their lived experiences represented a truthful "research report" about their lives. The audience showed great support for these young women through their applause and cheering.

Stage 6: Post-Performance Activities

As is often the case in EDT, both *Pre- and Post-Performance Questionnaires* were administered in order to measure change of attitudes in the audience as a result of witnessing the ethnodrama.

In the *Pre-Questionnaire*, there were ten statements which audience members answered in pencil on paper as "Strongly Agree," "Agree," "Disagree," or "Strongly Disagree."

1. Adolescents in placement do not think about the consequences of their actions.
2. Adolescents in placement are concerned about their futures.
3. Adolescents in placement want to be regarded as the "black sheep" of their families.
4. Adolescents in placement worry about what others think of them.
5. Adolescents in placement do not have good problem-solving skills.
6. Adolescents in placement are angry most of the time.
7. Adolescents in placement lack confidence.
8. Adolescents in placement want to be isolated from others.
9. Adolescents in placement want to help others.
10. Adolescents in placement need more opportunities to control and direct their own lives.

In this this project, there was no formal discussion or forum with the audience, but a *Post-Questionnaire* was distributed immediately after the curtain call. It consisted of three questions: (1) what did you think about the play?; (2) what did you take away from the play?; and (3) what new information did you learn about adolescents from the play? A total of 30 audience members responded to this questionnaire. Here is a condensation of their responses, revealing the following themes (in italics):

Appreciation for the authentic voice: many respondents stated the need to listen more carefully to kids under youth protection, but the most common response was that the girls had expressed themselves *authentically*. The audience stressed the importance of how the performance allowed the girls to speak "in their own voice." One 40-year-old female audience member, answering the second question on what she would take away from the play, stated: "To slow down and think, because it is not just another girl/boy that we are 'dealing' with but rather another human who has a voice and a vision of where they would like to go." As one 42-year-old male responded: "It sounds like it has [come] from their heart, their hearts, their voices. It pains me to hear how we fail them, miss our objectives, that we don't often reach them ... I loved the way they used themselves as the main props ... Courageous."

Another common theme that was presented in the responses was the audience members' understanding of *the girls' desire to be respected*. The opening scene of the play had presented the negative frame of this theme: all the ways the girls felt disrespected while receiving services from Batshaw Centres. It was obviously something they needed to give voice to, and the audience perceived the magnitude of its importance to them. A 60-year-old female stated that "I learned they are human, make mistakes, but deserve to be respected and loved just like everyone else."

A third significant theme was: *the need for change in the system*. Many audience members expressed their understanding that "the child protection system does not work perfectly and needs change." For example, one 26-year-old female audience member succinctly stated: "To help an individual grow they need to have healthy relationships. The system is here to help them not hinder. Let's make their experiences into a more positive one." An ethnodrama is meant to catalyze such questions, and this one certainly did. A 45-year-old female stated: "What's missing in the way the system works. Some good things but lots of room for improvement." This theme was corroborated through a previous interview with the Youth Empowerment worker who stated:

> Is Batshaw Centres perfect? Of course not, nothing is perfect. I feel like there is a lot in place to help youth and families, but it is not perfect. Also, people have to be willing to accept the help that is offered to them, which not everyone is willing or able to do.
>
> (Dupuis, 2012)

We felt from our analysis of the responses to the post-performance questionnaires that we had, at least to a small degree, succeeded in our goal for this EDT project of changing perspectives towards youth in the system; there had been some new awareness created in the audience, via viewing the play, in how they perceived these female adolescents in Youth Protection. In terms of our goal of catalyzing changes in the system, a plan was put in place, soon after this project, to use the only video documentary of the play, previously mentioned, as a training tool for new staff at Batshaw. We look at this as a valuable, positive effect of our research. We will discuss what we *learned* from the full experience of this project in the Conclusion section at the end.

Stage 7: Closure

Just as the post-performance work is crucial to the research and social activist functions of EDT (see Figure 1.4), closure is of paramount importance to the therapeutic process. These young women had spent the last six months, engaging in art therapy and drama therapy experiences, sometimes reviewing their traumatic pasts. They needed the opportunity to review their whole experience and to process their feelings about it.

On Tuesday, April 3, the group met for a final closure process at the Dorval Residence. One of the girls couldn't make it, but the rest were present. Overall, the girls said they were proud of their accomplishments with the project and were glad they had participated in it.

The following week, on Tuesday, April 10, Batshaw paid for the staff and the cast of the project to celebrate the completion of the project with dinner at a Chinese restaurant, nearby the Dorval Residence. This was the formal conclusion to the project.

Shortly afterward, the main staff contact person sent some comments from the parents and the girls that summarized their experiences of the project:

> Parent #1: "I cannot believe what my daughter can accomplish."
> Parent #2: "When I saw her up there she made me cry."
> Parent #3: "I think we should have more programs like this."
> Participant #1: "The program affected me in a positive way."
> Participant #2: "My social worker saw a different side of me."

Follow-up with Georgia and Teresa

On April 24, I did a follow-up interview with Georgia, in which she expressed her gratitude for being able to say what was inside of her as regarding her Batshaw experience. She felt this was the main value of the project:

> Yeah, because when the audience was there, I felt like I was telling them how I feel, how I feel to be in Batshaw. It helped me like bring out, my, my feelings. But, it didn't help me like a really good way, you know, like if it would have helped me to get out of Batshaw, no problem. But, *it just helped me express my feelings. That's all it did.*

Also, on the same day, I did a final interview with Teresa. Her responses seem to suggest some real therapeutic benefits from being in the project. She says:

> I feel even more determined because like I was singing on stage … Now like I'm just determined to really work hard on my music cause it's like my passion, and I don't want to rip it up this time. I want to be out there … And I want to let people like … I want to see if people will understand, you know.

In her pre-rehearsal interview, she had explained that she had destroyed much of the artistic output of her childhood, songs, poems, stories, etc., just "ripped them up and threw them away." This would seem to parallel her former self-destructive and suicidal tendencies. So, this post-project statement would seem to be a hopeful note.

Unfortunately, because of scheduling and other issues, a full closure could not be done individually with each girl. Neither was the group closure as complete as what had been offered to the participants in the "It's a Wonderful World" project (Chapter 2). In reviewing this project in retrospect, and, especially, in considering the work as "trauma-informed drama therapy" (Sajnani & Johnson, 2014), this appears as a major deficit and one that needs to be sensitively addressed in the implementation of EDT projects.

Stage 8: Evaluation, Analysis and Dissemination

I have given a few examples of the post-performance questionnaire responses. We also analyzed the pre-performance questionnaire responses.

Statistical Analysis of Pre-Performance Questionnaire

The Pre-Performance Questionnaire developed by Dr. D'Amico was based on an extensive literature review of the general attitudes, including negative and stigmatizing attitudes, that the general public hold of youths in care. A four-point **Likert scale** was used. A total of 33 (n=33) out of 50 participants responded (23 females; nine males and one undisclosed). Table 3.1 presents the descriptive statistics arising from the questionnaire.

Evaluation of Project Goals

As the primary goal had been to empower the youth-in-care by providing them with the opportunity to express their personal voice and narratives, we can see this *experience of authentic expression* evidenced in both Georgia's

Table 3.1   Statistical Analysis of Pre-Performance Questionnaire Responses

Question: Adolescents in placement	Strongly agree	Agree	Disagree	Strongly disagree	Mean	Standard Deviation
1. Do not think about the consequences of their actions		10 (31%)	20 (63%)	2 (6%)	2.75	0.568
2. Are concerned about their futures	10 (30%)	20 (61%)	3 (9%)		1.79	0.600
3. Want to be regarded as the 'black sheep' of their families	1 (3%)		17 (53%)	14 (44%)	3.38	0.660
4. Worry about what others think of them	7 (21%)	20 (61%)	5 (15%)	1 (3%)	2.00	0.707
5. Do not have good problem-solving skills		14 (42%)	16 (49%)	3 (9%)	2.67	0.646
6. Are angry most of the time		6 (18%)	25 (76%)	2 (6%)	2.88	0.486
7. Lack confidence	2 (6%)	20 (61%)	10 (30%)	1 (3%)	2.30	0.637
8. Want to be isolated from others			21 (64%)	12 (36%)	3.36	0.489
9. Want to help others	2 (6%)	25 (81%)	4 (13%)		2.06	0.442
10. Need more opportunities to control and direct their own lives	9 (28%)	19 (60%)	2 (6%)	2 (6%)	1.91	0.777

Source: Permission from Dr. Miranda D'Amico and *The Drama Therapy Review*.

statement above and in the post-questionnaire responses that demonstrate that the audience really heard and reacted positively to the girls' portrayals of their frustrations and challenges. These responses reveal an understanding of the girls' desires and their developmental and psychosocial needs. This is particularly important as it validates the central aim of the ethnodrama method as a "form of public voice ethnography that has emancipatory and educational potential" (Mienczakowski, 2001, p. 469). It also relates ethnodrama to the psychotherapeutic objectives of drama therapy, especially as they are employed in therapeutic theatre. The drama and art therapy methods utilized in this project were adapted to the therapeutic goals for the young women. The script was created in the same light as a script for a therapeutic theatre production, i.e., "the play must be developed with therapeutic intentions and goal-setting" (Snow et al., 2003, p. 75).

Another goal was to measure whether witnessing the ethnodrama changed the audience's perceptions towards these girls. This was meant to be accomplished through a comparison of the responses to the pre- and post-questionnaires.

Evident from the results of the pre-performance questionnaire is the fact that the respondents were by and large positive and avoided making extremely negative assessments of the statements presented. The respondents generally disagreed with statements that portrayed the youth-in-care as not thinking about the consequences of their actions, not being concerned about their futures, as not having good problem-solving skills, as being angry most of the time and as wanting to be isolated from others. Noteworthy and challenging popular notions of youth-in-care as the "black sheep" of their families is that most of the respondents (97 percent) disagreed with the statement. Given that this questionnaire addressed attitudes, but did not explore the underlying knowledge that leads one to having this kind of attitude, it is something that needs to be further explored. The relatively small sample size and the nature of the study does not make it possible to conduct more extensive analyses or explore alternative explanations. What is apparent, however, is that the respondents are part of a community that supports the youth and, perhaps because of their personal involvement and awareness, have a more positive and constructive view of them. Another plausible explanation that may occur is that in an unintentional manner, the respondents may try to portray themselves or their organization in a more favorable light, what is referred to as "a social desirability bias."

A goal had also been established to catalyze post-performance discussions that might induce changes needed in the Batshaw system. Although a central aim of ethnodrama is to change a health-care system (Mienczakowski, 1995a, 2001), regrettably, we did not have the time to fully explore and dialogue on this matter with staff at Batshaw Centres.

Perhaps the greatest limitation of this study was that we never established an effective tool to measure the young women's change in self-perception. This would have been very useful to demonstrate the emancipatory effectiveness of ethnodrama via a pre- and post-comparison. Did they see themselves differently *after* the performance? They probably did, but we had no way to accurately *measure* the girls' change in attitude towards themselves. This has been a perennial problem of the EDT process: not having really sophisticated tools to measure the therapeutic benefits of the specific project. This will be addressed in Chapter 10.

Dissemination

As EDT always represents a serious research endeavor, there is an expectation, usually established in both the proposal to fund agencies and the application for ethics approval, that there will be dissemination of the research findings.

Publications

In the next two years, after the completion of the project, we presented a 65-page Report to Batshaw Youth and Family Centres and to the Centre Jeunesse de Montreal Institut Universitaire. This was later condensed into an article published in the *Drama Therapy Review*, Volume 1, Number 2, 2015 (pp. 201–218). With the kind permission of the co-author and the journal's principal editor, these sources have been used, in part, to create the present account of the project in this chapter.

Presentations

In May 2012, I was invited to give a brief presentation on the Batshaw Project at the International Research Congress on Integrative Medicine and Health in Portland, Oregon. It was framed as a "Focus on the Treatment of Trauma in the Creative Arts Therapies." I got permission to show a short section of the research video documentary, but with the faces of the young women pixelated, so they were not identifiable.

In November 2012, I presented, along with several members of the research team for this project, at the 33rd Annual Conference of the North American Drama Therapy Association in New Haven, Connecticut. Our topic was: "Integrating Ethnodrama and Drama Therapy: Trauma and Other Issues Therapeutically Performed."

In April 2013, I was invited to present on the Batshaw Project for the Research Roundtable on the Arts Therapies at the Expressive Arts Therapies Conference, Alexandria, Virginia. This panel was exploring the types of research methods that can be used in the creative arts therapies. It was a good opportunity to espouse the value of this performance-based ethnographic research approach.

I notate these presentations in some detail to give students and professionals who wish to get involved in EDT research an idea of the avenues that are open for the dissemination of this kind of research and to emphasize the importance of presenting one's research in this field.

Conclusion

We have covered a great deal of territory in this chapter. EDT is an ambitious endeavor, integrating research, therapy, theatre and social activism into one method. The goal has been to demonstrate to potential users of this method what the map of the eight stages looks like *in action*. This begins with the ethnographic research function of uncovering the lived experience of the chosen *ethnos*. Who are these people, emotionally, psychologically and socially? Interviews and creative arts therapies techniques were utilized to create personal narratives. Out of the application of these tools, a script was developed to lucidly reflect an authentic portrait of the group. Through the Informant Validation approach, the group had the final say on what was true and what was not in their "self-portrait." For the EDT to be effective, the group must embrace ownership of the script and the performance. This latter was challenging in this project because of the extreme resistance of adolescents, especially in this situation of court-enforced incarceration.

Lessons Learned

In relation to the four functions of EDT, there were many valuable lessons learned in this project. Each domain provided a specific set of challenges. Sometimes, these challenges were met and sometimes we floundered. However, each experience gave us something to build upon in terms of improving the method as a whole.

Theatre

As will be discussed in Chapter 8, in regard to ethics in EDT, there were some tensions created between the theatrical ambitions of the director and the adolescent females, who seemingly rebelled against the director's desire for "making them into great actresses!" This needs to be looked at very carefully. It was a lesson about *really knowing your population and the kind of challenges they will bring*. Here, it was the degree of resistance to be expected in adolescent groups. The game plan cannot be too grandiose. In this case, too much pressure was placed on these young women, so the production values had to be kept very minimal and the group decided to present their performance only as a staged reading. However, in the end, I think I can honestly say that the informants seemed to truly appreciate having the opportunity to voice their feelings and perspectives through performance. This was their feedback to us.

Research

The research element was quite successful in terms of documenting the perspectives of the specific audience, who seemed very empathic and supportive of the way these young women expressed themselves in the performance.

However, this was not true of the measuring of the participants' change in regard to their own self-image. We recognized that *there was no real research tool developed to measure the efficacy of the therapy process – an area that really needs to be addressed for the EDT process*. Only self-reports were available and these at a very minimal level.

Social Activism

In terms of the social activist function, there were areas to be addressed: (1) changing the stigmatization and prejudiced view towards a marginalized group and (2) changing the system in which the marginalized group is held and treated. In terms of the former, the play production needed to be brought out to the general public. Working with only the staff and family as audience, we perceived the *severe limits for any potential measurement of changing perspectives in the general population*. Scheduling and funding did not allow for this. So, this goal was harshly impeded. As it was, more discussion was needed with the audience and, especially, with the Batshaw administration and staff. A few minimal steps were taken, such as using the research documentary video to train future staff at the agency. This can be regarded as a small positive outcome.

Therapy

Change is the ultimate goal of the EDT process, as it has always been for the ethnodrama process. As Mienczakowski clearly states, the central purpose is to "pursue emancipatory outcomes for specific health consumers" (1995a, p. 46). In this case, our focus was youth-in-care, who may have experienced major trauma in their lives and were presently held under "Youth Protection," which is required to provide care for their safety, their educational needs, rehabilitation, as well as address their social and psychological issues. In adding the creative arts therapies, coordinated through the therapeutic theatre paradigm, EDT aimed to create positive change in the emotional and psychological well-being of the participants. Although this will always be part of EDT's mission, in this case, we learned once again *how difficult it is to measure therapeutic change*. We will discuss this challenge further in Chapter 10.

References

Batshaw Youth and Family Centres. (2011–2012). Annual Management Report, 2011–2012, Montreal, Quebec: Batshaw Youth and Family Centres.

Corradetti, C. (2012). *The broken narrative: Mourning the separation loss of adolescents in residential care* (Unpublished master's thesis). Concordia University, Montreal, Quebec, Canada.

Denzin, N. (2001). The reflexive interview and a performative social science. *Qualitative Research*, 1(1), 23–46.

Dunne, P. (2012). Giving voice to adolescents through drama therapy assessment. In D. R. Johnson, S. Pendzik, & S. Snow (Eds.), *Assessment in drama therapy* (pp. 287–307). C. C. Thomas Publisher.

Emunah, R. (1985). Drama therapy and adolescent resistance. *The Arts in Psychotherapy*, 12, 71–79.

_____. (1994). *Acting for real: Drama therapy process, technique and performance.* Brunner/Mazel Publishers.

_____. (2020). *Acting for real: Drama therapy process, technique, and performance* (2nd ed.). Routledge/Taylor & Francis.

Gil-Kashiwabara, E., Hogansen, J. M., Geenen, S., Powers, K., & Powers, L. E. (2007). Improving transition outcomes for marginalized youth. *Career Development for Exceptional Individuals*, 30(2), 80–91.

Mienczakowski, J. (1995a). *The application of critical ethno-drama to health settings* (Unpublished doctoral dissertation). Griffith University, Nathan, Australia.

_____ (1995b). The theatre of ethnography: The reconstruction of ethnography with emancipatory potential. *Qualitative Inquiry*, 1(3), 360–375.

_____. (2001). Ethnodrama: Performed research – Limitations and potential. In P. Atkinson, A. Coffey, S. Delamont, J. Lofland, & L. Lofland (Eds.), *Handbook of ethnography* (pp. 468–476). Sage Publications.

Mienczakowski, J., & Morgan, S. (2001). Ethnodrama: Constructing participatory, experiential and compelling action research through performance. In P. Reason & H. Bradbury (Eds.), *The handbook of action research: Participative inquiry and practice* (pp. 219–227). Sage Publications.

Mitchell, S. (1994). The theatre of self-expression: A "therapeutic theatre" model of dramatherapy. In S. Jennings, A. Cattanach, S. Mitchell, A. Chesner, & B. Meldrum (Eds.). *The handbook of dramatherapy* (pp. 41–57). Routledge.

Murchison, J. M. (2010). *Ethnography essentials: Designing, conducting, and presenting your research.* Jossey-Bass.

Sajnani, N. & Johnson, D. R. (Eds.). (2014). *Trauma-informed drama therapy: Transforming clinics, classrooms and communities.* C. C. Thomas Publisher.

Saldana, J. (Ed). (2005). *Ethnodrama: An anthology of reality theatre.* AltaMira Press.

Saldana, J. (2011). *Ethnotheatre: Research from page to stage.* Left Coast Press.

Scannapieco, M., Connell-Carrick, K., & Painter, K. (2007). In their own words: Challenges facing youth aging out of foster care. *Child and Adolescent Social Work Journal, 24*(5), 423–425.

Snow, S., D'Amico, M., & Tanguay, D. (2003). Therapeutic theatre and well-being. *The Arts in Psychotherapy, 30,* 73–82.

Snow, S., & D'Amico, M. (2012). *The application of ethnodrama to adolescent girls under youth protection: Pilot project with Batshaw Youth & Family Centres, April 2011–April 2012.* Concordia University, Montreal, Centre for the Arts in Human Development.

Snow, S., & D'Amico, M. (2015). The application of ethnodrama with female adolescents under youth protection within a creative arts therapies context. *Drama Therapy Review, 1*(2), 201–218.

van Manen, M. (2016). *Researching lived experience: Human science for an action sensitive pedagogy* (2nd ed). Routledge.

4
The "Sex Ed." EDT Project at CAHD

However, the sexual needs of this population and how those are to be realized remains a highly controversial legal issue.

(Simon Foley, 2012)

Finding the Theme

As with any EDT project, a theme must be located. But how is this to be done? Basically, there are two ways: the research team can suggest a topic to the group; or the group, itself, can suggest a theme they want to work on. As will be seen in Chapter 7, in my work with Chinese students at the Apollo School in Beijing, it was always the group who located the subject matter to be processed in the six-day EDT workshops. This created automatic "ownership" of the process as the group was emotionally invested in the theme. It was derived through a sociometric procedure (Garcia & Sternberg, 1989), so the topic was chosen via collective engagement and had meaning for everyone in the group. This is probably the most organic approach to finding a theme.

Since the first ethnodrama at CAHD in 2007, I had been exploring the use of a **participatory action research (PAR)** approach in our EDT projects. What this means, in essence, is that everyone involved is considered to be a co-researcher. As Chevalier and Buckles describe it, "We espouse the idea of partnering creatively, towards the *interfacing* of views, goals, skill sets and forms of knowledge and experience that can be brought to bear and evolve through action research" (2019, p. 27). Everyone involved in the project is a stakeholder in the research and its outcome. Of course, working with the population at CAHD, who have many intellectual, cognitive, and neurological challenges, this had to be a "qualified" PAR (Snow et al., 2017, p. 244). We had to make concessions around academic research language, so ideas and theories could be digested. Nonetheless, we made every effort

DOI: 10.4324/9781003083818-6

to hear their voices and take their ideas and opinions into account, and this began with the selection of the theme. In regard to PAR, McTaggart writes, "a group identifies an area where the members perceive a cluster of problems of mutual concern and consequence. The group decides to work together on a 'thematic concern'" (1997, p. 27). In the case of our project, the "thematic concerns" were the challenges of relationships, including sexual relationships.

For over a decade, previously, we had frequently heard the participants voice the importance of relationships in their lives. This came in creative arts therapies sessions, in supervision and in the weekly Friday "Rounds," where psychological and emotional issues of the participants are discussed. The professional team, from both research and clinical perspectives, thought the subject of relationships would be an excellent topic, so we presented it to the participants in Cohort 9. We had also witnessed, over the years, the lack of sexual knowledge in our groups, so the idea of specifically focusing on sexuality was also proposed. In this project at CAHD, we presented the idea of the theme to the 20 participants and then negotiated with them, over many months, on how to best articulate the subject. The final result was an ethnodrama entitled "The Amazing Adventure of Relationships."

In the previous chapter, the content was framed within the model of the *Eight Steps of Ethnodramatherapy*. In this chapter, we will look at the case study through the framework of the *Four Functions of EDT* (see Figure 1.4). In the triangulated model delineated in Chapter 1 (Figure 1.1), the functions of therapy, research and theatre were reviewed. This chapter will emphasize the fourth function – **Social Activism** in EDT. I will focus on the goal of the production: to significantly change the social attitudes towards sexuality in the lives of adults with developmental and intellectual disabilities. The social and political context of oppression in regard to this phenomenon (see the epigraph at the beginning of this chapter) will also be discussed. We will then proceed to describe and analyze the *Therapeutic Function*, looking at how the clinical process was implemented. The parallel *Research Function* will, subsequently, be explored. Finally, the important place of the art of theatre in the EDT process will be defined in terms of the *Aesthetic Function* of this integrative method.

The Function of Social Activism in EDT

As already pointed out in Chapter 1, the **social activism** function in EDT is a resonance derived from Mienczakowski's concept of "Emancipation," i.e.,

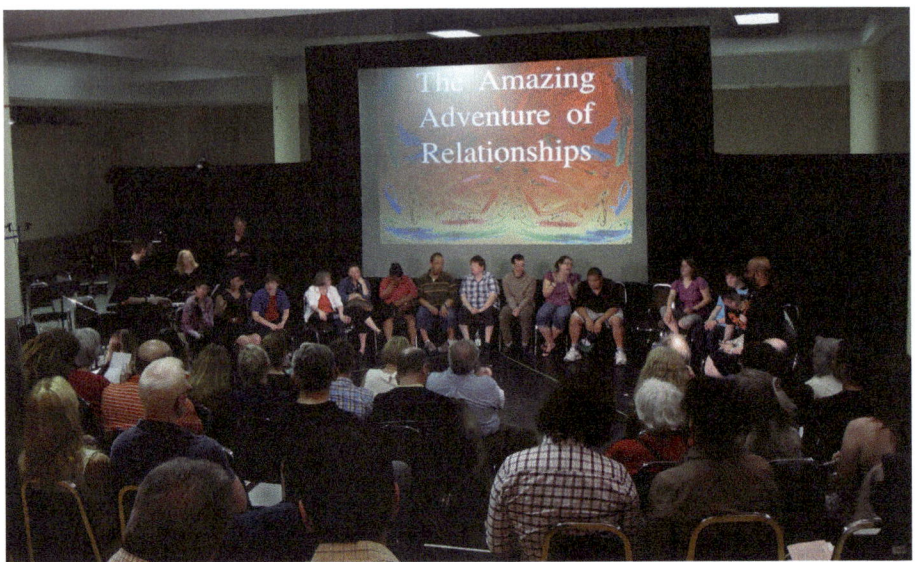

Figure 4.1   Audience and Cast for "The Amazing Adventure of Relationships" (photo courtesy of Eric Mongerson)

that the essential purpose of ethnodrama is to change systems and thinking that are oppressive to human well-being. In this project, in 2014, we were confronting the oppressive attitudes towards denying adults with developmental disabilities their rights as "sexual citizens" (Foley, 2012, p. 382).

In 2012, a powerful film, depicting the coming-of-age of a young woman with a development disability, including her exploration of sexuality, appeared in Quebec. This award-winning film was created by Quebecoise filmmaker Louise Archambault (Archambault, 2013). It was entitled *Gabrielle* as it depicted the life experience of Gabrielle Marion-Rivard, a young woman with **Williams syndrome**. This film catalyzed a lot of interest in and discussion of the topic of sexuality in the lives of adults with developmental and intellectual disabilities. We showed it to Cohort 9 when we began, as *co-researchers*, to investigate this theme.

We reviewed international literature in social work and disability studies to gain a better background knowledge on the subject. We discovered that in Ireland, in 1993, it was "a criminal offence for an individual with a mental impairment who is not living independently to engage in sexual relations unless they are married" (Foley, 2012, p. 384). The UN Convention on the Rights of Persons with Disabilities had shifted this perspective to allow for greater freedom of sexual expression by persons with developmental disabilities. This, then, created a conundrum for parents whose children with developmental disabilities lived at home. Did they control the ultimate say over their child's sexual expression? As Foley writes, "in order for many adults with Down syndrome living in the parental home to exercise their legal right to have a sexual life, they will be dependent on the proxy decisions made by their parents" (2012, p. 390).

Although this is a case in Ireland, the issues exposed are universal. Around the issue of sexuality, parents have great fears for their children with developmental disabilities. In a study on parents of children with ASD, it was noted the parents felt "generally, people are more likely to associate sexuality and disabilities in a negative and fearful way rather than the positive association for neurotypical individuals" (Nichols & Blakely-Smith, 2009, p. 77). We found these fears and apprehensions in the parents of Cohort 9 as well. Foley says parental protectiveness, based on fearful concerns and anxieties, can generate a state where these adult children become "protected prisoners" (2012, p. 387).

In a Dutch study of sex in the lives of adults with intellectual disabilities, based on 76 interviews, results confirmed that romance and sex were important issues for them: "Our respondents appeared to already have considerable experience with many facets of romantic relationships and sexuality, and they also appeared to have many needs of relationships and sexual activities" (Siebelink et al., 2006, p. 292). Another study on developing Sex Ed. programs for individuals with developmental and cognitive disabilities (DD/CD), restated the problem of social oppression in this area:

> The individual with DD/CD has been denied their right to sexual feelings and has been pictured as a perpetual child who is protected. Society holds to the myth that the individual with DD/CD has not developed interest in their own sexuality or the sexuality of others.
> (Swango-Wilson, 2009, p. 224)

In our 2014 EDT production at CAHD, our social activist mission was to throw light on this area of experience and desire in the lives of Cohort 9.

Wikipedia gives a simple, clear definition of social activism: "organized action taken by a group to improve social conditions" ("Activism," 2021). In our group, using ethnodrama in a PAR mode, we were following Mienczakowski's objective to establish a research program that "seeks to influence *change* among participants and audiences, while retaining potential to construct new understandings" (italics mine, Mienczakowski & Morgan, 2001, p. 220). In the later sections, we will show some of the changes that took place in both the participants and the audience. Our social activist mission in this project was to change oppressive attitudes towards sexuality as they are associated to persons with developmental disabilities and, possibly, to create a progressive model of sex education for this population. The audience responses to the four questions clearly demonstrate that many witnessing the ethnodrama gained significant new insights in regard to the issue: 91 supported sexual relationships for this population, with 142 expressing support, but with big concerns around **STDs**, pregnancy and other "risks." The need for better sex education was clearly validated.

One of the innovative elements of "The Amazing Adventure of Relationships" is that we brought in a professional sex educator, Stephanie Mitelman of Sexpressions, who specializes in this population, to give two half-day workshops during the rehearsal period. These were intensive experiences for the group, but they also served to make group members more comfortable with talking about issues like STDs and other very concrete aspects of sex. The experiment was so successful, we actually replicated the workshop as a scene in the production with a drama therapy student/actor playing the role of the sex educator. At this time, we were also in communication with the emergence of a new "Human Sexuality" program, at Concordia, with the idea of co-developing an innovative Sex Ed. program with this population in the future. However, due to a lack of funding and time constraints, this project was never realized.

Social activism is a central part of every EDT process, although the issue will be different each time. Here, we aimed to change ingrained attitudes and concepts about sexuality and developmental disabilities. The post-performance questionnaire responses reveal many such changes. Another positive outcome of this project was that several parents thanked us, afterwards, for opening up this topic, which had consequently allowed them more freedom and intimacy in discussing sexual issues with their adult children. The role of the social activist is one of the main roles for any person authentically undertaking the EDT process (Snow & Bleuer, 2020).

The Therapeutic Process

Assigning Therapeutic Goals

As mentioned in Chapter 2, early on we realized that the whole group at CAHD, including participants, professional and administrative staff and volunteers, constituted a *therapeutic community*. Therapeutic work and therapeutic goals were at the heart of our time spent together, and this included time allotted to the EDT projects. However, it should be pointed out that, although this "groupness" was extremely important, we also very carefully paid attention to each individual. Perhaps, nowhere is this better exemplified than in the files we used to establish therapeutic goals for each participant involved in an EDT process. These files consisted of several parts. First there was a recent photograph of the individual. Then, there was a short psychosocial summary of the person, giving their age and family background, as well as describing their diagnosis. Following these were a brief description of their personality, with both positive and negative traits, as well as successes and challenges during their two years at CAHD, and a short outline of their therapeutic goals for the regular clinical year. In terms of the latter, we built on these to establish the goals for the EDT project. The remaining contents of the file was the Rating Sheet, based on the participants' enactment in the "Drama Therapy Role-Play Interview" (DTRPI) (Snow & D'Amico, 2009), a 20-minute role-playing assessment administered to each EDT participant. Along with this was a description of observation of their individual DTRPI and, finally, a short statement of their therapeutic goal for the project.

The Clinical Assessment Tool

By 2000, with the aid of my colleague, Dr. Miranda D'Amico, I had developed an assessment tool, based on improvisational role-playing by the subject, that we utilized to help us find the "right" role for individual participants for the therapeutic theatre productions. This is fully described in our chapter, "Casting the Healing Role: Assessment in Therapeutic Theatre," in Johnson, Pendzik and Snow (2012, pp. 91–120). I will just give a brief synopsis of the DTRPI, here, in the form administered to Cohort 9 for the EDT project.

The subject is asked to play two different roles: a Cleaning Man or Woman, and a Teenage Boy or Girl. There is a table of props to be used for improvising a role play of these two characters. The interview administrator (it is called an "interview" and not a "test," to make it less intimidating) explains the role play, then asks the subject to choose costume and props; to look at themselves in a mirror as the character; to spend 30 seconds doing what their character would do in the workplace (Role-Play 1) or at home (Role-Play 2); then, to receive a phone call from an irate boss saying they were late to work (Role-Play 1), or a best friend who has had their feelings hurt by the Teenager (Role-Play 2); finally, they are asked to de-role and put all costumes and props back on the table. The written script for the administrator (who plays the Boss and the other Teenager) must be presented the same way for each subject, but the participants' parts are totally improvised. After the written and delivered lines of the administrator/role player, the subject improvises their lines (Snow et al., in Snow & D'Amico, 2009).

Role-Play 1 is meant to access four variables: "Ability to Follow Direction," "Focus of Attention," "Spontaneity" and "Assertiveness." Role-Play 2 measures all the previous variables, plus "Communication Skills." In rating the subject, afterwards, the administrator ticks off items related to the variables on a Checklist of 42 items. The score is then translated to the DTRPI Scoring Sheet that converts the score for each variable to a number on a 1 to 10 Likert-type scale (on previous models of the DTRPI it was 1 to 7). So, a very low score on "Focus of Attention would be a "1"; the highest score would be "10." The DTRPI is also videotaped and the scoring is done through observation of the taped "interview." The administrator may also write down special observations of the subject.

The observed and scored role-plays give the director of the EDT project much valuable information. They provide assessment of each individual participant: how they move, how they speak, their psychological and emotional state; their capacity to focus on a task; their general role-playing ability; their potential for creativity and spontaneity. In the early work at CAHD with therapeutic theatre and fairy tales, this information was immensely helpful in finding the "right" role for a person (Snow and D'Amico in Johnson, Pendzik and Snow, 2012). In our EDT work, where the participant is mostly playing themselves or characters in other people's actual life stories, the DTRPI still gave basic knowledge about a person's capacity and desire for theatrical performance, which is also related to the aesthetic function of EDT. In the end, the major value of this assessment was in helping us to define an appropriate therapeutic goal for each individual, as you will see in the following case vignettes. For the sake of confidentiality, pseudonyms will be used for each of two participants.

Establishing a Therapeutic Goal for "Betty"

Betty was a 23-year-old woman who had a "global intellectual delay." As a child, she had both gross motor and intellectual delays. She also demonstrated some unusual fears of curtains, birds and the color green. She has been reported to be easily emotionally overwhelmed and has been known to fabricate dramatic stories. She also expressed that she has a large degree of anxiety. There was some apprehension that she may have been a victim of neglect as an infant, a plausible cause for her states of anxiety. She had been a supportive, engaged member in her creative arts therapies groups in her two years at CAHD. Her goal for the clinical year was to build up her emotional expression and regulation skills; to develop coping strategies for her anxiety; and to further develop her self-confidence and self-esteem. She did extremely well on the DTRPI and received scores of "10" for both "Ability to Follow Directions" and "Capacity for Physical Embodiment in Role and Movement" (an adapted version of "Spontaneity" for this project). She was very empathic in the role of the Teenage Girl. The administrator made a note that she had "Basic Good Voice and Movement." This, later on, led the director of the EDT project to cast her in an important musical dance number and to give her a powerful monologue in the "Sex Ed." section, among other roles. Taking her whole background into consideration, her therapeutic goal for the project was: "to use the performance-building period and the actual performance as a way to decrease anxiety and to build self-confidence." Her self-evaluation of her experience in the ethnodrama will be reported in the section on "Therapeutic Effectiveness."

Establishing a Therapeutic Goal for "Donald"

Donald was a young man of 26 with a diagnosis of **Prader-Willi-Lockhart syndrome**. He was very intelligent, articulate and determined. For various reasons he had been placed in a crisis residence and was quite frustrated with this situation. Because of his diagnosis, Donald was quite overweight and experienced muscle weakness. His determination manifested in his making a lengthy commute to CAHD each day during the clinical year. In many groups, he preferred to sit in a sturdy chair for most of the session, including the drama therapy group. However, he was observant, often commenting on things he noticed. His overall therapeutic goals were building expression and regulation skills to support him in exploring his frustration and anger, and to develop reciprocal conversation skills for engaging with others. His DTRPI scores were very high in "Ability to Follow Direction" and "Clarity, Volume and Articulation of Speech" (also an adapted category for this project), but low in the area of empathy ("Communication Skills"). The director cast him as the narrator, due to his excellent speech and his need to be seated, most of the time. The test administrator observed that Donald, "Listens carefully, intelligent, *But*, with an attitude – 'this is stupid!'" Reviewing all of this information, his therapeutic goal for the EDT was defined as "to help him build his capacity for trust and to engage reciprocally with others, through the performance and the performance community." We believe Donald made great strides towards these goal in the months of the EDT project. This will be reviewed in the section on "Therapeutic Effectiveness."

Drama Therapy Techniques Used to Build the Ethnodrama

Between January and June 2014, we utilized many drama therapy interventions to catalyze the authentic voice and roles of participants, as well as to help them succeed in their personal therapeutic goals. We were also using the drama therapy methods to help us answer the three main questions of our investigation: (1) What types of relationships are available to adults with developmental disabilities, and how are they experienced? (2) What types of sexual relationships are available to this population, and how are they experienced? (3) In locating answers to question 2, how can we develop a best practice model of sex education for this population?

Below are three examples of essential Drama Therapy methods used in our rehearsal process.

Firstly, we had realized there would be many different attitudes around the discussion of sexuality, so we decided to poll the group via a sociometric exercise known as the *action spectrogram* (Sternberg & Garcia, 1989, pp. 115–116). Participants situated themselves on the side of a line running the whole length of the room, representing the full spectrum of who wanted to talk about sex and who did not. Then, each individual was asked to explain his or her position. This exercise goes to the heart of locating "authentic voice" in the group. The responses were very dynamic as participants expressed their personal opinions on this topic. Eventually, this became a two-sided choral number in the play, "Let's Talk about Sex," adapted from a popular song of the same name that one of the participants had brought to the group. This method, drawn from Moreno's **sociodrama** framework, helps the group to focus: "As group members literally see where each other stands on social issues, lively discussions ensue, and it becomes clear which issues feel most important to members to explore in action" (Sternberg & Garcia, 1989, p. 116).

Secondly, as mentioned in Chapter 2 and 3, the CAHD research team had discovered that playback theatre is a wonderful method for evoking stories in the EDT process. Playback is an improvisational role-playing method in which four or five actors and a musician spontaneously play back a story told by one of the group's members. However, playback theatre can also very much be seen as a drama therapy technique. As Salas states, "Most mental health clients are people who can clearly benefit from Playback's capacities to affirm subjective perception and experience, strengthen identity, increase awareness and compassion, express emotion and respond creatively to the expressions of others" (Salas in Emunah & Johnson, 2009, p. 448). We trained the participants to become playback actors and in this way many experiences about romance and intimacy were captured. One example of this was a story of how a female participant always used to watch horror movies on TV with her boyfriend; how they would get scared and cuddle. This personal story was told in the performance by this participant and, then others enacted it. This type of use of playback has a definite therapeutic effect (Salas, 1993). Playback catalyzed an openness about exploring personal stories and a way of deeply sharing one's personal experience in this group therapy setting. Our work in this project was much like Salas' "workshop-model" playback. As she states:

> Playback's intrinsic healing effects go further. Taking active part as an actor helps to develop spontaneity (in the Morenean sense of having full access to all one's resources). It also promotes expressiveness, receptiveness to others, self- confidence, self-esteem, creativity, teamwork, playfulness, and the capacity for aesthetic mastery and pleasure.
> (Salas in Johnson & Emunah, 2009, p. 447)

As our therapeutic goals were often built around "self-confidence" and "self-esteem," playback was a great therapeutic asset. Later on, as can be seen in Chapters 6 and 7, we utilized the methods of psychodrama to help participants *work through* psychological issues that had been revealed in their playback stories. In fact, the three methodologies of playback, sociodrama and psychodrama were to become central to EDT.

Thirdly, we did a lot of work with developing personal stories into monologues. This gave individual drama therapists and drama therapy interns a good amount of time to work in-depth with participants and to help them process the meaning of their story for themselves. An example of this is the story of a "first kiss" that was also developed into a dance.

It is important to note that the professional staff in other modalities of the creative arts therapies (art, music and dance/movement therapies) also made significant contributions to the development of the ethnodrama, using their own specialized therapeutic tools. One of the innovative contributions to this type of research at CAHD, as was discussed in Chapter 2, has been the use of gathering data via *all* the arts. Facilitating this variety of avenues for self-expression helped ensure meaningful participation by all participant co-researchers. Images, narratives, motifs and relevant experiences were recorded and reviewed for potential inclusion in the script. The dance created to interpret the "first kiss" monologue, developed by a participant with Down's syndrome, became one of the most energetic performances in the play (Figure 4.2). It combined the efforts of the art therapist, the music

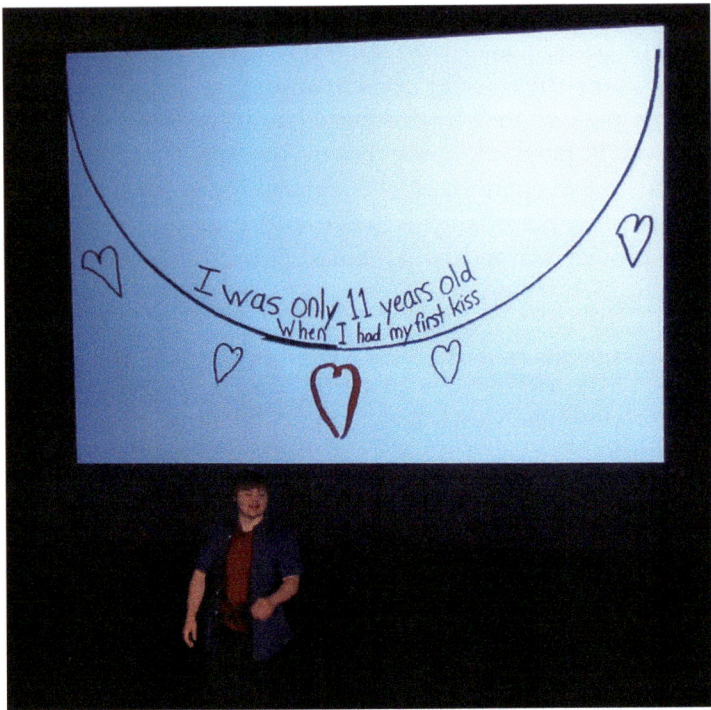

Figure 4.2   Dance of the First Kiss (photo courtesy of Eric Mongerson)

therapist and the dance/movement therapist to aid the participant in producing a powerful, emotionally resonant performance. The art image was
used as scenography; the dance image became a humanizing portrait of romance for this population.

Personal Interviews with Each of the Informant/Performers

In order to gain a deeper understanding of each participant's attitude towards
romance and sexuality, personal interviews were conducted with all 15 in-
formant/performers. A preamble was established so the interviewees knew
that all was done in the utmost confidentiality and that they could stop the
interview, at any time, if they felt uncomfortable. Here are the basic questions that were used:

1. Is romance part of your life?
2. What part does sex play in your life?

3. Is there anything you would like to share about your own sexual experiences?
4. What was your experience in sex education? Could you describe it for me?
5. What do you feel you really need in a sex education program? What would a great program look like?

Because the interviewees functioned at many different levels, cognitively and intellectually, the interviewers were given a great deal of license in regard to phrasing the questions, the order in which they were given and the use of follow-up questions to catalyze greater clarity in the responses.

Although these pre-performance interviews were handled with great sensitivity and clinical awareness, most of the really relevant and useful material actually emerged from the playback theatre sessions and the creative arts therapies groups.

Therapeutic Effectiveness

The pre-performance interviews provided some information and ideas for the play. However, it was the post-performance interviews that produced evidence of therapeutic effectiveness. For instance, in the follow-up interviews with Betty and Donald, it was clear they were able to speak about sexual issues with greater freedom. Here is Betty's response to the question, "Do you feel you're more comfortable talking about sex, now, after having been in the ethnodrama?"

> Yeah, it makes me open, but like, I don't know, like, to discuss that with my parents … I was dating a boy. So, I figured, it's o.k. But then it got deeper. I said, "No, I got to tell my mom because, if, god forbid, anything happens she has to know." So, I went to my mom and my mom agreed that if he does that again and you get the kissing disease, or whatever, like herpes or whatever, what would you do? So, I'm like, "No, I don't want to even be kissed yet … I'm not ready, and he has to respect that." So, he didn't, and I broke up with the guy, and then the guy called me on the phone, and he's like, "why did you break up with me?" and I'm like, "Because you don't respect me, that's why'"… We've lost touch ever since, and I don't want to call him, and I don't want him to call me.

Donald gave a succinct reply to the question, "What did you learn about sexual experiences or sexual activity when you were listening to the things that your friends talked about during the play process?"

Good question. Um … [long pause]. That's a tough one. Umm … a lot of people didn't know what sex was. A lot of people did not know what sexually transmitted infections were. A lot of people did not know about the dangers of rape, the dangers of teen pregnancy, the uh, dangers of drinking and getting together with your partner, that can lead to pregnancy. I notice a lot of people did not know the dangers … and they should.

Although we never got to actually creating a model sex education class at CAHD, based on the responses to being in the ethnodrama, we certainly saw growth and evolving awareness of issues inherent in negotiating intimate relationships with safety and respect in many of the participants.

In watching the documentary video of "The Amazing Adventures of Relationships," with the participants, almost a year later, in spring 2015, it was clear how much ownership of the project they had and what a great value it was for them to be able to express themselves in their authentic voices on these intimate and sensitive subjects. We hear this reflected in the interviews of Donald and Betty who both expressed that they felt more confident. Donald remarked that by "talking about it, you become less shy about it." Betty stated, "It took courage, it took a lot, but, I'm really proud I did it, and I like it. And it helped us a lot because it was a play that I never thought I would have to do like that … I enjoyed, like, doing it."

In the end, we had no precise measurements in regard to the outcome of the personal therapeutic goals that had been established. We had only observations, like the ones above, that confirmed our belief in the therapeutic value of the project.

The Research Frame

Like the projects described in Chapters 2 and 3, the "Sex Ed." project had a similar protocol. Besides examining the therapeutic value for the participants, the research was aimed at measuring the "emancipatory" or educational value for the audience. This aim of EDT goes back to Mienczakowski's original conception of ethnodrama, "the reconstruction of validated ethnographic research as public voice theatre holds emancipatory and educational potential for informants, informed and general audiences" (1995a, pp. iii–iv). We had observed the value for our participants. We also wanted to see if public attitudes about sexuality in the lives of adults with developmental disabilities had been changed by witnessing our play.

Analysis of Responses to the Post-Performance Questionnaire for the Audience[1]

What follows is an analysis of emerging themes for answers given by the participating audience members to the post-performance questionnaire and, where relevant, verbatim quotes are included that substantiate the themes further. The results were analyzed qualitatively, and each question was transcribed verbatim. We followed the six step process as defined by Braun and Clarke (2006).

Question 1: *Do you think adults with developmental and intellectual disabilities should be able to have romantic relationships? Why or why not? Please explain.*

All answers were in full support of this statement – "yes, they should be able to have romantic relationships." Only one respondent stated some hesitation by answering "yes and no. Provided some support is involved. No, if there isn't (for sexual relationship)."

The themes that emerged from the answers (N=247) were: that individuals with developmental and intellectual disabilities have the same feelings as "normal" people; that it is a natural and inalienable right; that everyone deserves love; it is a basic human need; they should have the right to full lives.

One audience member answered, "of course! Every human has the right to be happy! Romance only facilitates that state of mind. Who is anyone to reject someone else of that pleasure?" Another further stated, "their disabilities do not define them, they have so many other qualities." "Without relationships/romance it would be easy to fall into a place of isolation and further those potential feelings in disabled adults." "Yes, they should be able to live these experiences to decrease 'accidents' and 'misunderstandings' that could arise in society. The more it is talked about and accepted, the better the structure that educates them will become." "The song stated it true!: 'We all have hopes – we all have dreams'…." "To deny a human need (i.e., Maslow's hierarchy) of security would be unfair to these people." Another of the audience members stated "as a mother of an 18-year-old with autism, I believe with all my heart that he should be able to be in a loving, romantic relationship and I hope he will be in such a relationship soon."

1 The author wishes to thank Dr. Miranda D'Amico, who designed this part of the research program, and the Editor of *The Drama Therapy Review*, where parts of it were previously published.

Question 2: *Do you think adults with developmental and intellectual disabilities should be able to have sexual relationships? Why or why not? Please explain.*

The majority of respondents were in support of this statement (N=91) with a larger group expressing support of the statement, but with some concerns (N=142). The themes that emerged pointed out that for individuals with developmental and intellectual disabilities: sexual relationships are part of basic human needs and are an expression of natural feelings; it was affirmed that if they have romantic relationships, then why not sexual ones as well; it is not realistic to think it can be avoided; they are not children and they may have dreams of having their own families.

One of the audience members stated it is, "hard to generalize – there are many not diagnosed who perhaps should not!" Another qualified, "sexual education should include the element of protecting your emotional and physical wellbeing for all!" "I personally know many 'normal' people less qualified to have any type of sexual relationship than most of the young adults I saw perform tonight, i.e., not intellectually or physically challenged."

A large number of respondents clearly stated that they supported the statement in question 2, but that they still had some concerns (N= 142) about the vulnerability of adults with developmental and intellectual disabilities because we need to: teach them how to protect themselves from the risks of Sexually Transmitted Disease and pregnancy; provide proper counseling and education about sexuality and sexual relationships; guide them to respect each other and boundaries; give instruction on personal space and private parts; ensure that this sexual education takes place in a caring environment with no risk of exploitation or danger.

One person stated that if the individual was emotionally ready and comfortable, "family, and educators should support the process of learning about his or her own body, understanding his or her personal limits and readiness, knowing how to have safe and pleasurable sex and how to choose the right partner(s)."

A recurring concern was that the nature of the relationship be understood by both parties: "sexual education should include the element of protecting your emotional and physical wellbeing for all!"

Question 3: *What should be the major components in an effective Sex Education class for persons with developmental and intellectual disabilities? Please describe, briefly.*

Responses expressed in question 3 included components to effective sex education class that take into account and emphasize: safety and limits; human sexuality; abstract concepts/psychosocial information; practical topics to also be included.

With regard to safety and limits, responses included adding lessons on: consensual sex and regard to others; personal space; good touch/bad touch. In concerns about setting limits – "yes means yes" versus "no means no"; safer sex and safe relationships (physical, emotional, also, internet safety – e.g., providing personal info, going on websites; sexual assault prevention knowledge and programs. "Exactly what was included in the "sex education" scene: relationships, description of sex, safe sex, emotional components." "Pregnancy wasn't mentioned in the sex education class scene, and this is an important topic to cover."

The second major point to the respondent answers to question 3 was that any component of the "sex education" class had to discuss aspects of "human sexuality" that is, individual diagrams of sexual anatomy and demonstration; sexual problems for men and women; sexual health and hygiene; STD details and how to prevent them; normal changes with puberty and hormonal issues; the different types of sex (i.e., oral); normal feelings of pleasure (i.e., masturbation, orgasms); pregnancy prevention and issues surrounding pregnancy (i.e., natural abortion, miscarriages).

The third theme of question 3 was concerned with what "abstract concepts/ psychosocial information to include" and here, the emphasis was on helping individuals with intellectual and developmental disabilities understand acceptance and rejection and how to cope with heartbreak. Helping them develop the confidence, self-assertiveness, self-respect and ownership of their own body along with choosing the right partner who respects them and is accepting of who they are. Included were issues of acceptance of sexuality and greater understanding of the rights and responsibilities associated with it. A major issue expressed in the audience answers was the challenge of helping individuals with intellectual and developmental disabilities describe their feelings around love and emotions, how to understand social cues and, importantly, how to differentiate lust, love, sex and romance. Useful suggestions were revealed in quotes such as, "There should be a place where the group can talk about previous breakups and how to deal with future relationships" and "a teacher who is present, loving, non-judgmental, non-directive and accepting of each person." "Don't shut them up."

One audience member informatively commented, "Studies prove full integration of students with both developmental and intellectual disabilities in tandem with non-disabled peers promotes better learning among the former groups."

With regard to the fourth theme, "practical topics to include," these included how to handle unwanted advances; how to talk about sex with a partner; how to meet someone (a romantic partner); how to say NO; how to have sex; how to ask someone on a date; how to navigate relationships; how not to feel weird about sex; how not to be swayed by flattering communicators; where to have sex; where to look for more information; what is same sex attraction and LGBTQ information and what social skills are needed for dating.

Quotes such as, "My own sex education was inadequate". "Exactly what was included in the "sex education" scene: relationships, description of sex, safe sex, emotional components." "Pregnancy wasn't mentioned in the sex education class scene, and this is an important topic to cover."

Question 4: *What was the most important thing that you learned from the play? Please describe briefly.*

Responses to question 4 were divided into three themes. Answers included: overall learning from the play; learning about the population; learning about oneself from the play. All participants answering this question (N=217) talked about gaining insight into how adults with intellectual and developmental disabilities think about the topic and its importance to their lives. Mentioned in their answers was that they also learned about drama and art therapy and its impact on the participants. Reaffirmed in their answers was the need for further sex education intervention as they felt that the confusion on what constitutes sexuality was very evident in scenes where physical contact such as holding hands was considered "sex"!

The quotes below illustrate the impact and lessons from the play:

"the warmth of the human spirit can transcend almost any disability"

"The most powerful part of the play was: the baseball diamond"

"a reminder of how simple love and sex can be despite the layers"

"learnt about the existence of sex education for this population"

"Was touched by their dreams, but somewhat sad at the same time"

"This field (ethnodrama) is powerful"

"This production touched my heart."

Overall, the audience expressed that they were reminded to be accepting, that the participants "are just like us" – that is, they have "bigger dreams than I thought" – and the need to develop clear guidelines to teach about sexuality for individuals with intellectual and development disabilities.

The Art of Theatre

The Aesthetic Function in EDT

The power and dynamics of the artistic components in EDT should always be carefully considered. The task in mounting an EDT project, alongside its therapeutic, research and social activist functions, is also *making art* (Figure 1.4).

This function includes the elements of beauty, poetics and entertainment. As Gordon Craig said in *On the Art of the Theatre*, "The Theatre affects the people in two different ways. It either instructs or it amuses. There are many ways to instruct and to amuse" (1956, p. 246). These theatrical outcomes are based on the artistic choices of the director, the production team and the company. Such decisions are made through the individual and collective vision of shaping the content of any theatre production. As has been witnessed, this content is often very unique in an EDT project, largely founded in the lived experience of the participants in relation to the particular theme. As Peter Brook has stated in regard to the vision of the dramatist, "the choices he makes and the values he observes are only powerful in proportion to what they create in the language of the theatre" (1968, p. 43). Theatre has its own special language through which to frame embodied discourse on given topics. Movement, sound, light, rhythm, images, costumes, props, music, masks, puppets, ritual and poetry are its elements. Out of these elements a whole theatrical experience is shaped.

Practitioners of ethnodrama have recognized that they are making theatrical art. Johnny Saldana's book, *Ethnodrama: An Anthology of Reality Theatre*, begins with a short poem as an ode to theatrical art:

the theatre

must never
be boring

indeed
must be
the opposite
of boring

so it may
delight and arouse
the senses
and the mind

may soothe
and shake
and shock

dig deep
really and
truly deep

in the earning
of a single clap
or bravo

(Prendergast in Saldana, 2005, p. xiv)

As Saldana mentions, later on, in his book, the works of ethnodrama are "comparable in intent to the performance interviews collected by Anna Deveare Smith (2000) … and the Tectonic Theatre Project's (2001) celebrated drama *The Laramie Project*" (2005, p. 3). These are works by noted theatre artists and give all of us practicing ethnodrama inspiring models of the *theatrical art* to aspire towards. Both Smith and The Tectonic Theatre Project have created innovative theatrical forms to produce their performances. As the TTP team suggests in their text on devising theatre, "Theatre as an art form has such magnificent potential! And *theatricality* as a language is endless in its ability to address the audience's imaginations, minds, and feelings" (Kaufman et al., 2018, p. 5).

In the period between 1982 and 2012, "the conception of performance expanded, moving theatre aesthetics into social, cultural and political domains" (Landy & Montgomery, 2012, p. 129). My own nearly decade-long excursion into performance studies led me to explore many of these new forms of performance and the accompanying new aesthetics. One specific form that emerged in this time was **Applied Theatre**, which often delves into politics and social activism. It is important then to review how this type of theatre, whose purpose is social change, relates to the aesthetic dimension of theatre. As Landy and Montgomery state, "Applied Theatre is a complex form that serves several goals and populations, that occurs within multiple cultures and community spaces, and that exists in a somewhat ambivalent relationship to the *art form* of drama/theatre" (italics mine, Landy & Montgomery, 2012, p. 166). This concept of "ambivalence" to art, presented, here, in relation to a theatrical endeavor is interesting. It indicates a possible prioritization of other functions, such as political, educational or therapeutic, above the objectives of theatrical art. In discussing work in "Drama Therapy and Social Theatre," Anna Seymour strikes a similar cord, in regard to theatre developed in schools, prisons and hospitals; she writes, "Inevitably it seems the work strayed into areas more commonly associated with therapeutic practice" (Seymour in Jennings, 2009, p. 29). If therapy, politics or social activism are more focused on, does this diminish the aesthetic function of theatre?

In EDT, the goal is to balance the four functions, so none takes priority over the others; each is looked at, as a different but dynamic component of the whole. This concept will be further discussed in Chapter 10, "The Integration."

The Theatrical Art Employed in "The Amazing Adventures of Relationships"

Scenic Design

It is very important in EDT to create artful and effective theatre design through lighting and stage construction. The theatre space, itself, plays an important role. I have been very fortunate to have had, as a colleague, Eric Mongerson, a Professor of Theatre Design at Concordia and a highly skilled professional theatre designer. He has served as a co-investigator on all of CAHD's ethnodramas since 2005. He has become very acclimated to the special requirements of this form of theatre. For this project, he actually designed a special 200-seat amphitheatre in a way to sensitively contain the intimate stories that were told and enacted (Figure 4.1). His notes reveal the conscious design that went into the "set":

> An intimate place to hold performance. Need to feel welcoming, not intimidating. A relaxed environment is needed. Intimate stories are uncomfortable for actors and audiences. In transitioning from drama therapy productions to ethnodrama, drama therapy never really went away. Exploitation – finding a balance. Keeping the environment safe psychologically and physically. The sense of performance should be felt but it should not be overpowering. The audience should be close to the performers but not in their face.
> (E. Mongerson, personal communication, May 26, 2015)

He also oversaw the lighting and slide projection elements (see Figures 4.3 and 4.4). He worked with the art therapist and the director to select the most relevant and theatrically powerful slides of artwork, created and consented for use in the play, by the participants. As in "It's A Wonderful World," these slides became a major component of the theatrical atmosphere.

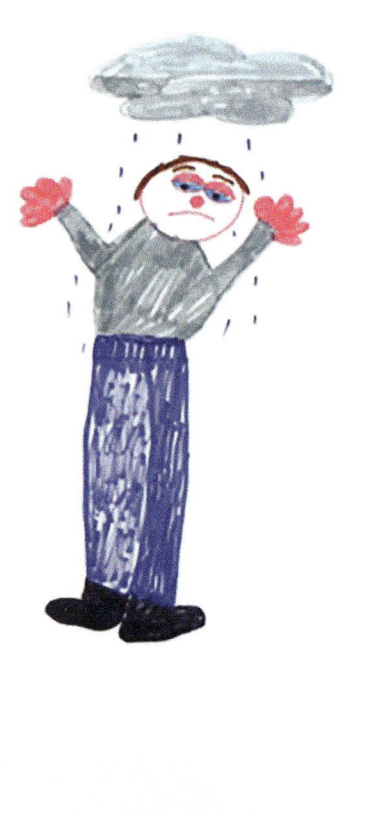

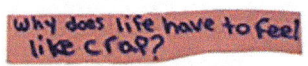

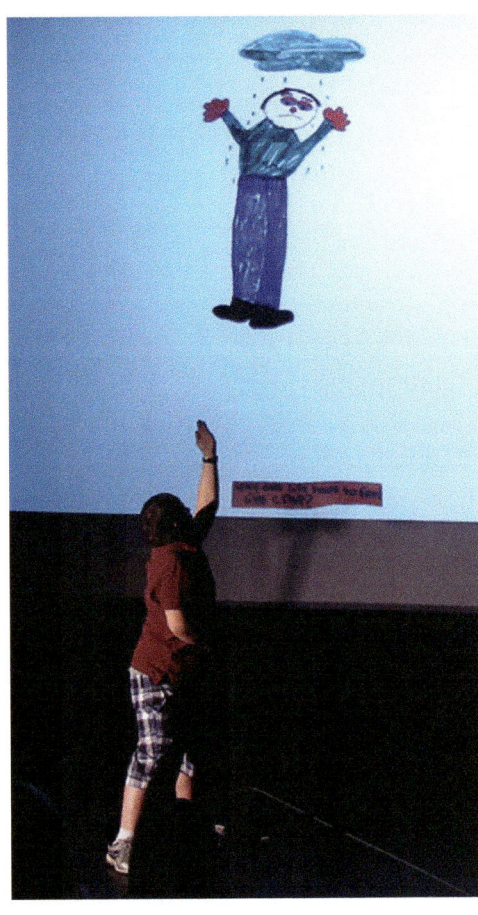

Figure 4.3   Image of Sadness (photo courtesy of Eric Mongerson)

Figure 4.4   The Dance of Sadness (photo courtesy of Eric Mongerson)

Music, Dance and Acting

The music and dance for the production were both enhanced by having professional artists guide the ensemble. The musical director, Shelley Snow, is also a music therapist who is able to sensitively evoke the most honest and touching performances from the participants, as described in Chapter 2. As a professional composer, she wrote the music for the score, coordinating it with the theme of the piece and the unique abilities of the performers. She brings in professional musicians for the band, like Gary Schwartz, a professional Jazz musician and part-time faculty in the Music Department at Concordia, who has worked with us on many productions. Millie Tresierra is a professional actor–dancer who has also worked on our shows many times in the past. Although not a dance therapist, she brings great sensitivity to working with the population. She helped one nonverbal participant to create a very moving dance, just guiding his powerful natural instincts for movement. Many audience members remarked on the emotional power of his dance (see Figure 4.4).

The high quality of the acting performances in our productions is frequently commented upon by the audiences. Two factors are at play, here, I believe. All the participants have had two full years of drama therapy sessions at CAHD before they begin the EDT work. They are thus very comfortable with improvisation, role-playing and creating characters. Secondly, we have screened them through the DTRPI, so we have previously located roles, methods and performance responsibilities that they will feel safe and comfortable with. They are also assisted in learning their parts by many students and volunteers at CAHD, with the intention of helping them to give their best possible performance.

The use of professional artists in our productions often brings up the questions of the real "authenticity" of the performance. As Nisha Sajnani questioned in her doctoral dissertation on our first ethnodrama, "the *overt* message celebrated through such performances is one of the empowerment of the marginalized group, the *covert* message (i.e., that they are not capable) is held in the shadows, as a conversation that cannot be held simultaneously, and that therefore goes unexamined or challenged (2010, pp. 70–71). Although, I will address this question in depth in the chapter on ethics, I will state here that my basic philosophy is that we are trying to bring the *art of theatre* to its highest level with the budget, the staff, the time, and the performers that we have, and our goal is to still keep all of this in the context of a therapeutic community. It is why I still place my EDT work in the domain of therapeutic theatre.

Artistic Synergy of Art Image, Storytelling and Dance

To give one example from our script of how the collective devising of the ethnodrama came together in an artistic synergy, here are three artistic components brought together in one moment in the play: art image, narration of a story from a transcribed interview and a dance interpretation of these first two.

From the Script:

[Slide 18: **Feeling All Alone**]

NARRATOR: And sometimes family members can make us sad and disappoint us.

NARRATOR comes away from the NARRATOR'S spot and does the following speech.

NARRATOR: I had a friend whose mother attacked his brother and really hurt him. She was an alcoholic, we think. Later, she got put in the Douglas Psychiatric Hospital. I don't know what happened to his brother, but my friend was always really sad.

(*Music in. The dancer performs a dance to portray the sad feelings expressed in the art image and the story, as depicted in Figure 4.3. His movements evoke the emotional pain in these experiences, as shown in Figure 4.4.*)

Although impossible to recapture in written description, I believe this is an excellent example of the kind of synergy that can take place in the EDT process.[2]

A Final Note

The art of theatre is so important. As Renée Emunah suggests, it can interface beautifully with and actually enhance the therapeutic function, "There is a reciprocity between actor and audience: the audience becomes empathic witness for the actor, contributing to the actor's healing; and the actor bestows upon the audience the gift of inspired live theatrical art" (2015, p. 80).

---

2 A documentary video of the performance of "The Amazing Adventure of Relationships" was made and is available through CAHD at www.concordia.ca/finearts/research/cahd.html .

In EDT, all the four functions should work in harmony to not disturb or compete with each other. The research, through its PAR framework, should provide valid outcomes that are insights into correcting a situation of social oppression or prejudice. In our case we saw new possibilities for sex education and sexuality in the lives of adults with developmental disabilities. Some parents thanked us for opening up this topic and allowing them a new space for communication with their child. The therapy should provide new self-expressiveness and self-confidence in the participants. We saw this in the cases of Betty and Donald. The art of theatre allows for profound emotional and poetic communication with the audience. It instructs while it entertains through song, dance, music, storytelling and artwork in the scenography. Finally, the social activist function opens up important questions about social structures that are unhealthy to people who live in that society.

Those who practice EDT should always be open to questions that come from the audience. This happened to our team in a surprising way at the 2017 Annual Conference of the North American Drama Therapy Association. We gave an afternoon workshop on this project, entitled, "Whose Sex Life Is It, Anyway? An Ethnodramatic Exploration with Adults with DD/ID." After a panel presentation and showing of the video documentary, there was time for discussion with the audience. Towards the end, Dr. Jason Butler, the Director of the Drama Therapy Program at Lesley University, asked a very provocative question, something along the lines of, "You asked them to reveal and describe their sex lives to you (the professional staff of therapists and theatre artists), did you do the same for them?" An awkward pause. No, we had not. Looking at how seriously we took the PAR approach, why had we not been more forthcoming ourselves? This was a question for some serious contemplation. It will be discussed, specifically, in Chapter 8 on ethics in EDT.

References

Activism. (2021, April 23). In Wikipedia (in italics). en.wikipedia.org/wiki/Activism

Archambault, L. (2013). *Gabrielle*. Canada: micro_scope.

Braun, V. & Clarke, V. (2006). Using thematic analysis in psychology. *Qualitative Research in Psychology, 3*, 77–101.

Brook, P. (1968). *The empty space: A great theatre director gives his views on the making of drama*. Penguin Books.

Chevalier, J. M., & Buckles, D. J. (2019). *Participatory action research: Theory and methods of engaged inquiry* (2nd ed.). Routledge.

Craig, E. G. (1956). *On the art of the theatre*. Theatre Arts Books.

Emunah, R. (2015). Self-revelatory performance: A form of drama therapy and the-atre. *Drama Therapy Review, 2*(1): 71–85.

Foley, S. (2012). The UN convention on the rights of persons with disabilities: A paradigm shift in the sexual empowerment of adults with Down syndrome or more sound and fury signifying nothing? *Sex Disability, 30,* 381–393.

Garcia, N., & Sternberg, P. (1989). *Sociodrama: Who's in your shoes?* Praeger.

Kaufman, M., McAdams, B. P, Fondakowski, L, Pierotti, G., Paris, A, Simpkins, K. Maize, J., & Barrow, S. (2018). *Moment work: Tectonic Theatre Project's process of devising theatre*. Vintage Books.

Landy, R. J., & Montgomery, D. T. (2012). *Theatre for change: Education, social action and therapy*. Palgrave Macmillan.

McTaggart, R. (1997). Guiding principles of participatory action research. In R. McTaggart (Ed.), *Participatory action research: International contexts and consequences*. State University of New York Press.

Mienczakowski, J., & Morgan, S. (2001). Ethnodrama: Constructing participatory, experiential and compelling action research through performance. In P. Reason & H. Bradbury (Eds.), *Handbook of action research: Participative inquiry and practice* (pp. 219–227). Sage.

Nichols, S., & Blakely-Smith, A. (2009). "I'm not sure we're ready for this ...": Working with families toward facilitating healthy sexuality for individuals with Autism Spectrum Disorders. *Social Work in Mental Health, 8,* 72–91.

Prendergast, M. (2005). Prologue: The theatre. In J. Saldana (Ed.), *Ethnodrama: An anthology of reality theatre* (pp. xiv–xvi). Altamira Press.

Sajnani, N. (2010). *Permeable boundaries: Toward a critical collaborative performance pedagogy* [Unpublished doctoral dissertation]. Concordia University, Montreal, Quebec, Canada.

Salas, J. (1993). *Improvising real life: Personal story in playback theatre*. Kendall/Hunt Publishing Company.

_____ (2009). Playback theatre: A frame for healing. In D. R. Johnson & R. Emunah (Eds.), *Current approaches in drama therapy* (2nd ed., pp. 445–460). C. C. Thomas Publisher.

Saldana, J. (Ed.) (2005). *Ethnodrama: An anthology of reality theatre*. Altamira Press.

Seymour, A. (2009). Dramatherapy and social theatre: A question of boundaries. In S. Jennings (Ed.), *Dramatherapy and social theatre: Necessary dialogues* (pp. 27–36). Routledge.

Siebelink, E. M, de Jong, M. D. T., Taal, E., & Roelvink, L. (2006). Sexuality and people with intellectual disabilities: Assessment of knowledge, attitudes, experiences and needs. *Mental Retardation, 4*(4): 283–294.

Snow, S., & D'Amico, M. (2009). *Assessment in the creative arts therapies: Designing and adapting assessment tools for adults with developmental disabilities.* C. C. Thomas Publisher.

_____ (2012). Casting the healing role: Assessment in therapeutic theatre. In D. R. Johnson, S. Pendzik & S. Snow (Eds.), *Assessment in drama therapy* (pp. 91–120). C. C. Thomas Publisher.

Snow, S., & Bleuer, J. (2020). Ethnodramatherapy. In D. R. Johnson & R. Emunah (Eds.), *Current approaches in drama therapy* (3rd ed., pp. 250–283). C. C. Thomas, Publisher.

Snow, S., Maeng-Cleveland, J., & Steinfort, T. (2009). The development of the drama therapy role-play interview. In S. Snow & M. D'Amico (Eds.), *Assessment in the creative arts therapies: Designing and adapting assessment tools for adults with developmental disabilities* (pp. 99–162). C. C. Thomas Publisher.

Snow, S., D'Amico, M., Mongerson, M., Anthony, E., Rozenberg, M. Opolko, C., & Anandampillai, S. (2017). Ethnodramatherapy applied in a project focusing on relationships in the lives of adults with developmental disabilities, especially romance, intimacy and sexuality. *Drama Therapy Review, 3*(2), 241–260.

Swango-Wilson, A. (2009). Perception of sex education for individuals with developmental and cognitive disability: A four cohort study. *Sex Disability, 27,* 223–228.

5

The Experience of Caregivers for Loved Ones Who Have a Mental Illness

The play was an honest and strong reflection of my experience as a caregiver. It brought tears to my eyes through the shared moments of other stories. I am not a lone caregiver fighting the system. Many of us are increasingly seeking to be heard. The play is another voice for us.

(P.M., Audience Member for *Through the Eye of Caregivers*, 2015)

Orientation

The political power of ethnodrama as a form of "Public Voice Ethnography" (Mienczakowski 1995b) was made manifest in this project. The purpose was to draw an authentic portrait of this group of family caregivers who are not often studied or written about and, through public performances, to make the general public more aware of this aspect of mental health. To accomplish this purpose, we aligned ourselves with AMI-Québec Action on Mental Illness, a major advocacy group in Montreal that focuses on educating the public about issues in mental health, as well as providing services for caregivers and individuals with mental illnesses. This began a whole EDT program in social activism in regard to mental health: "The Ethnodrama Mental Health Education Series." The overall project was funded by Team Start-up and Accelerator grants from the Office of the Vice-President for Research and Graduate Studies at Concordia University and took place between 2014 and 2021.

The benefits of this chapter for students and professionals who may wish to practice EDT lie in several of the special therapeutic and research techniques that were used to make this project an effective vehicle for mental health education. In fact, this production was closest to Mienczakowski's earliest model of ethnodrama (1995a; 2001). His play was entitled *Syncing Out Loud* and consisted of an in-depth look at the experience of schizophrenia. The informants were persons with schizophrenia who functioned

DOI: 10.4324/9781003083818-7

at a high level. Mienczakowski's team focused on "uncovering the experience of psychosis through detailed ethnographic and phenomenological research processes" (Mienczakowski, 2001, p. 470). In their original format, the performers of this play were nursing, health science and theatre students. In our case, the play was entitled "Through the Eyes of Caregivers"; the informants were carers for loved ones with mental illnesses; and the performers were drama therapy students with training and experience in acting along with professional actors (Figure 5.1).

As a whole, the preparation and presentation of "Through the Eyes of Caregivers" is really an embodiment of Mienczakowski's original ethnodrama method. In this approach, *the informants are not the actors*. This is an enormous difference. In ethnodramatherapy, the informants *are always* the performers, so they can also go through a therapeutic process with measurable results. This is the ideal. However, several new techniques were employed in this production that eventually became part of the EDT process.

1. At the very beginning of this project, in April 2015, we began to utilize psychodrama methods to deepen the personal narratives presented to us by informants. For several years, I had been exploring a transitional process, whereby a story told in playback theatre could be converted into a psychodrama format. Psychodrama is a powerful therapeutic tool in which a storyteller, called the *Protagonist*, tells and acts out his/her story, with the help of *Auxiliary* actors who play the roles of important people in the Protagonist's life. For 40 years I had studied many of the techniques of psychodrama (Blatner, 1973; Kellerman, 1992; Leveton, 1992; Moreno, 1946). This project afforded a perfect opportunity to add them to the evolving EDT process.
2. In June 2015, I facilitated a half-day workshop at Concordia University for 20 caregivers brought together by AMI-Québec. We used playback theatre to evoke and capture narratives from the group. The playback team was made up of graduates and students in the drama therapy program. We warmed the participants up to sharing their experiences as caregivers through drama therapy and sociometric methods. Some of the stories improvisationally performed that day became part of the script.
3. This project provides a vital example of the use of interviews in the EDT process. From Fall 2014, interviews were done with the board of AMI-Québec, other caregivers and participants in the June 2015 workshop. Then, there were follow-up interviews. This provided a dynamic source of reliable information on the caregivers' experience, so that we could build an authentic portrait of it.

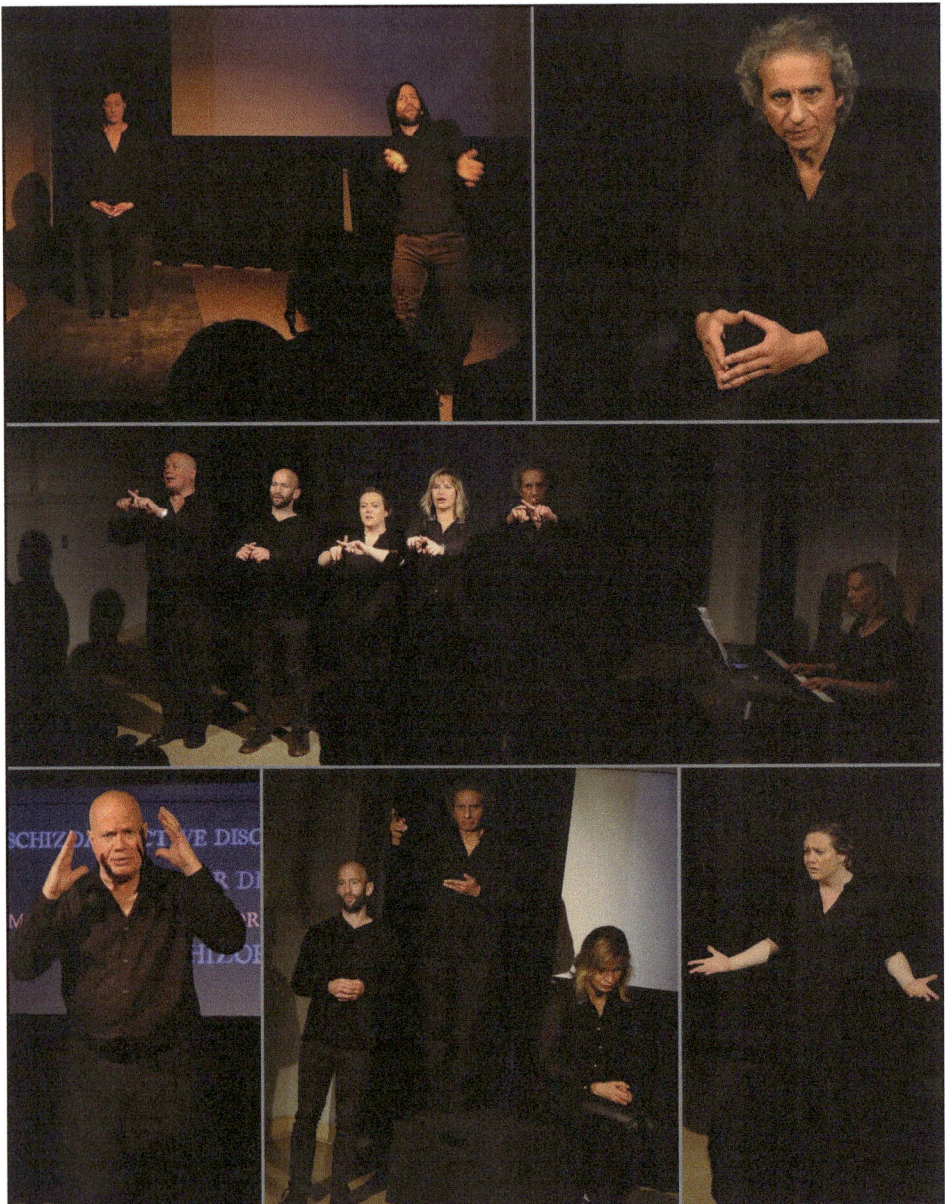

Figure 5.1   Performers in "Through the Eyes of Caregivers," from left to right: Mindy Sirois, Simon Driver, Alejandro Moran, Stephen Snow, Calley McConaghy, Katia El-Eter, Shelley Snow (at piano) (photo courtesy of Eric Mongerson)

4. In touring "Through the Eyes of Caregivers," we really began to realize the value of acquiring new data from our post-performance discussions with the audiences. Many audience members were caregivers themselves and provided us with new stories and perspectives on caregiving. We would often take their suggestions and adjust the script and performance, accordingly.

5. The quantitative evaluation of the audience responses to pre-and post-questionnaires is an excellent model of a statistical analysis that provides evidence of the educational impact of an ethnodrama. It demonstrates very clearly the importance of research in the EDT process for the future and, specifically, in the area of educational efficacy.

Collecting the Data

Phenomenological Ethnography

In gathering data on the lived experience of caregivers, like Mienczakowski (1995a; 2001), we used "ethnographic and phenomenological research processes." In fact, combined, these represent a form of "phenomenological ethnography," which constitutes our major research framework.

To begin with, phenomenology is a very accessible and concrete way to capture the "lived experience" of human beings. As Betensky writes, "Founded on the philosophical anthropology of man as being-in-the-world, phenomenology asserts the centrality of man's subjective experience, its intentional character, and its accessibility to consciousness" (1995, p. 13). In his dissertation (1995a), Mienczakowski reiterates this conception, adding how it helps with the location of themes:

> The phenomenological position maintains the concerns and agenda of the individual, and their interpretations of the contexts of their own existence, are the fundamental agenda through which social contexts should be interpreted. The phenomenological reduction of themes, as applied to the data collection of this study, involved collaboratively prioritising the agendas of respondents (Giorigi, 1985), in order to discover themes and phenomena of common interest or experience.
>
> (p. 162)

This was the approach that we used in this project and in every EDT project, thereafter. We are harnessing performance ethnography to give us the most authentic reflection of the lived experience of a specific *ethnos*, in this case, those family members who care for loved ones with a mental illness. We deeply, earnestly, sensitively, wanted to know the phenomena of their experience.

This is *ethnographic* research as we are studying a group, in depth, to understand their experience in life around a specific topic. With the adolescent girls in Youth Protection, (Chapter 3), the research focus was how they experienced themselves and life inside "the system." As Katz and Csordas write, "Phenomenology is a natural perspective for ethnographic research that would probe beneath the locally warranted definitions of a local culture to grasp the active foundations of its everyday reconstruction" (2003, pp. 284–285). In the Caregiver project, we wanted to know how the caregivers (the "local culture") experienced their everyday lives as caregivers.

And so, the interview is a crucial tool. As Mienczakowski writes, "the research approach specifically drew on the techniques of observation and interviewing" (1995a, p. 156). Of course, we were practicing **participant observation** during the whole preparation process, observing, taking notes, looking for repeated motifs of experience; however, it was the interview that was the major instrument for our ethnographic investigation. Murchison (2010) recommends an informal approach to begin with and the use of open-ended questions. This can lead to the spontaneous emergence of very valuable material from the informant, "an interviewee will take an interview in an unexpected direction and open up a whole new avenue of insight and analysis. The job of the ethnographer as interviewer is to create opportunities for this" (2010, p. 109). This was our experience, again and again. Listen empathically and sensitively to the informant and the truth of their *lived experience* will be revealed. This was the quintessential principle of our work, prior to creating the script. To repeat Denzin's perspective, "I want to re-read the interview, not as a method for gathering information, but as a vehicle for producing performance texts and performance ethnographies about self and society" (2001, p. 24).

The Early Interviews

Interviewing the Board of AMI-Québec

On November 4, 2014, I interviewed the board of AMI-Québec, accompanied by my research assistant Shannon Rzucidlo, who audiotaped and transcribed these interviews. Mienczakowski agrees with Murchison, that open-ended questions are the best means to spur an effective interview,

"In order to allow respondents to explain themselves in their 'unique ways of defining the world' … open ended interviews were preferred" (1995a, p. 160). These were the type of questions we asked the board, almost all of whom were caregivers themselves. Here is a short sample of the questions:

Q1: What does it mean to you to be a caregiver?

Q2: What do you derive from being a caregiver? What do you get out of it?

Q3: What are some of the challenges that you constantly face?

Q4: Some brought up stigma. Is that part of the challenge, as well?

Q5: If you were to write a movie script or a novel about your experience as a caregiver, what would the title be?

Just to give a little feel of the responses of this group, these are the verbatim responses to the last question, asking for a title for their experience:

MALE VOICE 1:	"A Hell of a Job" [roaring laughter]
FEMALE VOICE:	"Not for the Faint of Heart" [roaring laughter]
FEMALE VOICE:	"Rollercoaster Boogie" [roaring laugher] … "or rollercoaster something"
MALE VOICE 1:	"Maybe a positive one, 'Rewards … if it Works'"

The group had already explained the weight of the responsibility they felt as caregivers: "A constant weight on the shoulders … it doesn't go away." "And you can't escape from it. I mean, you have to do it. You're not paid for it. You're not compensated in any way. And you have no choice about it. You feel you have no choice about it …" "It lasts a lifetime." "You can't quit. If you do, you're dropping the ball and you're back to square one."

In answering **Q3**, one board member made the following statement that eventually became a monologue in the play. She is discussing the challenges she has faced with her brother and his wife, both of whom have schizophrenia:

> One more challenge is *expectations*. So not to scare anyone, however, my brother doesn't brush his teeth, he doesn't do his laundry, and I have to let that go. Because that's how he is choosing to live. I'm not going to be the one who's going to go in there and make sure he does all that. That's just not going to happen. And so, I don't expect that. When I go to visit him – and that's why one of my sister's won't go, because him and his wife, they both have schizophrenia, they are chain smokers, and my sister won't visit because of the cigarettes – and so I know that when I go in there I will come out smelling like I just smoked a pack of cigarettes. And that's o.k. And I'm going to sit on a couch that is falling apart.

And that's how they live. And I just have to … the challenge to let go
of all my expectations of how a person should be living. Because they are
living their life, and they are happy together, and they get through each
day. And for me, that's a success.

(A. N., personal communication, November 4, 2014)

This is a good example of an interview-to-monologue, later performed by a
drama therapy graduate student/actor, which was done almost verbatim and,
as Mienczakowski notes, "the physical interpretation on stage are in the authentic language of, and therefore recognizable and interpretable by informants" (2001, p. 469). In the end, this speech was validated by the caregiver
from the board. For the audience, it maintained the ring of authenticity.

The evening spent interviewing the board of AMI-Québec was well spent.
It gave a full background in the essential experiences of caregivers and provided material that would later be developed into monologues and scenes.
It truly demonstrated the value of getting things, "straight from the horse's
mouth"!

Interviewing a Mother Whose Son Has Paranoid Schizophrenia

I had known C.P. as a friend and colleague in the Theatre Department at
Concordia, where she was an administrative staff member. I also knew she
was connected to AMI-Québec and had a son with a serious mental illness.
On April 2, 2015, I did an in-depth interview with her, based on many open-
ended questions, such as: "What is the most important thing you would want
the general public to know about what it is to be a caregiver?" As Murchison
suggests, this led into a "whole new avenue of insight and analysis." C.P. told
a painful story of her son's repeated hospitalizations, due to seriously delusional thinking that often would get him in trouble with the authorities. In
one instance, he came to believe he had won 11 Nobel prizes. Around this
theme, C.P. gives a report of one such instance that was used as a monologue
in the play:

> I was at work when I received a phone call from him, saying: "Mom, guess
> what? I am in London!" I responded, "Great! What are you doing there?"
> He said, "Well unfortunately, I only have $200 dollars in my pocket, but
> I am going to Bristol. I'm going to meet the physicist who won the Nobel
> prize with me." So, I had to contact the physicist. I found the world-
> famous physicist on the internet. I sent the physicist an email and said,
> "I am the mother of a son who is 20 years old and has schizophrenia, and
> he may come knocking at your door. He is not dangerous in any way, but
> don't open the door or encourage him in any way." The physicist emailed
> me back, a couple of days, later. My son went to Bristol, stayed on the

bus, and came back to London. I think he had done "a very intelligent thing."

(C.P., personal communication, April 2, 2019)

In the play, the story was adapted for a male actor, who told the story as the boy's father. It was the first monologue in the play and began with the line, "Let me tell you what it's like to be the caregiver for someone with a mental illness." It was performed with surprise, humor and poignancy, and was a good representation of the kind of challenge parents face with a child who has major delusional thinking.

Deepening the Process with Psychodrama

In many ways, playback theatre is a form of interview – the Conductor interviews the Storyteller to get the essence of his/her personal story. "The interview ends with a brief summation and perhaps a suggestion for staging. Then the conductor's job is over for the time being" (Salas, 1993, p. 34). The Storyteller stays in their seat and watches the actors bring their story to life.

It is important to know, although there is not space enough to go into full detail, here, that the Caregiver project began in fall 2014, as a playback theatre project. The idea was to create a playback theatre company, *Pro Bono Playback Theatre Company*, with nine actors and a musician, which would eventually perform people's stories about mental health challenges in their lives. The group was made up of mostly first-year students in the MA program in Drama Therapy at Concordia. This ensemble stayed together until Spring 2015. However, a crisis in the company developed after the group performed a scene in a public playback performance about a person who had a friend with schizophrenia. The actors felt performing this story about a homeless, mentally ill man (one of the actors was required to play this role) was unethical. They refused to go on with this work, and many dropped out of the group, altogether. This "failed experiment," this crisis, demanded that I find a new way to work with playback.

It may also be important to note here that playback is very related to psychodrama. Jonathan Fox, the creator of the method, was training as a psychodramatist when he invented playback theatre (Fox, 1987). The essential difference is that the Storyteller is not a Protagonist, as in psychodrama, where the participant plays her or himself in the enactment. This is a very different vantage point and is related to Landy's concept of **distancing** (1993; 1996). In psychodrama, one of the goals is to move the Protagonist towards experiencing **catharsis** (Blatner, 1973). There are different perspectives on what exactly catharsis entails in terms of psychodrama.[1] Here, I am looking at the moving towards catharsis in psychodrama as an "underdistancing" experience for the Protagonist. In Landy's important theory of distancing, he reviews how the overdistanced client protects themselves with intellectual defenses, whereas the underdistanced one is often overwhelmed with emotion. As he writes, in regard to the therapy process, "Overdistancing becomes a cognitive process of remembering the past; underdistancing, an affective process of reliving or reexperiencing a past event" (1996, p. 17). Psychodrama purposefully moves to remove the Protagonist's defenses, to get down into the raw emotional material of experience. Psychodrama has been called "psychic surgery." It is a very direct and rapid approach, and it provokes great emotion in the Protagonist via the "affective process of reliving or reexperiencing a past event." It has been my experience that there is always the need to have a box of tissues nearby whenever facilitating a psychodrama. On the opposite side, the Storyteller in playback is literally quite removed, watching the enactment of his/her life from the Teller's Chair. This can constitute a more **distanced**, observational attitude. Psychodrama is a therapeutic technique; playback theatre has healing properties, and sometimes people spontaneously experience catharsis, but, in general it is not a therapy format, unless designed as such for clinical work in a mental health institution (Salas in Johnson and Emunah, 2009), or as in our ethnodramatherapy projects.

After the rupture in the *Pro Bono Playback Theatre Company*, I wanted to find a new format, to process individuals' stories of their mental health challenges more sensitively, in a deeper more therapeutic fashion. We would work with only one individual Storyteller/Protagonist at a time. There would be four playback actors, a musician, and myself, as Conductor/Director (this being the term in psychodrama for the facilitator/therapist). The individual would present their story, first, for a playback enactment. This was safer and more distanced for them. If it felt right, then, I would ask them if they would like to become the Protagonist in their own story and, if they said, "Yes," we would process the same experience as a psychodrama. We did four of these in May and early June 2015.

A good example of this type of integrated approach was our work with caregiver J.P., on June 4, 2015. In playback, J.P. told the story of how her daughter went through a depression. She and her husband did not take it too seriously at first, thinking it was just teenage development. Then, her daughter tried to take her life, on three separate occasions. The first time, at

---

1 Please see the Glossary for a review of essential definitions of catharsis.

the hospital, they almost lost her. Then, a year later, there was another attempt. Again, the daughter attempted suicide and was rushed to the hospital. J.P. says, "And I just about collapsed because at the point I was so confused." Finally, the daughter made a third attempt, actually going to the internet to find out how to do it. But, when she saw the blood, she said, "I can't do this to my mother."

In the playback re-enactment of this, J.P. chose the actors to play her daughter, her husband, the clerk at the hospital admittance desk and the doctor. She watched and was moved as the musician and the four actors re-created these crises and the visits to the hospital. I asked her if she would like to re-enact the scene with her daughter on the third attempt, as a psychodrama. She said she would. Under her instructions we set up the scene where her daughter said, "I can't do this to my mother." She played herself and also got to **role reverse** with her "daughter," to feel what her daughter was feeling in that moment. It was a powerful experience for her. Tears flowed. I took her for a **walk and talk**, to give her a little distance from the moment. She said how much she loved her daughter. I asked if she would like to do a **future projection**, away from this overloaded crisis moment, where she could talk calmly with her daughter and tell her how much she loved her. Acting this out with her **Auxiliary** daughter, catalyzed another cathartic moment. At the end, everyone in the group, shared with J. P. their own experiences of family crises and closeness. I thanked her for her deep sharing of this experience that she allowed us to process as a psychodrama.[2]

What was captured here, that could not be so clearly relayed by the telling of the story or a playback performance of it, was the deep emotional resonance of a family feeling helpless. It was a major theme we discovered for the first experiences of caregivers, "feeling helpless." J.P. wraps it up, beautifully. "Nobody told us about getting help, anywhere. No one. No one! So, he [my husband] said, 'Let's find help!' So, we started with AMI-Québec." J.P.'s experience became a major monologue in the play. In real life, her daughter recovered, and the two of them started an advocacy group for education on mental health (STEPP vers la santé mentale).

A week, after the session, J.P. wrote me this email:

> Thank you so much for the opportunity to participate in the drama/psychotherapy session for caregivers, last week. I truly enjoyed meeting the

---

2 References to the psychodrama techniques in bold can be found in Blatner (1973), Leveton (1992), Kellerman (1992) and Garcia & Buchanan in Johnson & Emunah (2009).

troop of young drama and music therapists (in the making). They are very good and endearing.

I must admit that while I did not expect to feel anything, I know that the work we did made a shift inside of me. The next morning, I felt it in my bones that something has shifted (as I have normally felt when I have done deep work on myself). Also, on the week-end I had a marvelous dream, being a child disguising myself as a doctor to make people laugh meanwhile laughing my heart out in the dream and after waking up for a good five minutes. It felt great to reconnect with that part of me. Thank you.

(J.P., personal communication, June 10, 2015)

Since this time, the psychodrama techniques have become a regular part of the EDT process.

The June 27, 2015 Workshop for Caregivers

This workshop, from 1pm to 5pm on a Saturday afternoon, was a deep cauldron and profound sharing of caregivers' experiences. There were 14 caregivers with various backgrounds attending, along with four actors and a musician from the *Pro Bono* company, and myself, as the facilitator.

I warmed the group up using classic drama therapy warm-ups. For instance, we did a *name game*, followed by an embodied version of it, in which the members of the group said their name with an accompanying gesture. Then, the whole group reflected this back to them with sound and movement. We did this at a fast speed and slow speed to feel the difference, Next, I guided them in *emotional greetings* (Emunah, 1994, p. 150). This exercise is a brief introduction to improvisational role-playing where the members get in pairs, back to back, and, when they turn around on cue, they greet each other in a feeling state. We used "shyly," "suspiciously," "like professionals at a conference," and "like dear childhood friends who have not seen each other in five years!" By this point the group was relaxed and in a playful mood.

Sociometry, a science of measuring aspects of relationships in groups, and created by J.L Moreno, is a most relevant method in a group process like this (Moreno, 1953/1993). I utilized a sociometric exercise I often use (Garcia & Sternberg, 1989). I asked the group to form four subgroups, with one of the playback actors as the guide. The subgroup had to locate three challenges as caregivers that they felt they had in common. After some discussion, the group's guide presented these, and I put them on the long blackboard on the wall at the end of the room. Once we had located these multiple themes,

I asked each group to choose the one that was most important to their group. The final results were: "Communication," "Self-Care," "Worry" and "Boundaries." The process of distillation allowed me to see what baseline areas were of concern for this group. In aiming to locate the deep commonalities of experience of a group, it is invaluable to the EDT process.

The goal was now to use playback theatre to reflect actual personal experience of group members in relation to the four established themes. When we began with "Boundaries," M.P., who was very warmed-up to the moment, told a harrowing story of her son, who has **paranoid schizophrenia** and had become homeless, trying to break into her house. She experienced both great fear at his threatening her life and guilt at having to call the police to protect herself. This story was performed as a *fluid sculpture* (see Chapter 2). Afterwards M.P. was in tears and group members went to comfort her. Through this powerful, authentic story and the playback team's skillful rendering of its emotional content, the space was opened for deep discussion of the four thematic challenges. After each *fluid sculptural* representation of a theme, the group shared their own experiences around the same issue – a cauldron of experiences was cooking! Three of the stories told in this part, later became either scenes or monologues in the play.

As in the traditional playback format, the *fluids* were followed by actual *scene* creation. From our previous playback/psychodrama sessions with individuals, we had developed a model for such a scene with C.P., who also has a son with paranoid schizophrenia. It was a story about stigma. She was with co-workers waiting for the bus on a beautiful Fall day. Her colleagues were all boasting about how great their children were doing. Suddenly, they turn to her and ask her about her son. She says, "Well, my son … actually he doesn't do anything. He has schizophrenia. He is not capable of doing anything." Long embarrassed pause, and the group changes the subject. Then, the bus comes. The performance of this story catalyzed other sensitized stories about family members with schizophrenia or who were "misdiagnosed" as having schizophrenia. Most of these stories became scenes in our ethnodramatic theatre production.

This half-day workshop turned out to be both inspiring and useful. At the end, I facilitated a strong closure (Emunah, 1994, pp. 43–45), as so much strong emotion had been expressed. Among other exercises, I used a technique I had learned in a sociodrama workshop, years ago. The whole group forms an outer circle and an inner circle. The outer group faces in and the inner group faces out. They take the hands of the partner facing them. Three questions are asked. After the partners discuss it, the outer circle turns one person to the right. The three questions were. "What did you learn from today's experience?"; "What surprised or fascinated you the most?"; "What lovely thing are you going to do to take care of yourself, this weekend?" After much poignant and playful interplay between partners, the group ended. I said: "Thank you all, so much! Shannon will check in with you to set up a one-to-one interview."

The Follow-Up Interviews

After the workshop on June 27, and contacts made with other caregivers, there was a need to do in-depth, follow-up interviews. Through the psycho-drama and the playback methods, we had begun to dig deeply into the rich texture of experience of these many caregivers. Now, we needed to fill in the details, so we could properly script the play. C.P. and J.P. had already been interviewed in the Spring, so now, in the next few months, Shannon or I interviewed ten of the other 14 attendees at the workshop. Only two were not given a follow-up interview. Shannon transcribed all these interviews, so I could review them with a fine-tooth comb.

Here is one example of the process. W.O. was a nurse from Ireland, working in Montreal. She had a brother with schizophrenia, who had gone missing back home in Ireland. She was very upset about this and presented the basic story in the workshop. She explained how she got into a big fight with her other brother and ended up feeling very distressed and depressed about her situation. In the workshop presentation, she had given a statistic about the high rate of schizophrenia in Ireland, and another group member chirped in, "What's in the water?" This caused a momentary incident as W.O. was very upset about this comment and angrily rebuked the other person. It was an important moment for us as a group, around the need to learn to be sensitive about how we use language in regard to mental health issues. In her interview, she gave the whole background about her relationship with her brother who has schizophrenia:

> [he]was the second to the last. [He] ... I do believe he may have devel-
> oped schizophrenia when he was about 21. I was gone from the house
> then, I was studying in London, and he came over there and I met him. I
> had no understanding or knowledge of mental health in the times. And
> I came to Canada. If there is anything I regret in my life, it is that I left,
> then, because, he was in really, in nearly full-blown schizophrenia at that
> stage. He wrote me two letters, and I kept them. I gave them back to him
> recently. I was always writing, trying to contact him, but I could never
> find him, because he didn't have a phone. And I eventually caught up

with him. I went to London once from here when I was 40 and made contact with him. I didn't know about schizophrenia, then, either. And he used to tell me things that I know could not possibly be true. But I listened to them. But it was very stressful, because I don't think he had anywhere to live, and he told lies, lots of lies.

(W.O., June 25, 2015)

W.O. goes on to tell the story about the brother she loves who becomes homeless and, then, no one knows where he is. She fills in all the details of her big fight with her other brother, who got furious with her and yelled at her. She speaks of having a "heaviness of the soul" and feeling "worthless." She says,

[He] … told me he was missing. And he is screaming and shouting at me. Telling me that "you never sent his address, I would have contacted him." I said, "that is not how I live." He was screaming. He is out of touch. Suddenly, after so many years … he suddenly wakes up and decided to contact him. I feel that I have wasted my life!

She expresses her depression around these complex and conflictual family relations related to a loved one with a mental illness.

To give a sense of the transition from in-depth interview to playscript, here is how this material looked on the page, for the actor to perform:

Monologue #6: Willy's Story

[with a slight Irish brogue]

My brother has schizophrenia. He lives in Ireland, and I live in Halifax. A whole ocean separates us. Now, a short while ago, Freddie, my brother with schizophrenia, disappeared from the place he was living. None of us knew where he was! My brother Pete calls me from Ireland. He had never been involved. I personally had put in a lot of long-distance effort. I had been telling him for years that Freddie has schizophrenia. "You have to understand that and be more involved and be more caring. Be caring." So, Pete starts screaming and shouting at me. "You never sent me his address!" And, of course, now, he is lost to us, he doesn't have an address. But, Pete keeps yelling over the phone, shouting all kinds of terrible things at me. Suddenly after all these years, he wakes up and wants to have contact with our sick brother. And it just made me feel horrible. I felt worthless, absolutely worthless. I even felt suicidal in a way. I felt a heaviness of the soul. I felt "how is it worth it to be living? What's the point?"

(*MUSIC*)

I had reviewed over 20 pages of the transcribed interview with W.O. I had listened carefully to the cadence of her voice on the digital recording. Like Anna Deveare Smith, as a playwright, I was trying to capture the "spirit" of W.O., as a character. However, for reasons of confidentiality, I had changed the gender of this character, as I did with several others in the script. This is very different from Deveare Smith who uses verbatim transcriptions to create her monologues. She has developed a powerful method of locating character via their language. As she writes, "If I were to inhabit the speech pattern of another, and walk in the speech of another, we could find the individuality of the other and experience that individuality viscerally" (Deavere Smith, 1993, p. xxvii). Still, in directing the actor who spoke in language very close W.O.'s words, I aimed to capture the unique experience of suffering in that individual. Like Saldana, I believe there is much to be learned from Deveare Smith's approach in order to "portray what was invisible about that individual" (1993, p. xxxii). This is our goal as theatre artists in EDT: to translate the unique experiences of individuals into a viable and aesthetic theatrical experience.

Translating the Data into Theatre

A huge amount of material had been collected via interviews, participant observation and workshops in playback and psychodrama. Out of this raw material, a script and subsequent performance was to be created. This is the central task of the ethnodramatist and the ethnodrama director. In this case, both were myself.

Scripting the Ethnodrama

As Saldana writes, "The basic content for ethnodrama is the reduction of field notes, interview transcripts, journal entries, etc., to salient foreground issues – the 'juicy stuff' for 'dramatic impact'" (2005, p. 16). Saldana has also been highly influenced by the work of Anna Deavere Smith and looks carefully into how she locates the most relevant and resonant moments in her interviews and then translates them into the script. "These portions of an interview tend to be the richest and most significant, and thus find their way onto the page and onto the stage" (Saldana, 2011, p. 19).

It is very important to note, here, also, how Saldana, the major North American interpreter of Mienczakowski's ethnodrama, distinguishes between

"Ethnodrama" and "Ethnotheatre." The first is all about the scripting process, the creation of a script. As he writes: "Simply put, this is dramatizing the data" (2011, p. 13). On the other hand, "Ethnotheatre" is about the integration of performance ethnography with the art of theatre. All of the preparatory ethnographic research, in the end, is "fieldwork for theatrical production work" (2011, p. 13).

Undoubtedly, having both the role of playwright and theatre director, as I did for this project, has its disadvantages and challenges. However, it can also provide the advantage of seeing the potentials for dynamic staging as the script is being created. It can lead to a unity in the script and subsequent performance. For instance, in this case, I had previously worked in several professional theatre productions as a narrator, so I decided to create and take the role of narrator in our production of "Through the Eyes of Caregivers." It was a way to tie everything together. It also came out of my personal motivation to focus on this topic: my own father had a **bipolar disorder** that, at times, severely impacted our family life. So, I knew something about this topic personally.

The opening narration in the play went like this:

Narration #1

Good Evening and Welcome. As you know, you are about to see a short play on the topic of mental illness. It's a play about how mental illness affects peoples' lives – both the person with the illness *and* their family. After the play is over, we will have a discussion on the issues that arise, with you – the audience. Now, of course, plays have been written about this subject, *before* – just think for a second … (*testing the audience*) … What comes to mind? … *One Flew East* … *One Flew West* … (*audience responds*) … *One Flew over the Cuckoo's Nest*. Exactly! The Hollywood version of mental illness! As glamorous as Jack Nicholson!

We are taking a *very* different approach. Our play is grounded in reality. The stories and scenes you are about to see are based on the *actual* experiences of persons who have been, or presently are, *caregivers* for a loved one with a mental illness.

I am the narrator of the play. I must confess, the subject of mental illness is very personal for me. It's not an abstraction, like for those people who can speak of "The Myth of Mental Illness." No, mental illness is very concrete for me because I experienced it within my own family. When I was junior in college, I was with my father in the psychiatric hospital after he had gone through an acute psychotic episode, and I saw, firsthand, how it affected our whole family. It was the real thing – not the Hollywood version.

In many ways, mental illness is the *central character* of our play. Why do I say this? Because mental illness *touches* each and every one of us. It really does! The statistics show that one in five people experience some form of mental illness in their lifetime. One in Five![3] Think of it! This means that, in almost any extended family, someone is bound to be afflicted with it. This means a great many people have loved ones, for whom they become a caregiver. And *this* is how we are going to tell the story of mental illness, tonight – "Through the Eyes of Caregivers."

These narrations were woven in between monologues (like the ones already presented) and scenes, most of them based on the interviews. Previously to this, I had written over a dozen play scripts, so I had a pretty good sense of dramatic construction and timing. The aim was to give as wide a variety of lived moments of mental health challenges as possible. It was a kind of theatrical pastiche of the DSM-V. We sought to touch each of the major disorders: schizophrenia, bipolar, depression, suicidality and anxiety. All were based on authentic individual experiences, and, were, sometimes, *very* challenging.

We decided to work with M.P.'s story about her son threatening to burn her house down, while she was inside. This was confronting the difficult and complex issue of violence and mental illness. We wanted to confront this truthfully, but we also did not want to increase stigmatization against people who are mentally ill. The narration tried to keep a balanced and honest view. We used a slide of statistics to back the words being said:

Narration #7

Really bad stuff can happen. It is simply the truth. Like that pilot in Germany, a few years ago, who was allegedly depressed, had been treated in a hospital and then went to work anyway and flew his plane into the side of a mountain – killing all of his passengers! [*Slide #11*] However, the facts are that most people with mental illnesses are *not violent*. They are not the

---

3 Here, I am using statistics from Canadian estimates supplied by AMI-Québec. In the next chapter, I use estimates from the World Health Organization that state *one in four* people will experience a mental health challenge in their lifetime.

killers so often portrayed in the media. They are not automatically violent because they have a mental illness. The statistics show this. [*Slide #12*] But, bad stuff can and *does* happen. I worked in a big state psychiatric hospital, in the U.S., for several years. One time, on my ward, a patient snuck up behind a very petite female recreation therapist and smashed her over the head with a chair, seemingly for no reason at all. She was hospitalized and out of work for months. Bad stuff can happen, and we have to be cognizant of that potential – a person with a mental illness *can be* erratic – and we have to deal with this phenomenon in a realistic manner – no matter how challenging that may be sometimes.

The scene that followed was taken almost verbatim from M.P.'s interview (personal communication, July 20, 2015), and shaped into dialogue.

Scene #4: Natalie's Story

(*NATALIE*; *GENE*, *her son*; *TWO COPS*)

NATALIE: My son has a lot of problems. He started smoking marijuana in Grade 8. In Grade 10, he got arrested for selling hash. He was expelled. I got him out of trouble, *every time*. Then, by 19, he became very sick. He would get angry and hit the wall with a baseball bat. He was diagnosed with paranoid schizophrenia, and he was also addicted to drugs. For 12 years, I tried to help him. I would rent him places to live, shop for furniture, set it up, clean his house and bring him food, too. I tried to give him some structure. So, I said: "You do not cook, here – he had a big fire in his previous apartment and *this* was a brand new condo I had purchased for him – you smoke outside, and no strangers can come here." He slowly broke every one of these rules. I felt helpless. All he was doing, all day, was smoking in bed. The nice table I got for him, next to the bed, was filthy with sticky drinks, sodas, empty bags for chips, cigarette butts, everywhere. It was so damn filthy. It was disgusting. And he was using all his money for weed, for marijuana. At this point, I realized that there is nothing I can do for him, anymore. I had had it. It's twelve years that I caregave for him, and I told him, "You have to leave, I am renting this place." So, after that he was homeless. Sometimes, he would come to my house to ask for money for food, for cigarettes, but basically he was out on the street, scrounging about for weed, and I don't know what else …

(*MUSIC. GENE enters and dances an embodied expression of his desperate state of being.*)

NATALIE: Then, last summer he wanted to live on my balcony. He made a little fire, caused a burn on the patio veranda. I felt I could not deal with it anymore. I said, "You can't come here, anymore. I don't want you to come." I didn't want to see him because you never know what he is going to do. Then, one day, last January, he came out by the back door. I would not let him in. He said he wanted money. I said I could not give him any. He became very threatening …

GENE: (*pacing back and forth by the back door*). Mom! Mom! I am going to start a fire! I am going to burn your house down. You hear what I say. I am going to burn it down. You gotta help me, or I swear I will burn you up in there!!!

NATALIE: I was shaking. For a moment, I felt helpless. Then, I found the guts to go upstairs and call the police. *I pressed charges against my own son!* I can't tell you how horrible that felt. I felt so guilty. I kept saying to myself, "Would he really do this?" But, I was also terrified. So, the police came and took him away …

(*Sirens. TWO COPS enter and go through a mime of arresting and handcuffing GENE. They mime putting him in the cop car. Sound of sirens. Lights change.*)

NATALIE: They took him to a detention centre first, then to the Pinel Institute. Later, he was transferred to the Montreal General. He is there under the Tribunal Administratif du Quebec. I have not seen him since last January. And I cannot see him, because I am the one that pressed charges. And I thought, "Really, I cannot help him." (*Begins to cry.*) My heart breaks every time I see a homeless person, now. I'm always afraid I am going to run into my son on the street. I always want to keep a little bit of hope … but after all these years. It's such a tragedy to see your son at 31 years old – as if he were dead. If someone actually dies, you have your mourning, you reach a stage of acceptance. But this – to live. He's a living corpse to me.

Altogether, the play had nine narrations, 14 monologues, five scenes and two songs.[4] It lasted about one hour and was always followed by a discussion with the audience, after they completed the post-performance questionnaire.

---

4 There is not space to present the whole script, here. However, the author would be happy to send a copy of it to any interested party. Please contact him at stephen.snow@concordia.ca.

Validation of the Script and Performance

After the June 27 workshop, the ensemble took a break, and I went to work on the script. A full draft was completed on September 2, and we went into rehearsals, 6pm to 8pm, on Tuesday nights, starting on September 8. We were preparing for a preview performance at the North American Drama Therapy Association conference in White Plains, New York, on October 17.

Our presentation was entitled: "Performance as an Empathy-Building Tool: Experimental Integration of Playback and Ethnodrama." At this point, it was a 30-minute piece with eight monologues, two scenes, three narrations and one song, all with musical accompaniment. After the play, the audience answered a brief questionnaire. In this way, we were able to get feedback, early on, that the play impacted the audience emotionally and educated them about the experiences of caregivers. The questions were quite simple, like, "Did viewing the *ethnodrama* presentation help you to have greater empathy for persons who are caregivers for loved ones with a mental illness? Please explain why or why not." Through the feedback from the responses, we gained confidence we were on the right track.

Because we were commissioned to present this preview, within a short rehearsal period, the validation process was out of the traditional sequence, which would have been to have shown the script and the performance to the informants, *first*. However, when we returned to Montreal, we went right back into rehearsals and further developed the script. The new script was ready on October 30, and we prepared for a validation preview with an audience made up of most of the caregivers from the June 27 workshop, along with Ella Amir and some of the board members of AMI-Québec. This took place on November 10. The feedback was, again, very positive. There was a clear sense from the group that we had authentically translated their stories into theatrical art. This prepared me and the ensemble for our first full public performances on November 21, 22 and 23, 2015.

Touring the Play: Gathering New Data

New Material for the Script

After the November 2015 performances, we took the play on tour until June 2017 (Figure 5.2). Altogether, we did 11 performances of "Through the Eyes of Caregivers." These included special performances for Laurentian Care in Mont-Tremblant, for Creative Art Therapies Week in Montreal, and for Laurier Macdonald High School in Saint-Leonard.

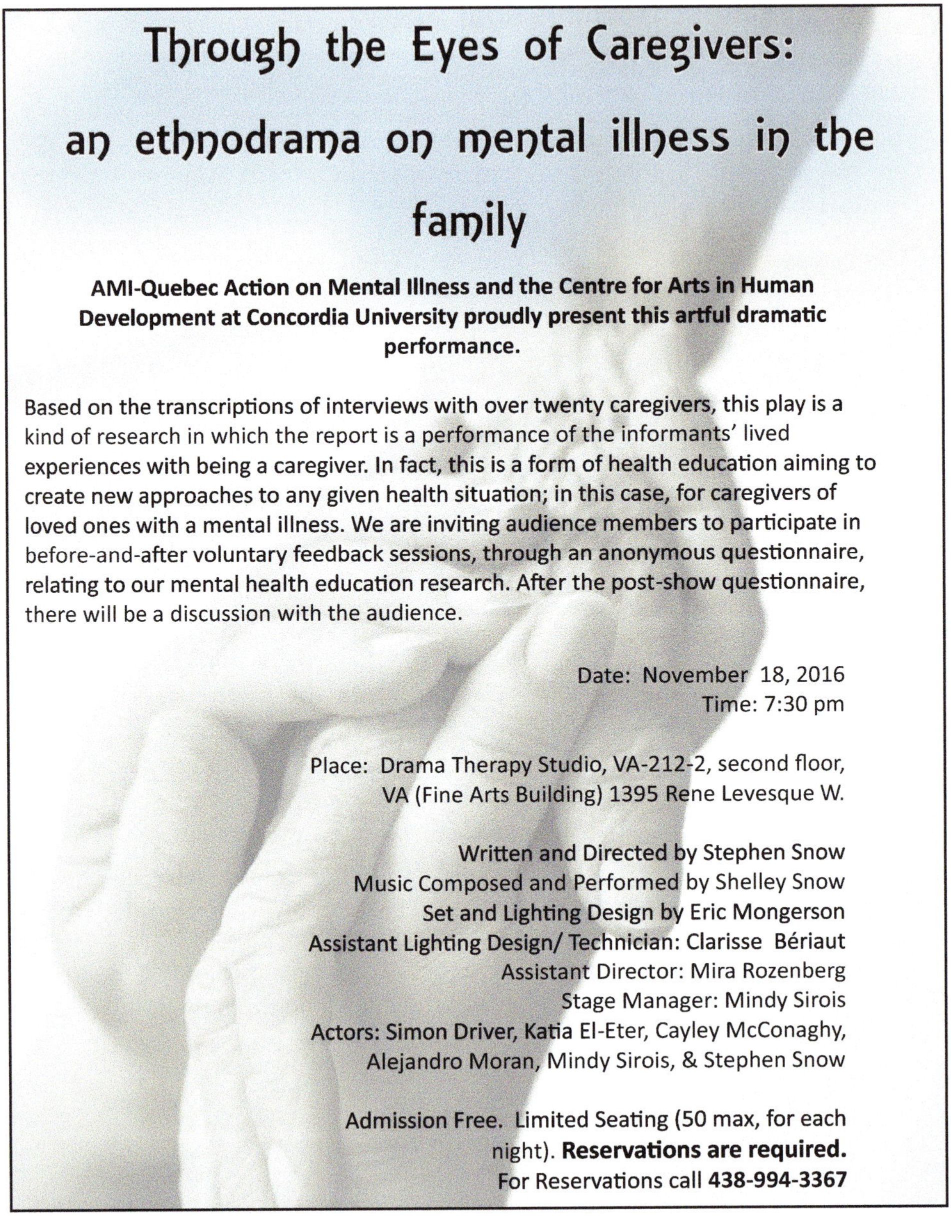

Through the Eyes of Caregivers:

an ethnodrama on mental illness in the

family

AMI-Quebec Action on Mental Illness and the Centre for Arts in Human Development at Concordia University proudly present this artful dramatic performance.

Based on the transcriptions of interviews with over twenty caregivers, this play is a kind of research in which the report is a performance of the informants' lived experiences with being a caregiver. In fact, this is a form of health education aiming to create new approaches to any given health situation; in this case, for caregivers of loved ones with a mental illness. We are inviting audience members to participate in before-and-after voluntary feedback sessions, through an anonymous questionnaire, relating to our mental health education research. After the post-show questionnaire, there will be a discussion with the audience.

Date: November 18, 2016
Time: 7:30 pm

Place: Drama Therapy Studio, VA-212-2, second floor,
VA (Fine Arts Building) 1395 Rene Levesque W.

Written and Directed by Stephen Snow
Music Composed and Performed by Shelley Snow
Set and Lighting Design by Eric Mongerson
Assistant Lighting Design/ Technician: Clarisse Bériaut
Assistant Director: Mira Rozenberg
Stage Manager: Mindy Sirois
Actors: Simon Driver, Katia El-Eter, Cayley McConaghy,
Alejandro Moran, Mindy Sirois, & Stephen Snow

Admission Free. Limited Seating (50 max, for each
night). **Reservations are required.**
For Reservations call **438-994-3367**

Figure 5.2   Poster for Performance in November 2016 (Permission from Cayley McConaghy for design)

There were a few changes in the cast, as time went on, as well as some changes in the script. As Mienczakowski points out, in regard to touring his play in 1995, "the performances were also used to further the data of the study" (1995b, p. 361). For instance, on our tour, after one post-performance forum, a young caregiver pointed out we did not have any material in the script that dealt with a child having to care for a parent with a mental illness. Very shortly, I located such a person and interviewed them about their relationship with a father who has **borderline personality disorder**. This interview was transformed into a monologue in which the parent's gender was changed. It went like this:

Monologue #3: Janine's Story

God, I feel so angry at my Mom! It's just a week ago, and I still feel so angry and hurt. I had just turned 21, and my Mom invited me and my brothers over for a supposed "Happy Time." It turned into the Birthday party from Hell! Now, my Mom has this personality disorder. I know this because, before they got divorced, my Dad made her go to see a psychiatrist. She never lets him forget this. For the past three years, she has just demonized my Dad as the Cruelest Man on Earth. He was just trying to help her because she can be so irritable and moody. She was officially diagnosed with borderline personality disorder by the psychiatrist. My Dad told me that. But, then you just forget 'cause she can really be very sweet at times. So, this night, I fell into the trap. I had written a poem that I wanted to share with everyone on my birthday. My Mom just lit into it. She had this sarcastic laugh and just kept putting me down. She has always had the ability to make me and my brothers feel like shit. But this night, I finally stood up to her. I started crying and yelling at her. I tell her *this is the way she has made me feel my whole life*. It was the first time I fought back, and she did not know how to deal with it. She just can't take any responsibility for what she says. And she refuses to go into any kind of therapy. She says everything is my Dad's fault and I know that is bullshit. She's the one that has mental health issues, and someday I hope she can really come to terms with that!

The ability to keep adapting the script, based on new information from audiences, demonstrates the elasticity of ethnodrama as a research method and its organicism as a form of theatre. We shifted and transformed material for the play continuously, as we received new input from audiences.

Responses from Audiences

People were moved by witnessing the struggles and challenges of caregivers and gained insight into what it means to live such a life. This is documented in many comments (see epigraph for this chapter) that we received from audience members:

> Often unfamiliar with the illness and unprepared for the road ahead, families affected by mental illness in a loved one are faced with multiple

challenges: learning about the illness, learning how to support an ill relative while sustaining their own well-being, and maybe most difficult – adjusting their expectations and accepting the limitations often presented by mental illness without losing hope.

"Through the Eyes of Caregivers" is a realistic depiction of the family experience. It is an effective educational tool to sensitize service providers and the public at large to the experience many families of the one in five individuals diagnosed with mental illness are going through.

(E.A., Ph.D., Executive Director of AMI-Québec
Action on Mental Illness)

Caring for a family member or friend with mental health issues means facing stigma, misunderstanding, and grief, but sometimes also unexpected personal growth. As such a caregiver, personally, this powerfully-presented ethnodrama has educated me on many diverse issues in other caregiver lives. What's it *really* like to be a caregiver in mental health and what are caregiver vulnerabilities and strengths? How do caregivers see themselves in the context of others? How can we share our human qualities of peer support? You have to see this play to get a better understanding! Great knowledge-building tool. I think everyone should see it!

(C.P., Caregiver)

Heartbreaking but hopeful stories from loving companions on the journey. Come and compare experiences...

(J.M., Recently retired after 40 years as chaplain at
the Douglas Mental Health University Institute)

I was very moved to witness the play, "Through the Eyes of Caregivers." It was a profound experience. It brought to light in a visceral and theatrical way, the suffering, joy and pain experienced by families and individuals who are caring for a family member suffering from mental illness. Therapeutic theatre of this calibre is life enriching, healing and raises awareness.

(B.H., Creative Arts Therapist/Psychoanalyst)

"Through the Eyes of Caregivers" allowed me to experience moments that were profoundly touching. Being myself a caregiver, I recognized several intense situations in my life. Through the play and these characters, I felt I could share my experience and could be better understood. This play highlights the discomforts, ostracism and fear of mental health. It awakens our minds to the painful reality often difficult to understand for those who are not directly confronted with it. "Through the Eyes of Caregivers" is one hand extended to the other. It raises the veil about the lives of caregivers and their loved ones living with a mental health problem. It is a cry from the heart, and it is a call to the opening of our humanity. And in today's times, this is what we need most, our HUMANITY!

(M.L., Caregiver)

Final Show

We ended the tour on June 9, 2017, in Concordia's Cazalet Theatre. With the consent of the cast and audience, we videotaped the show and post-show forum for a future documentary on the project.[5] The house was packed. For this occasion, we also brought together a special panel for the forum, consisting of two psychiatrists, the director of a mental health advocacy agency, a high school student advocate for mental health, a caregiver and myself. It was the most vigorous post-performance discussion we had on the tour. Two caregivers and one of the psychiatrists ended up talking in the parking lot, adjacent to the theatre until 2am in the morning!

This evening, we also administered a full pre- and post-questionnaire with the audience. These consisted of questions meant to reveal the audience's attitudes toward mental illness and, in the end, to see if there was a change in their attitudes. We had administered these questionnaires, sporadically, throughout the tour, as will be explained in the next section.

Analysis of the Impact of the Play on the Audiences

Over the course of the tour, we collected pre- and post-questionnaire responses from 111 audience participants. Their mean age was 41.91 years; 77 were females, 34 males, with 70 self-identified as English speakers, 17 French speakers and 21 English–French bilingual speakers. Their backgrounds included 37 mental health professionals; 54 caregivers; 50 who, themselves, had experienced mental health challenges. Some were in more than one category and 25 said they felt they belonged to none of the given categories.

---

5 This documentary, *For Those Who Care*, will be available in 2022. Please contact the author for information on how to view this documentary. Contact him at stephen.snow@concordia.ca.

What Was Being Measured?

The whole procedure to measure the impact of the play on the audiences was constructed on four categories.[6] We wanted to learn how our audiences thought about: (1) Stigma in regard to mental health issues; (2) Self-evaluation of one's potential to be a caregiver for a loved one with a mental illness; (3) Respect for mental health patients' need for autonomy; (4) Attitude towards caregiving. These four **subscales**, developed through prior pilot testing, were set up to assess the audience members' beliefs and attitudes about mental health, mental illness and caregiving (see Table 5.1). For each subscale, we created a single validating item that defined the main idea of the scale in a general way. Before the play began, audience members were greeted by a researcher who explained how to fill in the personal information and consent sections of the questionnaire. Then, the audience was asked to fill out the questionnaires and, after the play, a second questionnaire in order to provide pre-post measures. There was also a final questionnaire for comments on the play that the participants could fill out during the post-show forum or mail in from home. All the questions, except for the qualitative response to the play were related to a Likert-type, 6-point scale, with "6" indicating the greatest agreement and "1" the most disagreement.

Results

Analyses of the pre-show responses demonstrated that the four subscales all achieved a satisfactory degree of internal consistency, with **Cronbach's alphas** from .64 to .81. All subscales also correlated significantly with the uniquely constructed validity item, with **Spearman rho** ranging from .51 to .70, all $p < .001$.

The results from the qualitative evaluation of the play, itself, were all very positive, giving evidence that the play was a useful education tool; that it portrayed the lives of caregivers with accuracy and realism; and that the audience liked the play and would recommend it to others. The pre–post comparisons revealed statistically significant shifts in the direction of increased respect for a patient's need for autonomy and greater awareness of the challenges of caretaking. In the end, our research on the educational value of the play indicated it had a measurable impact on the audiences.

---

6 This entire procedure was set up by my colleague, Dr. Norman Segalowitz, of Concordia University's Department of Psychology. I am grateful for his lending his expertise to this project.

Table 5.1   Questionnaire Items Retained for Final Analyses of Audience Responses

*Stigma	• I would be embarrassed if my family thought I had a psychological disorder. • I would be embarrassed if people knew that I dated a person who once received psychological treatment. • I would not knowingly become friends with a mentally ill person. • I would be embarrassed if a person in my family became mentally ill.
*Self-evaluation	As a carer for a family member or a friend with a serious mental illness, I (would) … • feel uncertain about what I have to do as a carer. • feel confident about my abilities as a carer. • find I am able to cope with the situation. • feel able to evaluate how I am doing as a carer.
*Respect	As a carer for a family member or a friend with a serious mental illness, I (would) … • need to know about everything that goes on in this person's relationships with other people. • feel the need to know what this person is thinking about most things. • believe that this person should have interests different from mine. • have better insight into what this person is thinking and feeling than they do.
*Caregiving attitude	As a carer for a family member or a friend with a serious mental illness, I (would) … • feel ashamed. • find this person to be a burden. • be resentful for having to care for this person. • look forward to caring for this person.
The Play	1. I would recommend this play to others. 2. I was able to personally identify with some of the situations presented. 3. Overall, the play accurately portrayed the experience of carers (5.29 – score out of 6 for this item). 4. The play changed my understanding of the role and experience of carers. 5. This play is likely to change other people's understanding of the role and experience of carers. 6. As a result of seeing this play, I am more likely to seek out information on what it means to be a carer for someone with mental illness. 7. Overall, the play addressed real situations. 8. Overall, I enjoyed the actors' performances, special effects and staging. 9. I liked this play. 10. This play can be a useful tool in mental health education.

*Pre- and post-test Cronbach's α and 95% confidence intervals: Stigma: pre =.74 [.59 .89], post =.74 [.66 .82]; Respect: pre = .64 [.53 .76], post =.60 [.48 .72]; Caregiving attitude: pre = .70 [.61 .79], post =.73 [.65 .81]; Self-evaluation: pre = .72 [.64 .81], post =.81 [.75 .87].

The Main Takeaways

Again, for those students and professionals who would like to practice the full EDT format, it must be reiterated that the major element missing in this project was an in-depth therapeutic process. This was because the informants were *not* the performers. However, there are several valuable "takeaways" that help the prospective ethnodramatherapist to understand the development of EDT and how it has been finally formulated (see Chapter 10).

The use of psychodrama to deepen the emotional resonance in scenes and to provide the informant with a therapeutic experience is an important new contribution from this project. The use of sociometry to gauge the interests and interconnections in a group is another. This is an excellent way to locate vital themes. The heightened utilization of the ethnographic interview is well articulated here in regard to the preparation of the script and shows how important the interview process is to EDT. As the tour took place over 14 months, we really got to see how new data from audience responses would create new scenes and monologues. We began to realize the valuable "elasticity" and "organicism" of the ethnodrama approach. Because of being able to collaborate with highly skilled colleagues in quantitative research, we were able to attain an excellent model for the analysis of the educational impact of the play. Once we can do the same type of analysis for the longitudinal therapeutic component of EDT, we will have a fully integrated method.

References

Betensky, M. G. (1995). *What do you see?: Phenomenology of therapeutic art expression.* Jessica Kingsley Publishers.

Blatner, A. (1973). *Acting-in: Practical applications of psychodramatic methods.* Springer Publishing.

Denzin, N. (2001). The reflexive interview and a performative social science. *Qualitative Research 1*(1), 23–46.

Emunah, R. (1994). *Acting for real: Drama therapy process, technique, and performance.* Bruner/Mazel Publishers.

Fox, J. (Ed.). (1987). *The essential Moreno: Writings on psychodrama, group method, and spontaneity by J.L. Moreno, M.D.* Springer Publishing.

Garcia, N., & Buchanan, D. (2009). Psychodrama. In D. R. Johnson & R. Emunah (Eds.), *Current approaches in drama therapy* (2nd ed., pp. 393–423). C. C. Thomas Publisher.

Garcia, N., & Sternberg, P. (1989). *Sociodrama: Who's in your shoes?* Praeger.

Katz, J. & Csordas, T. J. (2003). Phenomenological ethnography in sociology and anthropology. *Ethnography, 4*(3), 275–288.

Kellerman, P. F. (1992). *Focus on psychodrama: The therapeutic aspects of psychodrama.* Jessica Kingsley Publishers.

Landy, R. J. (1993). *Persona and performance: The meaning of role in drama, therapy, and everyday life.* The Guildford Press.

Landy, R. J. (1996). The use of distancing in drama therapy. R. J. Landy (Ed.), *Essays in drama therapy: The double life* (pp. 13–27). Jessica Kingsley.

Leveton, E. (1992). *A clinician's guide to psychodrama.* Springer Publishing.

Mienczakowski, J. (1995a). *The application of critical ethno-drama to health settings.* [Unpublished doctoral dissertation]. Griffith University, Australia.

_____. (1995b). The theatre of ethnography: The reconstruction of ethnography with emancipatory potential. *Qualitative Inquiry, 1*(3), 360–375.

_____. (2001). Ethnodrama: Performed research – Limitations and potential. In P. Atkinson, A. Coffey, S. Delamont, J. Lofland & L. Lofland (Eds.), *Handbook of Ethnography* (pp. 468–476). Sage Publications.

Moreno, J. L. (1946). *Psychodrama, First Volume.* Beacon House.

Moreno, J. L. (1993). *Who shall survive?: Foundations of sociometry, group therapy and sociodrama.* American Society of Group Psychotherapy and Psychodrama. (Original work published 1953).

Murchison, J. M. (2010). *Ethnographic essentials: Designing, conducting, and presenting your research.* Jossey-Bass.

Salas, J. (1993). *Improvising real life: Personal story in playback theatre.* Kendall/Hunt Publishing.

_____ J. (2009). Playback theatre; A frame for healing. In D. R. Johnson & R. Emunah (Eds.), *Current approaches in drama therapy* (2nd ed., pp. 445–460). C. C. Thomas Publisher.

Saldana, J. (Ed.). (2005). *Ethnodrama: An anthology of reality theatre.* Altamira Press.

_____. (2011). *Ethnotheatre: Research from page to stage.* Left Coast Press.

Smith, A. D. (1993). *Fires in the mirror: Crown Heights, Brooklyn and other identities.* Anchor Books.

6

A Community-Oriented EDT Project on Mental Health

The effects of mental illness can present far-reaching challenges for the entire family, including care recipients and caregivers, as well as for care providers and the health-care system at large.

(Ella Amir, Executive Director of AMI-Québec Action on mental illness, 2011)

The Community Framework

As mentioned in previous chapters, the group in the ethnodrama process needs to have a depth of common experiences to be looked at as an *ethnos* – a "culture" to be studied. In this way, the process is always focused on a community. In this 2018 EDT project, however, we worked a bit differently; we brought together a very diverse community to focus on *one topic*: mental illness. Every member of this group became a stakeholder in the research investigation. As Chevalier and Buckles state in regard to participatory action research (PAR), "The community of all partners or members is the unit of identity" (2019, p. 29). What interconnected the members of this group was their essential humanity in the context of a global question: "What is mental health? What is mental illness?" This chapter will provide the reader with insights on how significant the PAR approach is to the EDT process. A small community banded together in the frame of our PAR exploration, so that each could contribute to the data that would be performed in our ethnodrama: "Nobody's Perfect: A Theatrical Exploration of Mental Health." Each major frame for the EDT process will be explored: research, therapeutic, aesthetic and social activism. We begin with the community framework.

Our Group

We were embracing the point of view of the World Health Organization that *one in four people* on this planet will be affected by mental illness at

DOI: 10.4324/9781003083818-8

some point in their lifetime (2001). Considered from the angle of the extended family, this means just about everyone has some connection to issues of mental health and that everyone is potentially vulnerable to experience mental health challenges. This was the rationale for developing a more "community-oriented" style for this project. Our group was made up of a diverse segment of the community, and the plan was to take this play on tour as mental health education for the community. The cast of 21 included 12 participants with development disabilities from CAHD, an 86-year-old male retiree, a young adult female with cerebral palsy who was also our Visiting Scholar from Florida, three graduate students from Concordia's Drama Therapy Program, an undergraduate student from the theatre department, and three young adult volunteers at CAHD. Every member of the cast and the production was considered a research informant and co-researcher. We made use of the PAR approach in the dynamic sense that is cited by McTaggart, "action research is the way in which groups of people can organize the conditions under which they can learn from their own experience and make this experience accessible to others" (1997, pp. 27–28). Everyone in the group, from the stage manager to the musical director, from the adult participant with a developmental disability to the octogenarian volunteer, from the student to the professor/director, were interviewed on their perspectives and personal experiences with mental illness.

A Global Theme

> Initial estimates suggest that about 450 million people alive today suffer from mental or neurological disorders or from psychosocial problems such as those related to alcohol and drug abuse. Many of them suffer silently. Many of them suffer alone. Beyond the suffering and beyond the absence of care lie the frontiers of stigma, shame, exclusion, and more often than we care to know, death.
>
> (World Health Organization Report 2001, p. x)

Before beginning this project, we had done a literature review on the status of mental illness in the world. Some of the statistics we found were staggering. The one quoted above is such, and this was from 2001! It suggested that, globally, *"One person in every four will be affected by a mental disorder at some stage of life"* (italics mine, WHO Report 2001, p. x). More recent data from 2017 reveals some "792 million people lived with a mental disorder … including 264 (Depression); 284 million (Anxiety disorder); 107 million (Alcohol use disorder); 71 million (Drug use disorder) … totaling 970 million (with any mental or substance use disorder)" (Ritchie & Roser, 2018, p. 1).

With nearly a billion people facing such mental health challenges, it must be asked: are we facing a pandemic in mental illness, worldwide?

This led us to look at the need for public education on mental health. Fortunately, we had a psychology undergraduate student on our research team who did an independent study on this topic. She focused on the need for such education in Canada. After researching the new movement in the world, and specifically in Canada, towards what is known as "Mental Health Literacy," she concluded:

> public health education may play a crucial role in helping individuals identify the early signs of common disorders such as depression, anxiety, or substance abuse; as well as modify beliefs associated with symptom interpretation, and so reduce delays in treatment seeking to favor more positive outcomes.
>
> (Moldoveanu, 2017, p. 4)

The goal for our new EDT project was to increase public knowledge about mental health, and, most significantly to reduce the stigmatization of mental illness. This has also been the intention on our previous ethnodrama on the lived experiences of caregivers (Chapter 5). In fact, our literature review on stigma for that production had shown how stigma "extends to the families of those who are living with a mental illness … [and] may delay how quickly family caregivers seek help, and often worsens the challenges families are already dealing with" (Mental Health Commission of Canada, 2013, p. 14).

The perniciousness of the stigma attached to mental illness became one of the major themes of "Nobody's Perfect" and the play opened with a scene portraying the stigma issue.

A Group Psychotherapy Process

The essential underlying structure of EDT is a group psychotherapy process. It is what distinguishes it from the performance-based research format of ethnodrama per se (Mienczakowski, 1995a, 1995b, 2001). It is what holds the group in place as a *therapeutic community*, exploring its own experience. As with all group psychotherapy, the essential element of group coherence is established through building a deep level of trust and empathy.

EDT is a type of therapeutic theatre (TT) and follows the definition of TT that we established in 2003 in the article "Therapeutic theatre and well-being" (Snow et al., 2003): *"therapeutic theatre is the therapeutic development of a play in which roles are established with therapeutic goals in mind; the whole* *process of the play production is, in fact, **a form of group psychotherapy**"* (bold mine, p. 74). The group psychotherapy component is what creates the intensive communal framework in EDT.

As Yalom states in relation to group coherence:

> Highly cohesive groups have greater levels of self-disclosure. Positive patient outcome is correlated to group popularity, a variable closely related to group support and acceptance. These findings taken together strongly support the contention that group cohesiveness is an important determinant of positive therapeutic outcome.
>
> (1985, p. 55)

In our group process, we were asking people to reveal intimate moments from their life experiences around the issue of mental illness. So, the disclosure level was very high. Everyone connected by sharing experiences on this one topic. Even with differences in age, ethnic backgrounds and cognitive abilities, all connected on an emotional level.

Moreno, one of the founders of group psychotherapy and the creator of psychodrama, sociometry and sociodrama, gave great consideration to how individuals connect with each other in a group. He writes, "The socio-emotional crosscurrents of plus and minus sign, attractions and repulsions, which flow between individuals and groups are forms of energy distribution" (1993, p. 253). Moreno built a complex body of theory and practice on how to promote positive energy in a group, to create a vital *therapeutic community*. This is known as sociometry. We utilized both sociometric methods and psychodrama techniques in developing this ethnodrama, as will be evidenced in other sections of this chapter.

Finally, I also conceived of the "community framework" for this project, as highly related to Victor Turner's concept of *communitas*. He defines this concept in the frame of ritual studies, "The kind of communitas desired by tribesmen in their rites … is a transformative experience that goes to the root of each person's being and finds in that root something profoundly communal and shared" (1969, p. 138). It was this deep sharing that was the subtext of our research-based ethnodrama production. I am greatly indebted to Turner for his articulation of this important concept and for his early development of performance ethnography as a research method.

The Research Framework

As with all EDT projects, we began with an application for ethics approval and an application for funding. As cited in Chapter 5, this project was Phase

II of a three-part research project on mental health, for which we had secured funding from the Accelerator Grant program at Concordia University in 2018. The more difficult task was securing the ethics approval certificate. Working with a vulnerable population (adults with developmental disabilities) who would tell their personal stories about their own mental health challenges would undoubtedly be questioned, and it was. Again, this is an important area for potential ethnodramatherapists to understand. Your applications for ethics approval (an absolute necessity) when working with sensitive issues and an at-risk population *will be* challenged.

Applying for Ethics Approval

As I wrote in the Summary Protocol Form on February 15, 2018:

> At this point, we will be fundamentally applying the *Ethnodramatherapy* method, as I have developed it over the past decade. This Ethnodrama will be quite like the 2014 "Relationships" Ethnodrama, as we will be doing interviews and focus groups with the participants around some very intimate topics. As before, I will be using Drama Therapy methods, such as Playback Theatre, Sociodrama and Psychodrama, as well as a variety of projective methods to explore personal experience and self-narrative. So, I am sure this puts the proposal in the *greater than minimal risk* category.
> (Snow, Concordia University SPF Form, 2018, p. 6)

I established the methodology for the same population that had previously been approved for an ethics certificate in 2007 and 2014. I go on to explain that this will be an "integrated" research-based theatre project, with several other kinds of people involved as a *therapeutic community*, all answering questions around the thematic inquiry: What is mental health? What is mental illness? And what do we most essentially need to know about them?

The Research Protocol Questioned

On March 19, 2018, I received the following email from the University's Human Research Ethics Committee, stating that our protocol had received "Conditional Approval." It continues:

> However, please be aware that recruitment or direct interaction with participants is not permitted and the Certificate of Ethical Accessibility is not issued until your responses to the following committee comments have been made and Full Approval is awarded.
> (M. Toca, personal communication, March 19, 2018)

The email listed seven issues that absolutely had to be addressed. I explore two of these issues here, to give the prospective practitioner of EDT a real sense of what an Ethics Committee might object to. I follow each with my response to the HREC:

> 4) Since the cohort attended the program for the last couple of years, we suppose a relationship was established, where participants trust and look up to the researcher, which leads to the possibility of *perceived coercion*. Please explain how this is addressed and how participants can freely indicate they wish to not be part of the project yet still be in the group/course/play.
> (M. Toca, personal communication, March 19, 2018, italics mine)

I responded by explaining how we develop a *therapeutic community* at CAHD and went on to describe how our Advisory Team, which included a participant from the cohort and a parent of a participant, would always be available to address any concerns of the project participants. Then, I precisely articulated the process of consent to participate in the project:

> We have written the Consent Form, with the intention to make it very accessible to our 12 participants. It is written in very simple language. We will spend over one hour going over this in detail to be sure participants understands its meaning. We will make it clear that it is their choice to be in this research project. If any of them do not wish to be in the research, we will accept that. If they wish to be in the play, but not in the research, then (as described above) we will find a way to make that possible.
> (S. Snow, personal communication, March 25, 2018)

Another vital ethical concern of the committee represents a perennial issue in regard to doing participatory action research with a group that has intellectual and cognitive challenges:

> 7) The UHREC raised a concern that participants are told they are co-researchers, when in reality they seem to have very little influence on the research. The committee was especially concerned since you are dealing with a vulnerable population and a sensitive subject. As such, please clarify if participants are being given credit as co-authors of the play.
> (M. Toca, personal communication, March 19, 2018)

In my 2-page response to this question, I explained that we had been utilizing a qualified version of PAR with this population in past productions (Snow et. al, 2017) and would continue to implement our adapted version of PAR with this project. Our aim was for the participants to be "respected and important members of the Research Team," and that we continued to struggle with the complex dynamics of applying PAR in a project like this:

> Recently, there has been research on developing more inclusive PAR projects with adults with developmental and intellectual disabilities, so they can be involved in "identifying problems, collecting and

analyzing data, and using the results to take action" (Kramer, Kramer, Garcia-Iriarte, & Hammel, 2010). As the authors of this study, "Following Through to the End: The Use of Inclusive Strategies to Analyze and Interpret Data in Participatory Action Research with individuals with Intellectual Disabilities," state: "Conducting analysis with groups of people with intellectual disabilities rather than individuals creates an inclusive process of social support and helps to *counterbalance the power differentials typically held between researchers and people with intellectual disabilities*" (italics mine, 2010, p. 271). We are very aware of this potential "power differential" and aim to create authentic communication among all co-researchers. However, the totally inclusive ideal of research for our projects is still in the process of development. As stated in our 2017 article, for the time being, the use of PAR will have to be qualified.

(S. Snow, personal communication, March 25, 2018)

And, in fact, the play was in the end credited as "Conceived and Written by Stephen Snow in Collaboration with The Nobody's Perfect Theatre Company."

It should be clear to the student or professional who wishes to practice EDT that it takes preliminary research in order to do the actual research! For our project, we needed to learn how to adapt the PAR approach: (1) for 12 members of the group who have developmental disabilities: (2) for the whole, very diverse group, with individuals with many different backgrounds. The former brought up ethical issues, related to the "power differential." This problem was already cited in Chapter 2, where Sajnani (2010) criticizes the potential masking of the power dynamics in the EDT process:

> the absence of any representation of the relationship between caregivers, service providers and the participants causes the audience to temporarily "suspend their disbelief" about the capacities of their relatives, peers and clients on stage … Thus, though the *overt* message celebrated through such performances is one of the empowerment of the marginalized group, the *covert* message (i.e., that they are not capable) is held in the shadows, as a conversation that cannot be held simultaneously, and that therefore goes unexamined or challenged.
>
> (pp. 70–71)

I repeat this citation, here, as it points to one of the greatest research ethics challenges in using PAR with a vulnerable group who have cognitive impairments. Again, this will be fully addressed in Chapter 8, which is focused on the potential ethical challenges in EDT.

Adapting Participatory Action Research for EDT

PAR is a wonderful approach. It is used worldwide today for groups of scientific researchers and citizens to explore collaboratively pragmatic solutions to problems that concern a specific community, i.e., "'the study of a social situation with a view to improving the quality of an action within it…'" Elliott in (Chevalier and Buckles, 2019, p. 22). It democratizes the research process by making all members of the team equal stakeholders by aiming to give all members an equal voice in the research dialogue. As McTaggart writes, "Participatory action research establishes self-critical communities of people participating and collaborating in all phases of the research process: the planning, action, observation, and reflection" (McTaggart, 1997, p. 35). The group chooses a "thematic concern" and then, together, develops a research protocol to find answers to the research questions that have been proposed. The social scientists – sociologists, ethnographers, political scientists – bring their academic expertise, but the people who live in that community and/or are engaged in the issue bring their own expertise in the form of their *lived experience* of the "thematic concern." The process of dialogue between these two groups is crucial to the success of a PAR project.

In developing the ethnodrama method, Mienczakowski embraced PAR as a natural framework for performance ethnography research which has emancipatory goals. His development of the "Informant Validation" method, previously described, is a perfect example of sharing the power of creating the "Research Report, i.e., the ethnodramatic theatre production. In his article with Stephen Morgan, "Ethnodrama: Constructing Participatory, Experiential and Compelling Action Research through Performance" (2001), he states that "Ethnodrama's contribution to action research lies in its potential to engage actively healthcare recipients, healthcare professionals and audiences in consensual deconstruction and dissemination of knowledge" (Mienczakowski & Morgan, 2001, p 225).

However, specific problems arise when there are potentially large "power differentials" between the academic research team and the "citizen research team," due to cognitive and intellectual challenges. McTaggart cites an essential democratic value in the PAR process, "Through dialogue among participants, regular checks are made to ensure that the agenda of the least powerful become an important focus of the group's work" (1997, p. 34). In adapting PAR to our "Nobody's Perfect" project, we made a great effort to allow the participants with developmental disabilities to have full voice in answering all the research questions. They did this through dramatic enactments, artwork, music and dance. They only participated minimally in discussions of the academic research team, although there was always one member of their cohort invited to be present at these meeting. So, there were not "regular checks" with the whole group. I agree with the author of another PAR study done with individuals with developmental disabilities, "Our experience with the participants in the TLC project led us to redefine the circle of participants" (Sample, 1996, p. 331). The author describes how some with less severe cognitive difficulties could understand the concept of research with its sophisticated intellectual and abstract constructs. Others could not. The author concludes, "If PAR is designed to assist marginalized, disempowered and disenfranchised groups to study their needs and design action to meet them, then the PAR model is perhaps the most appropriate research approach for this group" (Sample, p. 331).

The quote above represents a self-advocacy model of PAR. Although we had used this model in the past, the "Nobody's Perfect" project was about community and building a community to research the topic of mental health. It was no longer a so-called "Special Populations" piece, it was looking at the world as a "Special Population" where one in four people will experience a mental health challenge in their lifetime. Everyone in our group had thoughts about this and we interviewed everyone with equal respect in regard to their perspectives. I believe this was a strength in our adapted PAR approach to this production.

Digging in: The Interview Process

As with all EDT projects, interviews were a crucial part of our research procedure. We did both formal and informal interviews with the CAHD participants and created a formal pre- and post-performance questionnaire for the audience.

The formal pre- and post-interviews for CAHD participants were devised by Dr. Miranda D'Amico. It was meant to ascertain personal growth and psychological change in the performers with developmental disabilities, as they went through the EDT process. Here are the pre-performance questions:

1. What do you think the ethnodrama "Nobody's Perfect" is about?
2. What do you think you will learn from the ethnodrama "Nobody's Perfect"?
3. How do you feel about performing on stage in front of an audience?
4. So far, how has this ethnodrama and acting made you feel about yourself?
5. 5. What do you think the audience will learn from the ethnodrama "Nobody's Perfect" – what will they learn about you as an actor?

These were administered during the rehearsal process for the play. After the three performances, a post-test was administered.[1] The post-performance questions were the same as the pre-, but wording was in the past tense. Results of these questionnaires and the audience questionnaires will be reported in the "Outcomes" section.

We also did informal interviews with both the CAHD participants and other members of the cast. These usually were transformed into either monologues or scenes. For example, I did a long interview with Alyssa about her issue with "negative thinking." It was a very personal and honest statement of her struggle with an issue that many people have to deal with. The transcription of her interview was edited into the following monologue that she performed, herself, in the play.

ALYSSA: So, since high school, I have had a problem with "negative thinking." You know, thoughts come in my head that are negative. Like somehow I am not worth it in this world. I tell my parents and friends, and they get upset. They say, "Oh, Alyssa, you have to think more positively!" Well, it's not always easy. I can get really negative sometimes. It scares my Dad, but I can't help it. I really wish I knew what to do about it.

I say some of the interviews were informal as they happened, spontaneously, right in the middle of the rehearsal process. For instance, We were doing improvisations on stigmatization and "othering" and our Visiting Scholar, Andrea DeCrescenzo, who is in a wheel chair and has a companion dog named Winchester (who also became part of the cast), began telling a story of how when she was in the elevator on her way to the dentist, one day, a woman got in and began patting her on the head and treating her like a child (Figure 6.1). Andrea was furious, but felt she could not say anything to this elderly female. I interviewed Andrea like a Conductor in playback theatre and, on the spot, I cast other members of the group as Andrea, the elderly woman, the dog and Andrea's mother who was present in the elevator. Later on, we processed this as a psychodrama where Andrea, in "surplus reality," really got to tell the woman off. Eventually, this material was edited into the following scene in the play. The Protagonist became the Storyteller (Andrea already served as Narrator of the play). As she told this story, she cast the roles with

---

1 The author would like to thank Ms. Cassandra D'Amico for administering and transcribing all of the CAHD participants' interviews.

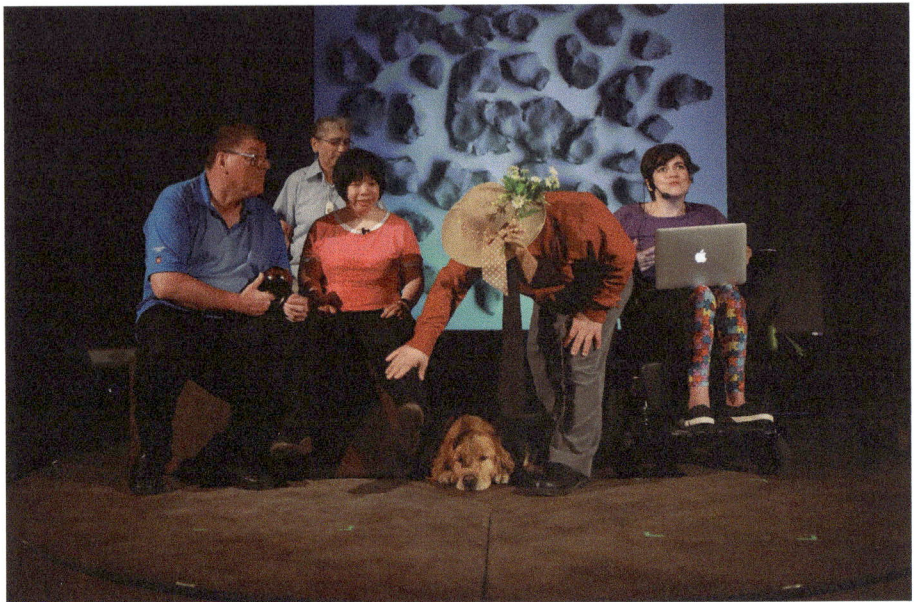

Figure 6.1   A Scene of "Othering" (photo courtesy of Dougy Hérard)

other members of the ensemble, including the role of herself, her mother, her dog, and the oblivious older woman. This more distanced approach still contained the authenticity manifested in the original psychodrama.

NARRATOR: I will tell the story and assign you your parts. So, I was going to the dentist with my mother and my dog Winchester, who, as you know, I always travel with. We get into an elevator, together, to go up to the dentist's office.
              Mack please be Winchester, Rita be me, and Gina be my Mom. Rick you can be the elderly woman who gets on the elevator, later.

(*Rita, Gina, Mack, in role, get on the elevator.*)

RITA: I think I waited too long to go to the Dentist.
GINA: I guess *so!*
NARRATOR: Suddenly this kind of elderly woman gets in beside me (RICK, as the elderly woman in a hat, mimes touching RITA, all over) and, *without asking my permission,* starts

touching me all over my head and body. It was so embarrassing. I couldn't understand why she was doing it!

Now, at the time, I did not say anything. She was treating
me like a little doll, or something. I suppose I felt she was too
old to yell at her. However, if I had it to do it over again, I
would say: "Lady, don't you realize how disrespectful this is!
Please stop touching me right now!!!" Could you enact this
for me?

*(The Playback team now enacts this version, with RITA yelling the line at the
elderly lady. Then, they all take a bow.)*

NARRATOR: Thank you. Oh, that felt so much better. Mack, will you stay
with me for a minute, everyone else can sit down. Mack, do
you feel people treat you *differently* because you spent those
nine years in the Psychiatric Hospital?

So, this scene was about the unhealthy repression of anger in the context of
being "othered." Many other scenes and monologues evolved out of our informal interview process. Some of these will be represented in the "Aesthetic
Framework" section.

The Therapeutic Framework

Therapeutic Goals Set

In terms of measuring the therapeutic effectiveness of this EDT project, we
only focused on the12 participants with developmental disabilities. Each of
these cast members was videotaped as they undertook the Drama Therapy
Role-Play Interview (DTRPI). This was subsequently scored by a graduate
research assistant and placed in their file for the project. This assessment
method had been found valuable in past therapeutic theatre productions at
CAHD (Snow & D'Amico in Johnson, Pendzik & Snow, 2012). Each of
these cast members had been at CAHD for the past two years, so in developing their therapeutic goals we also relied on a synopsis of their chart for the
past two years and their entry psychosocial report. Through observation and
discussion with team members, we tracked their progress, especially over the
last two months of the project.

Case Example of "Rita"

Rita was an especially interesting example in the group of CAHD participants. Known as the "wise woman" in the cast, she could be very perceptive and come out with spontaneous sagacious statements. She was 24 years old at this time. Rita has Williams syndrome and diabetes. She had experienced some bullying in her past, but was basically calm, empathic and has a very supportive family system. Rita received the highest score on her DTRPI assessment in "Focus of Attention" and "Clarity of Speech Communication," but a very low score on "Assertiveness." We aimed to use her experience in the EDT process to bolster her self-confidence. Her main therapy goal was stated as, "to develop her confidence in her genuine abilities." It was Rita who came up with the title, "Nobody's Perfect." In one of the rehearsals, the cast was asked to choose the title for the production. We all struggled for a while when suddenly Rita came up with an idea. As she states in an interview, done a year and a half after the play production:

> So, I said, "How about 'Nobody's Perfect'?" Because it's about us doing a play and it's about us not being perfect … and it's o.k. to be who you are … you just gotta be brave and try and do your best … and be who you are as a human being.
>
> (Interview with Rita, October16, 2019)

That just about summed it up for everyone. All agreed. This was the title of the piece.

Drama Therapy Methods Utilized

We began the process with two months of workshops aimed at building trust, creating a genuine ensemble and enhancing the improvisational skills of the participants. As mentioned, because of a very challenging ethics review from Concordia University's Human Research Committee, we got backed up by a couple of months. As we continued to work on improv skills in February and March, we also formally named the play, "Nobody's Perfect! A Theatrical Exploration of Mental Health" and the group, the "Nobody's Perfect! Theatre Company."

Once April came, we began to utilize drama therapy processes, including psychodrama and playback theatre. We also implemented art therapy workshops, led by two Art Therapy interns. These provided much of the scenography for the play. Out of these process-oriented workshops, the themes of the play began to emerge. There were ten major themes and each defined a segment of the play: "Stigma," "Depression," "Mental Health Literacy," "Mental Health and Aging," "Anxiety," "Mental Illness and Violence," "Mental Illness in Loved Ones," "Dreams, Nightmares and Hallucinations," "Othering," "Resources, Resilience, Recovery." Each of these units were fleshed out with material based on personal experience and shaped into scenes, monologues, songs and dances. For example, when we began to explore material for the "Depression" section, a psychodrama was enacted with a volunteer Protagonist from the cast. The Protagonist told the story of how he became very depressed after the horrible death of a close friend due to an accident with a truck on an icy road. Auxiliaries were chosen by the Protagonist: the female friend who called with the news; a newscaster who reported the story on TV (surplus reality); and the ghost of his dear friend who had been killed. Both **role reversal** and **doubling** were used to process the enactment. The Protagonist was given the opportunity to speak with his departed friend. One of the most touching moments was when her ghost passed by his bedroom window and they waived goodbye to each other. With the Protagonist's permission this whole scene was used in the play. However, the Protagonist asked if another member of the cast could play him in the theatricalized version.

The entire ensemble had the potential to do a psychodrama or to be a Storyteller for playback theatre during this two-month workshop period. Volunteers, musicians, research assistants, stage managers, all shared their personal experience around mental health issues – solidifying trust in the group. There was an honesty and willingness to share that created a "Pool of Empathy" in the process. Stories were adapted in a way to honor the informant's interpretation of how their self-narrative fit into categories like "Depression" or "Anxiety." This was an exemplification of the PAR approach in action. More introverted members of the ensemble were afforded the opportunity for deep sharing in the art therapy groups.

As cited for previous ethnodramas (Snow et al., 2017, p. 247), the action spectrogram was employed in the process. One day, we simply asked everyone in the group to find their place in a line that went from one side of the room to the other. They placed themselves according to how much they felt mental illness affected their personal life. It helped to illustrate the various attitudes towards the topic in the group (Blatner, 1973, p. 99). Later on, this spectrogram was incorporated by the choreographer into a movement sequence. Our senior actor, an 86-year-old who is bilingual, would stand at the side of the stage and say both in English and French: "how does mental illness affect your life?" and the actors would move themselves into specific positions on the stage.

Jean's Story

Interviews were done with cast members in a sensitive therapeutic manner, especially with the adults with developmental disabilities, like Alyssa or Rita. I also transcribed interviews from three non-CAHD informants who addressed specific questions relating to mental health. One was the story of a young woman who had been placed in a psychiatric hospital without her consent. This story was transformed into a long monologue performed by the student from the theatre department. The second was the experience of the senior citizen actor who told the story of forgetting where he parked his car one winter's day when the streets were filled with snow. He told how he became extremely agitated and started to fear he was losing his memory, perhaps a symptom of the beginning of Alzheimer's-type dementia. It was both a funny and sad monologue with a poignant ending (see Figure 6.2).

The third monologue came from a taped interview in a focus group with the board of AMI-Québec Action on Mental Illness (our community partner in this project) and was essentially a brief story of a mother watching her son, who has schizophrenia, be "othered" by a stranger in her apartment building.

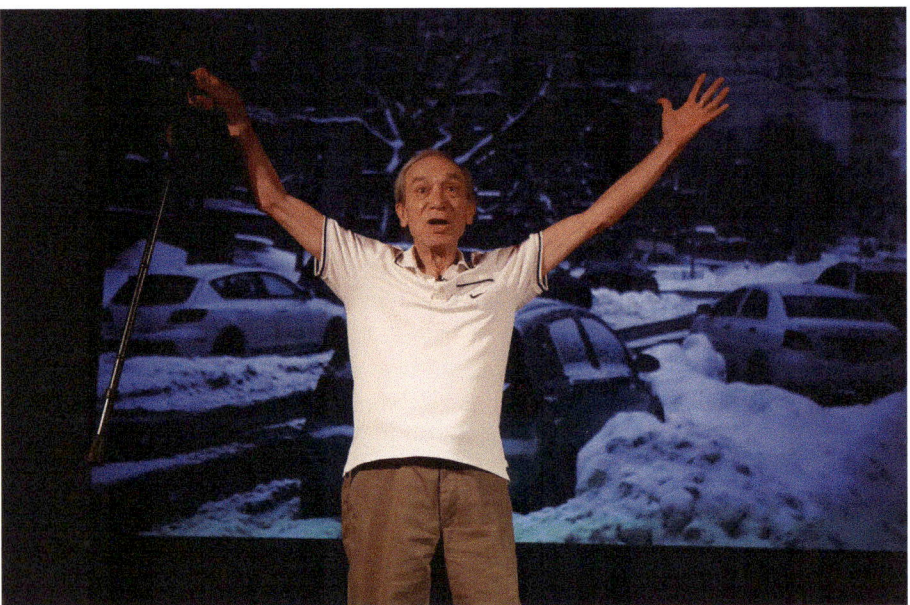

Figure 6.2   Senior Actor Performs a Monologue on "Dementia Worry" (photo courtesy of Dougy Hérard)

The mother was performed by one of the research assistants who was also a drama therapy graduate student. Drama therapy techniques were used to develop each of these monologues. All three became very powerful moments in the play. These monologues stood right beside many monologues based on the personal experience of actors. The frame was that anybody could play anybody else's story. This seemed to enhance the "Pool of Empathy" for performers and audience alike.

The Aesthetic Framework

Theatrical art is about shaping the content of the thematic materials into a flowing, embodied, dynamic representation of these themes. In ethnodrama, the content is based on the lived experiences of the informant/performers. The material is intimate, at times, self-revelatory, and, always, authentic. The task of the role of theatre artist in EDT is to authentically, poetically and aesthetically present these materials on stage through all the media of theatre. This theatrical representation should be "beautiful" and "alive." It is about carrying those moments that were spontaneously developed in rehearsal, and were so "alive," into performance, while at the same time artfully shaping them into exciting theatre.

Creating a Special Stage

The aesthetics begin with the stage, itself. It's look, its shape, its feeling. Once again, our long-time designer, Eric Mongerson, created a stage, specifically adapted to this particular production (Figure 6.3). First of all, there were several logistical challenges that needed to be satisfied. Our narrator was in a sizable electric wheelchair and travelled to the center for the stage with a dog beside her. A special ramp was created to accommodate this action.

Many of the performers had fragile mobility and balance. The two levels of the circular platform provided plenty of room for movement and special LED lights were installed all around the edge of the stage.

Beyond these logistical requirements, the circular form, adapted to a three-quarter amphitheatre for the audience, enhanced the "intimacy" of the performance. The circular shape of the raised stage gave the feel of an ancient ritual – the very roots of theatre. To accommodate projected scenery, a large screen was set up in back of the stage for the artwork to be rear-projected. At the beginning of the play, the actors did a shadow-movement enactment, and this was followed by the shadow puppet scene on "Stigma."

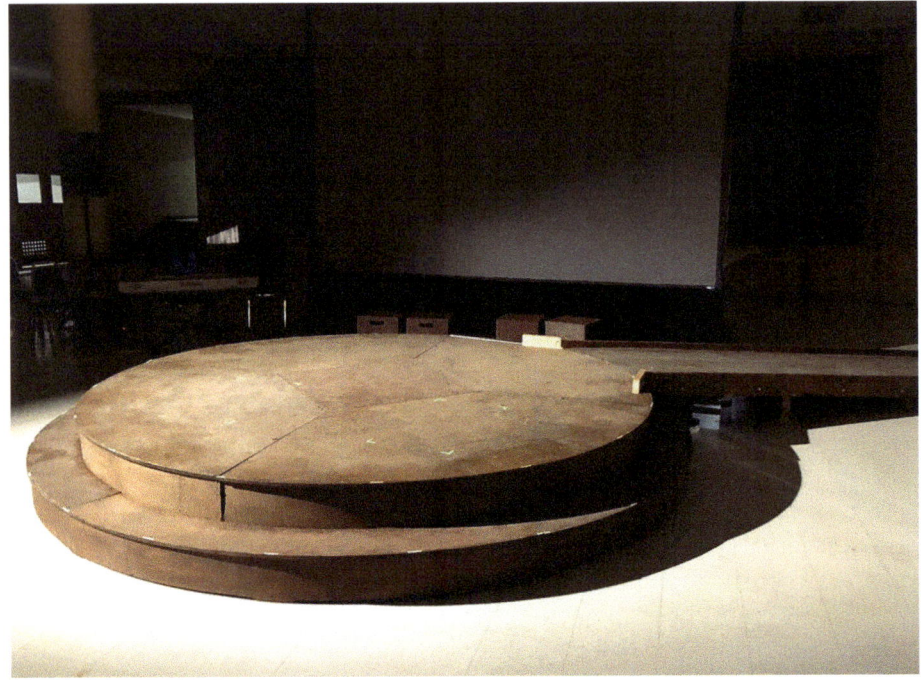

Figure 6.3   The Unique Stage Created for *Nobody's Perfect!* (photo courtesy of Eric
            Mongerson)

All in all, the designed stage functioned beautifully to hold and present the
unique content of this ethnodrama.

Artwork as Scenography

As in many previous productions (Chapters 2, 3 and 4), we utilized projected
artwork as scenography. These were pieces done by the CAHD participants
in their art therapy sessions.

They were often poignant and very aesthetically pleasing. They were matched
with the theme of a given segment, to create more atmosphere for that scene,
monologue, song or dance.

They often gave an emotional context for a unit of the production. Sometimes, performers appeared with their own artwork. The making of the art
also gave some of the introverted cast members a way to put their stamp on
a given theme about mental health and to reveal their personal talent in
graphic art.

Musical Art

We were fortunate to have Marie-Fatima Rudolf as our musical director and keyboardist. She is both a professional jazz musician and a music therapist. She could both nurture the musical skills of the participants and work with their psychological issues around performing. We had one outstanding singer in the CAHD participants. Everyone recognized his extraordinary singing talent. So, we created the central song of the show for him.

Here are the lyrics:

Song: Nobody's Perfect

Lyrics: Stephen and Shelley Snow

Music: Shelley Snow ©2018

(Introduction spoken before first verse of song):

> Nobody's Perfect!
> It's plain to see.
> Everyone struggles
> both you and me.

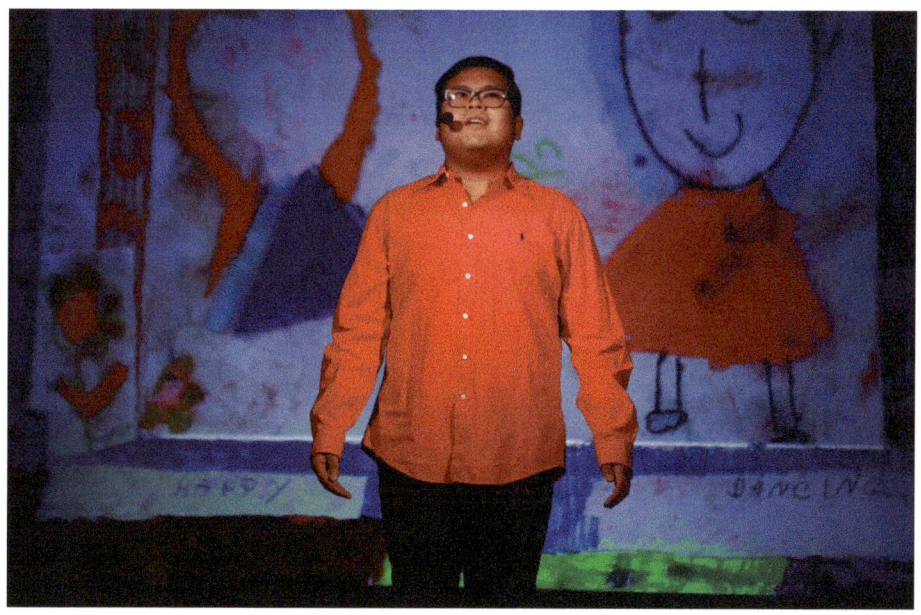

Figure 6.4   Actor–Singer Performs "Nobody's Perfect" (photo courtesy of Dougy Hérard)

Verses 1 and 2:

> We all have pain
> we all know sorrow;
> Sometimes today,
> sometimes tomorrow.

> We all have cares
> we all know woe;
> Sometimes it's fast,
> sometimes it's slow.

Chorus:

> *Nobody's Perfect!*
> *How could we be?*
> *We all have limits*
> *both you and me.*

> *Nobody's Perfect,*
> *it's plain to see;*
> *Everyone struggles,*
> *Both you and me.*

Verses 3 and 4:

> We all have troubles,
> we all know failure;
> Not all the time,
> but once in a while.

> We all have problems,
> we all have trials;
> They're sure to come
> for me and for you.

Bridge:

> Let's deeply care
> for ourselves

and each other.
Let's be aware
of strangers too.

Verses 5 and 6:

We all know sickness,
in mind and body.
We know disease
in heart and soul.

We all have pain
we all know sorrow;
Sometimes today,
sometimes tomorrow.

Bridge:

Let's deeply care
for ourselves
and each other.

Let's be aware
of strangers too,
of strangers too.

This was performed at the very beginning and at the end of the show, with a powerful artwork background behind it (see Figure 6.4).[2]

Choreography

We were very fortunate to have a talented choreographer who was also a research assistant and a drama therapy graduate student, Bill Yong. The group was made up mostly of non-dancers, so Bill devised a kind of contact improvisation dance style in which the whole group could participate in full chorus

---

2 Performance of this song and other parts of this show can be viewed online through the CAHD website at www.concordia.ca/finearts/research/cahd.html in the Research section under Ethnodrama Mental Health Education Series: video documentary.

choreography and, sometimes in just groups of four. Bill and Marie-Fatima worked very closely, together, and I believe this confluence of music and movement really helped the "flow" of the show. The aesthetic shape of the dances was just right for the content of this particular ethnodrama and the skill set of this diverse group of performers. It also provided opportunities to build the ensemble via unified rhythm and movement work.

Each of the production elements, set, lighting, music, dance and acting led to the total gestalt of the show. It was an aesthetic framework that very effectively supported the sensitive content derived from the EDT process.

The Social Activist Framework

The process was shaped around a social purpose: to educate the general public concerning issues of mental health and mental illness. The most immediate goal was de-stigmatizing public attitudes towards mental illness. This especially was our objective as social activists.

Reshaping Public Attitudes about Mental Illness

Many agencies, companies and individuals are working towards this goal, today: Bell has ads for mental health advocacy on TV and elsewhere. The famous Olympic swimmer Michael Phelps has a powerful testimonial on television on the value of therapy and that people should not be ashamed or afraid to seek treatment. In 2005, Canada adopted the Australian model for developing "Mental Health Literacy" in the public (Moldoveanu, 2017, p. 5). There is a very significant push towards de-stigmatizing mental illness. In the midst of what appears to be a worldwide epidemic in mental health, with 970 million people with some kind of mental or substance use disorder, there is an enormous need to end the historical stigmatization of mental illness. Why? The introduction to the 2001 World Health Organization Report, *Mental Health: New Understanding, New Hope* provides an answer:

> This landmark World Health Organization publication aims to raise public and professional awareness of the real burden of mental disorders and their costs in human, social and economic terms. At the same time, it intends to help dismantle many of those barriers – *particularly of stigma, discrimination and inadequate services – which prevent many millions of people worldwide from receiving the treatment they need and deserve.*
>
> (italics mine, WHO, 2001, p. xi)

Stigma is a gigantic factor in keeping people from the treatment they need and, therefore, exacerbates the "human, social and economic" issues surrounding mental illness. This is why the stigmatization of mental illness must be attacked, reduced and, ultimately, eliminated.

Our play, "Nobody's Perfect," addressed this issue in the opening scene, using a kind of allegory of schoolyard bullying, to show the insidious and harmful aspects of the stigma. This was performed as a shadow puppet show by the CAHD participants, with the assistance of Concordia students. Many audience members said they were very moved by this scene. Shortly after this scene, a member of the cast with a developmental disability asks the audience: "What do you do for your mental health?" This was preceded by a little ditty – "We brush our teeth for dental health, we exercise for physical health, but what do we do for our *mental health*!" Everything in the play was meant to show the many faces of mental illness, but also to "normalize" it. *One in four* will experience it in their lifetime. It is part of life, like the common cold or having diabetes. The world needs to be more open and sensitive to it. To catalyze more acceptance and empathy was the essential mission of our EDT process. The effects it had on the audience will be reported in the "Outcomes" section.

Ongoing Public Education on Mental Health

From the beginning, we planned to take our play on tour in order to spread the message of de-stigmatization and to educate the public about mental health issues. In Fall 2019, I wrote a grant application to *Aid to Research Related events, Publication, Exhibition and Dissemination Activities (ARRE)* at Concordia University for "Touring a Research-Based Performance for Mental Health Education." I received the funds, but, when I began reviewing how to develop the tour, I realized I only had half the funds necessary to remount and tour the production. This was going to be a bus and truck tour with 21 cast members and a dozen production crew. It was just too overweight, just too demanding. In the meantime, we planned to develop a documentary on the show, integrating clips with interviews and narration. In Fall of 2018, I decided we would cut everything down and develop a series of workshops for high schools, colleges and universities. We would take only 4 or 5 cast members, myself and my research assistant. The documentary would be shown, and we would administer pre- and post-screening questionnaires to the workshop participants. The documentary (see footnote 2) was completed in October 2019. We began contacting schools to make contracts for the workshop. However, we ran into two big problems. As there were students under 18 in the high schools, we had to have parental consent, as well as that of the students, themselves. Because of this new situation, we were required to apply for a new ethics certificate. The HREC was very wary of younger students being triggered by scenes in our play, like the one where a young woman discussed her suicidal ideation. This was very understandable, but their questioning procedure slowed down everything until we finally postponed the tour of the workshops until the new year. Then, COVID-19 struck, and there was no possibility of going to schools and universities in-person. A whole new strategy had to be developed.

The Webinar

By February 2020, everything at our university was online – classes, meetings, use of library, etc. It was at this point I began to envision doing our Mental Health Education Workshop as an online, Zoom webinar. I found that Advancement at Concordia was interested to sponsor this as an event for the Concordia community. I consulted with the HREC, as there was still a question of "vulnerable" persons with developmental disabilities – the co-researchers on the "Nobody's Perfect" project – being "guest speakers." I felt strongly that, as we had implemented a PAR process to develop the play and they performed in it, their voices should be heard. I wrote up a new "Consent, Waiver, Indemnity and Release Form" for them to sign. As the research element had been removed for the online webinar, the HREC accepted the consent form and, on August 17, 2020, I was granted a year-long extension on our ethics approval, necessary to produce the webinar with CAHD participants as guest speakers. The plan is to produce the webinar, using selections from the documentary, statistics from WHO and Mental Health Commission of Canada, along with guest speakers and questions from the audience. We hope to create four of these live online webinars, in the near future.[3]

Ethical Challenges Faced in this Project

The four essential roles for a director in the EDT are researcher, therapist, social activist and theatre artist (see Figure 3.1). The process is a complex network of functions that need to be balanced with skill, self-awareness and sensitivity. There are many times in which these roles collide and create

---

3 We finally produced the webinar on May 27, 2021. It was recorded. To view this recording, please contact the author at stephen.snow@concorida.ca.

major ethical challenges for a project. In this instance, one of these collisions involved a participant whose pseudonym is "Barry." Barry, a high-functioning, gifted and talented person with **autism spectrum disorder**, did not want to be involved in the ethnodramatherapy process. The team composed of myself and four creative arts therapies interns tried to engage him in the workshops, but he would respond by lying on the floor and sleeping or doodling on paper, seemingly uninterested in the group process. When asked to join he would often say, "I'm good." The team needed to use their therapist role to decipher whether his ambivalence to participate was part of a slow trust-building process that would eventually result in participation from which he would benefit, or whether he was being forced to attend by his caregivers signifying that the team did not have his free and non-coerced consent to participate in the process. His free consent was also of concern to the researcher role.

During the last week of rehearsals in the workshop space, Barry appeared to express his annoyance vocally. The cast was in full concentration mode, trying to get their lines and blocking down, aiming to artistically refine the ethnodrama they had created together. At a particularly focused moment in the rehearsal, Barry began to make loud disruptive sounds.

My countertransference overwhelmed me, and I angrily asked Barry to leave the space and not return. In this moment the theatre artist/director role was most present, most concerned about the upcoming production. The theatre artist perceived Barry as a selfish disrupter at a particularly sensitive moment of rehearsal. Upon reflection, it may also have been my frustration as a drama therapist of not having been able to engage Barry in the therapeutic process. It was clear that Barry was miserable being there, but it was still a *verboten* moment for a therapist. Later, I apologized to Barry and asked Barry if he would like to continue with the project or if he would prefer to terminate. Barry chose to end and expressed relief that this was the end of his suffering through the rehearsal process. He later attended the performance. This had been an experience where the role of theatre artist and drama therapist harshly collided. Mitchell warns of this potential conflict in the therapeutic theatre process:

> the dramatherapist is not there to theatrically realise their own vision and to use the "company" to fulfill their own artistic ambitions, but to be a convenor, a resource person, to facilitate in the best traditions of dramatherapy practice.
>
> (Mitchell in Jennings et al., 1994, p. 52)

And where was the social activist during this process? What were Barry's true needs? How could his voice, autonomy and personhood have been more respected? How did the process get so far without the team recognizing or validating that they did not have Barry's consent to continue? Another example of such a collision of roles is the case of "Mack," a participant with a mild intellectual disability who was also diagnosed as bi-polar. Mack was also older than most of the other participants from CAHD. Taking the PAR perspective that all participants are co-researchers in answering our research question about mental health, everyone, including back stage volunteers, was involved in the implementation of psychodrama, sociodrama and playback theatre. At one rehearsal, Mack revealed multiple experiences of trauma. These experiences were then explored through psychodrama, and were later produced as a very impactful scene demonstrating potential links between systemic trauma and mental health. While the scene formed an evocative and educational theatre performance, the process appeared to be unfinished and detrimental therapeutically. This performance experience overstimulated Mack, and he began to perseverate about this experience at his home, to the point that his caregiver asked for him to be removed from the project, after the three performances were completed. In retrospect, the therapeutic rupture was evident. I felt that the psychodramatic process required more containment and therapeutic processing than what was available within the performance timeline, and that the client was not adequately prepared or supported to continuously repeat his traumatic narratives as was required in the rehearsal and performance process. Again, this was the collision of the role of the drama therapist with that of the theatre artist. The scene was very moving in the performance, drawing parallels between the systemic impacts on mental health, but the inadequate process time and therapeutic containment resulted in the costs for the client being too high.

The Outcomes of the 2018 Ethnodramatherapy Project

As with all EDT projects, there was an intention to discover the therapeutic value for the participant performers, as well as the educational impact on the audience. However, in this project, we only attempted to measure the "therapeutic growth" of the CAHD participants, all of whom have some form of developmental disability.

Evaluating the Therapeutic Value

The first goal was at least partially realized by pre- and post-performance questionnaires of the actors. As an example, here are part of the pre- and post-responses of "Alyssa," who has a pervasive developmental disorder – not otherwise specified.

Pre-questionnaire:

Q1.   What do you think the "Nobody's Perfect" is about?

ALYSSA: "It's about people who are not perfect who have weaknesses and strengths of their own."

Q2.   What do you think you will learn from the ethnodrama "Nobody's Perfect"?

ALYSSA: "I will learn that I am not the only one that has a disability."

Q3.   How do you feel about performing on stage in front of an audience?

ALYSSA: "A little bit excited at the same time a little bit scared."

Q4.   So far, how has this ethnodrama and acting made you feel about yourself?

ALYSSA: "Pretty good."

        Post-interview:

Q1.   What was the ethnodrama "Nobody's Perfect" about?

ALYSSA: "In my opinion, the play was about people with a bunch of different disabilities and how people are not perfect. Like, everyone has different struggles."

Q2.   What did you learn from the ethnodrama "Nobody's Perfect"?

ALYSSA: "I learned that you cannot expect yourself to be better than everyone else because no one is better than everyone else. You're just good in your own way, but not necessarily perfect."

Q3.   How did you feel about going on stage in front of an audience?

ALYSSA: "At first, I was very shy. When I got up on the stage, I was literally really, really not wanting to be up there, but I did it anyways. The second night was not so much shy. The third night, a piece of cake. You get more used to it. Yes, I was used to it."

Q4.   How has this ethnodrama and acting made you feel about yourself?

ALYSSA: "Acting made me feel good about myself! Yeah!"

Dr. Miranda D'Amico, who developed and reviewed the questionnaires, writes the following:

> As exemplified by the above transcript from the pre- to post-test interviews, the EDT created the necessary conditions for the participant to engage in meaningful self-exploration of her feelings and behavior and enabled her to contextualize an acceptance of her skills and limitations. This was also corroborated by observations of the team and reports from her parents. Therapeutically, Alyssa significantly accomplished her goals in the EDT process.
>
> (personal communication, September 1, 2018)[4]

---

4 I want to personally thank Dr. D'Amico for her development of these questionnaires and the analysis provided above.

In an in-depth analysis of the transcripts of each participant in the group, all of the participants expressed that they developed a certain confidence in talking about themselves and their skills and acceptance of their limitations. Performing in front of an audience was at first daunting, but after the participation in EDT, it became the highlight of their experiences as they felt proud of their abilities. One participant, answering what he learned from the process, stated, "What I learned is that I like to talk about my skills and how not everything is always going to go right for me, and if ever there is a mistake I will be corrected. Not everything will be as I want it to be. Trying to expect for the best but sometimes that won't always happen." A very realistic response. Another replied to the question on what the audience learned, saying: "I think the audience learned that we all have challenges in life and that nobody's is perfect … What they learned about me is that I am an extremely nice person, and punctual and very, mostly good person and not someone who should be known as 'other.'" A very cogent anti-stigmatization

statement!

Analysis of the Audience Responses

So, what did the audience learn from the play production? For the June 16 performance, pre- and post-performance questionnaires were administered for the audience. These were based on the questionnaires originally developed for the Caregiver Project (see Chapter 5) and contained both quantitative and qualitative aspects.[5]

The quantitative measures focused on the performance's audience impact regarding changes in levels of stigma against and respect for the mentally ill. Five stigma and seven respect questions were used (all had good psychometric properties in the previous study). The questions, however, had to be adapted for a general audience and for a project that did not have caregiving as its main focus. As a result, once the data were collected, it was clear from analyses of the internal reliability of the two sets of questions (Cronbach's alphas) that some questions had to be dropped from the analyses, leaving only three questions in each set. As can be seen from Table 6.1, these sets have fairly good Cronbach's alpha values, although the post-test values are somewhat weaker. Overall, caution is in order in interpreting the results because

---

5 I especially want to thank Dr. Norman Segalowitz for developing the questionnaire materials for this part of the research and for the data analyses.

Table 6.1   Stigma and Respect Items in the Pre- and Post-Performance Questionnaires for
the "Nobody's Perfect" Study

Stigma items

---

(1) I would be embarrassed if a person in my family became mentally ill.
(2) The term "Psychological disorder" makes me feel embarrassed.
(3) I would not knowingly become friends with a mentally ill person.

Respect items
If I were a person in the social or family circle of someone with a serious mental illness,
I would ...
(1) need to know about everything that goes on in this person's relationships with
other people.
(2) feel the need to know what this person is thinking about most things.
(3) feel it necessary for someone to closely manage their activities.

Note: Questions were presented in 6-point Likert scale format where 1 = "Strongly Disagree" and 6 =
"Strongly Agree." Cronbach's alphas for the Stigma and Respect items were .74 [.63 .86] and .84 [.76 .92]
respectively (based on 46 participants' responses from the pre-performance questionnaires).

each measure is based on just three questions; nevertheless, the numbers are
clearly and statistically significant, i.e., in the right direction.

There were 46 audience participants (28 females, 17 males, 1 other), with
a mean age of 46.6 (SD = 18.5) years. Of these, 19 identified themselves as
mental health carers (that is, having a family member with mental illness
whom they cared for), ten as mental health professionals, ten with lived
experience and ten with no mental health experience (some, of course, were
in more than one category). However, only 27 completed both the pre- and
post-performance questionnaires. Because the analyses concerned the impact of the performance on the audience, the final data come from the 27
who completed all the questionnaires.

Participants' mean responses on the 6-point scales were calculated sepa-
rately for the pre- and post-presentation versions of the stigma and respect
questionnaires. For purposes of these analyses, all the data were adjusted so
that higher scores (maximum = 6) indicated more positive attitudes (i.e.,
less stigma, more respect). On the stigma scale, the mean pre-performance
score was 5.54/6 (SD = 0.49), that is, it was already on the high side,
indicating very little stigma in the members of this audience. The mean
stigma post-performance score was 5.75/6 (0.29), that is, less stigma. This
pre-post change difference of −.21 [95%CI: −0.37, −0.06] was statistically
significant ($t = -2.79$, $p = .010$). On the respect scale, the mean pre-
performance score was 4.53/6 (0.79) and the mean post-performance score
was 4.79/6 (0.78), that is, a gain in respect. This pre-post change of −.26

[–0.48, –0.05] was statistically significant ($t = 2.53$, $p = .017$), indicating a change in respect.

Thus, the results indicated that, after watching the performance, the audience stigma level decreased. That is, people claimed to be less embarrassed by the label of "psychological disorder" or "mental illness." Also, the results indicated that the audience members' level of respect for people with a mental illness increased. That is, people claimed to be more respectful of the personal autonomy of someone with a mental illness. Of course, it should be kept in mind that this small study has several limitations: The sample size was small, and the scales only had three items each. Also, a large number of audience members were mental health practitioners and mental health professionals have more knowledge than the "general public." Nevertheless, the results do point in a very encouraging direction.

We also explored the audience's reaction to the performance itself. After completing the post-performance questionnaire assessing levels of stigma and respect, the 27 audience members responded to ten items about the performance. The results are shown in Table 6.2. The play was obviously liked, as it received a 5.96 score out of 6. The scores for items 7 and 8 are noteworthy: Item 7 assessed the usefulness of the play as a tool for mental health education, and it received a score of 5.88. Item 8 addressed whether the audience member would recommend the play to others. It also had a score of 5.88. So, overall, there is a strong indication that the goal of mental health education had succeeded. The slightly lower scores for Items 2 and 3 probably indicate that the audience came in with a better than average understanding of mental illness and already had a positive attitude towards the mentally ill.

Another very significant area we explored was whether personal attitudes towards mental illness had changed from witnessing the play. This was framed as a set of prompt questions to which the audience could give a written response.

One such question was "Please describe the change(s), if any that you would like to implement in your life as a result of watching the play." Here are a few sample responses to this important question:

• "Being a bit more patient as well as improving my own behavior when interacting with … [persons with mental health challenges]."
• "Being more aware of not othering people with mental illnesses."

Table 6.2   Evaluation Items for the "Nobody's Perfect" Play

Item	Mean (max = 6)	SD
1. Overall, the play accurately portrayed the experience of the people depicted.	5.88	(0.33)
2. The play changed my understanding of the role and experience of people with mental illness.	4.28	(1.43)
3. The play is likely to change other people's understanding of the experience of people with mental illness.	4.28	(0.65)
4. As a result of the play, I am more likely to seek out information about mental illness.	4.64	(1.44)
5. Overall, the play addressed real situations.	5.64	(1.04)
6. Overall, I enjoyed the actors' performances, special effects and staging.	5.76	(0.44)
7. This play can be a useful tool in mental health education.	5.88	(0.33)
8. I would recommend this play to others.	5.88	(0.44)
9. I was able to personally identify with some of the situations presented.	5.16	(0.85)
10. I liked this play.	5.96	(0.20)

Note: N = 27. Items were presented in 6-point Likert scale format where 1 = "Strongly Disagree" and 6 = "Strongly Agree."

- "I am going to be more conscientious of what I do for my own mental health."
- "More accepting to differences of others."
- "Stress reduction and create more visibility of mental illness."

One person answered the question about "the ways in which the play helped change or strengthen any of your feelings or beliefs regarding mental illness," by summing it all up as, "There are many kinds of mental health issues. More are scarier than others because we are ill-equipped to deal with them. There needs to be more information in the public arena – like this play – for greater understanding."

The audience responded very positively to the diverse community of performers in "Nobody's Perfect"! Many said how moved they were to see so many different kinds of persons dealing with the issue of mental health. In the post-performance questionnaire, people described how they liked "the way the actors helped each other to tell and depict the stories." This "community theatre style" was an experiment for CAHD, but we would certainly consider working with this integrated format for EDT again.

Conclusion

For potential students of EDT, this chapter illuminates how significantly the PAR approach enhances such a community-oriented, research-based theatre project. PAR is naturally aligned with EDT. The processes of both are profoundly communal. This *communitas* functions on all levels: artistic, political, as research and as therapy. In terms of the latter, EDT can be authentically viewed as a group therapy process. If there are two concepts that go to the heart of EDT, they are "community" and "spontaneity." Significantly influenced by the philosophy and methodology of Moreno (1946, 1953/1993, 2019), it is the spontaneous flow of creative energy in the group process that particularly defines EDT. The next chapter will delineate how this "flow" was established in a shorter format: a six-day workshop model. In the end, it should be noted that EDT is not without potential dilemmas. The challenges to ethics have been described in this chapter. These are serious issues that must always be dealt with. As a highly integrative approach, EDT is vulnerable to such flaws. It is because it can be such a spontaneous and deep process that such vulnerability is always present. Probably, it is best to say that any given EDT project should always be looked upon as a "work-in-progress."

References

Amir, E. (2011). *The experience of family members in the context of mental illness: Caregiving burden, personality constructs and subjective well-being* [Unpublished doctoral dissertation]. Concordia University.

Blatner, A. (1973). *Acting-in: Practical applications of psychodramatic methods.* Springer Publishing.

Chevalier, J. M., & Buckles, D. J. (2019). *Participatory action research: Theory and methods of engaged inquiry* (2nd ed.). Routledge.

Kramer, J. M., Kramer, J. C., Garcia-Iriarte, E., & Hammel, J. (2010). Following through to the end: The use of inclusive strategies to analyze and interpret data in participatory action research with individuals with intellectual disabilities. *Journal of Applied Research in Intellectual Disabilities, 24,* 263–273.

McTaggart, R. (1997). *Participatory action research: International contexts and consequences.* State University of New York Press.

Mental Health Commission of Canada. (2013). *National guidelines for a comprehensive service system to support family caregivers of adults with mental health problems and illnesses.*

Mienczakowski, J. (1995a). *The application of critical ethno-drama to health settings.* [Unpublished doctoral dissertation]. Griffith University, Australia.

_____. (1995b). The theatre of ethnography: The reconstruction of ethnography with emancipatory potential. *Qualitative Inquiry, 1*(3), 360–375.

_____. (2001). Ethnodrama: Performed research – Limitations and potential. In P. Atkinson, A. Coffey, S. Delamont, J. Lofland & L. Lofland (Eds.), *Handbook of ethnography* (pp. 468–476). Sage Publications.

Mienczakowski, J., & Morgan, S. (2001). Ethnodrama: Constructing participatory, experiential and compelling action research through performance. In P. Reason & H. Bradbury (Eds.), *Handbook of action research: Participative inquiry and practice* (pp. 219–227). Sage Publications.

Mitchell, S. (1994). A "therapeutic theatre" model of dramatherapy. In S. Jennings, A. Cattanach, S. Mitchell, A. Chesner & B. Meldrum (Eds.), *The handbook of dramatherapy* (pp. 41–57). Routledge.

Moldoveanu, D. (2017). *Mental health education and the role of Ethnodrama* [Unpublished manuscript]. Department of Psychology, Concordia University, Montreal.

Moreno, J. L. (1946). *Psychodrama, First Volume.* Beacon House.

_____. (1993). *Who shall survive?: Foundations of sociometry, group therapy and sociodrama.* American Society of Group Psychotherapy and Psychodrama. (Original work published 1953).

_____. (2019). *Autobiography of a genius.* (E. Schreiber, S. Kelley, & S. Giacomucci, Eds.), The North-West Psychodrama Association.

Ritchie, H., & Roser, M. (2018). Mental health. OurWorldInData.org. Retrieved from https://ourworldindata.org/mental-health.

Sajnani, N. (2010). *Permeable boundaries: Toward a critical collaborative performance pedagogy* [Unpublished doctoral dissertation]. Concordia University, Montreal, Quebec, Canada.

Sample, P. L. (1996). Beginnings: Participatory action research and adults with developmental disabilities. *Disability & Society, 11*(3), 317–332.

Snow, S. (2018). *Nobody's perfect! A musical ethnodrama.* Summary Protocol Form, Concordia University, Montreal.

Snow, S., D'Amico, M., & Tanguay, D. (2003). Therapeutic theatre and well-being. *The Arts in Psychotherapy, 30,* 73–82.

Snow, S., & D'Amico, M. (2012). Casting the healing role: Assessment in therapeutic theatre. In D. R. Johnson, S. Pendzik & S. Snow (Eds.), *Assessment in drama therapy* (pp. 91–120). C. C. Thomas Publisher.

Snow, S., D'Amico, M., Mongerson, E., Anthony, E., Rozenberg, M., Opolko, C., & Anandampillai, S. (2017). *Ethnodramatherapy* in a project focusing on relationships in the lives of adults with developmental disabilities, especially romance, intimacy and sexuality. *The Drama Therapy Review, 3*(2): 241–260.

Turner, V. (1969). *The ritual process: Structure and anti-structure.* The Aldine Publishing Company.

World Health Organization. (2001). *World health report, 2001: Mental health: New understanding, new hope.* World Health Organization.

Yalom, I. D. (1985). *The theory and practice of group psychotherapy* (3rd ed). Basic Books.

7
Developing a Six-Day Workshop Model for EDT in China

It's awesome that you meet some strangers as a team, after a few days journey, these people "pregnant" together, welcoming a baby born: an opera (drama) concentrates all the stories of the team. Very valuable to the community & society. It's an amazing experience.

(T. T., participant in 2018 EDT Workshop in Beijing)

A Very Different Framework for EDT

This chapter is based on my field notes from four EDT workshops that I facilitated in China, between July 2018 and July 2019. They were presented under the title of "Theory and Practice of Ethnodramatherapy," with about ten Chinese students enrolled in each workshop. A Chinese translator was always present who translated everything into English for me and into Chinese for the workshop participants, especially those who did not speak any English.

With only six days to create an ethnodrama through the EDT method, a whole new approach had to be developed. Of course, the time factor was the biggest structural shift. As delineated in the last five chapters, the normal EDT process takes at least six months. With such a tight timeline in these workshops in China, all elements of the process had to be essentialized for only a few hours of learning and practice. The central purpose was to give these students an experiential introduction to EDT by breaking the whole process down into just a few units.

Another extraordinary aspect of the EDT process, in this particular situation, was that very politically charged and controversial themes were selected by the participants. There seemed to be a tremendous excitement about the freedom of self-expression and self-revelation. These themes will be reviewed in the following sections, and, also, how they emerged in each

DOI: 10.4324/9781003083818-9

specific workshop. As director of the workshops and the author of this chapter, I have great concern for the students' confidentiality and safety. For that reason, no identification will be made of any students' names nor will any other identifying factors be mentioned.[1]

Synaesthetic Spontaneity

Because of the extremely reduced time for the process, the group had to work very *spontaneously* across many media, including drama, dance, storytelling, poetry, artmaking and music. This involved participating in the senses of touch, sound, hearing and seeing, sometimes simultaneously, as we moved through the process of exploring experiences connected to the chosen theme. The end "product" or the ethnodrama/research report was not developed into a fully articulated script, but rather a scenario that simply contained the outline of units of action, without any dialogue (see Figure 7.3). The performance was based on the improvisation of these units.

A new concept emerged from this adapted process. I named it: **Synaesthetic Spontaneity**. Because of the quickened pace of creative explorations, participants dove into a multimedia pool of different sensory experiences, all based on working spontaneously in the moment. This pressure could at times have a very positive effect, pushing individuals to experience the arts in new ways and with new appreciation. This approach is highly indebted to the philosophy and methodology of J.L. Moreno (1946, 1953/1993, 2019) who was a pioneer in this realm. As he states, so eloquently, in *Psychodrama, First Volume*, "It is that quality which gives newness and vivacity to feelings, actions, and verbal utterances ... [it] has apparently a great practical importance in *energizing* and *unifying* the self" (1946, pp. 89–90). The major frame of Synaesthetic Spontaneity is the confluence of all the media and modalities of creative expression, occurring intensively over a short period of time (six days!), with the use of spontaneity, play and very little pre-conceptualizing in the process. This creates a unique synergy of sensory experience, with instantaneous choices based on intuition. As the great teacher of improvisational acting, Viola Spolin, writes, "The intuitive can only be felt in a moment of spontaneity, the moment when we are freed to relate and act, involving ourselves in the moving, changing world around us ... Intuition bypasses the intellect,

---

1 As will be seen, most of the themes that emerged in the workshops were very politically controversial, so confidentiality and anonymity are of great importance. For this reason, also, no individual or group photographs of students are included and quoted interviews will be cited as "Anonymous."

the mind, the memory" (1986, p. 19). This focus in spontaneous creation was the *modus operandi* in these workshops in China.

I was incredibly fortunate to have excellent translators in each of these workshops; individuals who also seemed to be very interested in the creative process. They could translate at lightning speed and, in this way, the spontaneous moment would not be lost. Many of them also came from mental health backgrounds, professionally, and were keen to nurture the therapeutic component of the workshops. The four functions of ethnodramatherapy (Figure 1.4) were still underscored in these workshops, even in the brief time frame.

I adapted a new ten-step approach in the workshops that I would present at the very beginning, so the students would have a good idea how the process would unfold. As you can see in Figures 7.1 and 7.2, I used a white board to present the title and components of each step along with their Chinese translation. Here are the ten steps that would occur in the workshop:

1. Form group: build trust via drama therapy exercises.
2. Locate common theme: use sociometry and sociodrama.
3. Use processes to explore the theme: sociodrama, playback theatre, psychodrama, as well as graphic arts, music, dance and interviews.
4. Collect authentic material for the script/scenario.
5. Build the script/scenario as a team.
6. Informant validation of the script/scenario.
7. Rehearsal process, up to performance, all based in improvisation.
8. Informant validation of the performance at dress rehearsal.
9. Performance of the ethnodrama script/scenario based on improvisation.
10. Public forum: post-performance discussion of issues and closure.

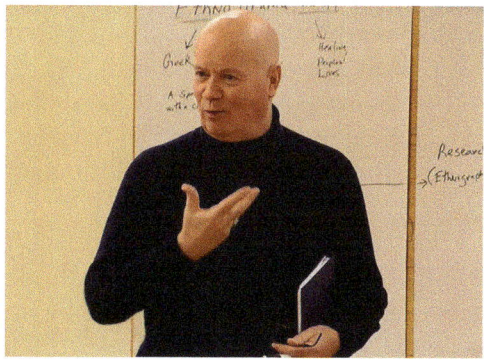

Figure 7.1   Author Leading EDT Workshop in China (permission from Dr. Li Weixiao)

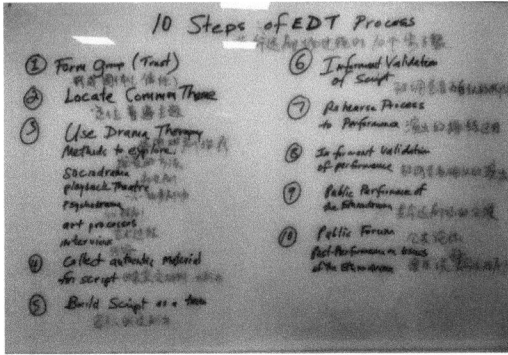

Figure 7.2   The Ten Steps of EDT Adapted for Six-Day Model in China (permission from Dr. Li Weixiao)

Certainly, this formula will look familiar to those studying this book with an idea to implement the EDT process sometime in the future. It was presented as a specific concrete outline to the Chinese students, so they could get a quick handle on how the whole process works.

Am I in a Bubble?

Sometimes, I had to pinch myself during these workshops in China. The students seemed so ready to go with the flow of sharing their intimate experiences. As often when working in another culture, I bring some of my own biases and pre-conceptions of how people will be. One tries to nullify such potential prejudicial thinking, but that is very difficult once such thoughts get introjected into the mind. For instance, I had expected some degree of resistance to self-expression, and especially to self-revelation. It was just the opposite. Many, if not most of the students, already had experience with self-expressive forms like playback theatre and psychodrama; some had even done developmental transformations (Johnson, 2009), the most improvisational method in all of drama therapy! Having only been to China three times (in one visit I facilitated two workshops), I have no demographic comparison for the students with whom I worked in the four workshops. I have known Chinese people who live in Canada. One person especially comes to mind; she lent me a book she wrote about her own painful experiences during the 1950s when Mao Zedong ruled in China. I think I have to consider the Chinese students I worked with as somewhat of a unique group. In the moment of facilitating the workshops, I had to ask myself at times, "Am I in a bubble?" I think the most honest answer is probably, "Yes." I was fortunate to have such accepting and free-spirited persons for the EDT process.

The Group Chooses the Theme

It is extremely important to emphasize that in these workshops, the group itself *chooses the theme* for their group exploration. It is not suggested, coerced or manipulated. It comes out of a specific sociometric process. It is likely especially true for groups from another culture that are not fluent or do not speak the facilitator's language, necessitating the presence of a translator. In many ways, this is a model of how the theme should be located in *all* EDT work.

The group is warmed up to each other through many traditional drama therapy exercises. Trust exercises like "Circle Falls" and the "Partner Blind Walk" (Emunah, 1994, pp. 171–173) can be utilized to build trust and group coherency. One exercise I often use is "Lemmings," which I learned from Jonathan Fox at a playback theatre training. The group bunches together in one mass. Then, a leader walks from one end of the room to the other, physicalizing a chosen expression in sound and motion. She stops, turns around and witnesses the whole group moving directly towards her in her own sound and motion. It is often quite emotionally powerful to observe this reflection of one's personal expression. After this, everyone in the group takes a turn. This is very playful and creates a great atmosphere for spontaneous creative expression.

Utilizing Sociometry and Sociodrama

This is the same as the warm-up phase that leads into the action phase in sociodrama (Sternberg & Garcia, 1994). The goal is to get the group ready to play and to comfortably connect up with each other. Then, I employ a sociometric exercise that I learned from Pat Sternberg and Nina Garcia, many years ago, at a National Association for Drama Therapy conference in the U.S. I will outline it in some detail, as it is a very powerful catalyst to uncover an authentic theme for a group. The group breaks up into three small subgroups of three or four people in each. They are asked to find three vital issues they have in common that they would like to explore. Sometimes, a prompt is given, like: "three issues very important to people in China, today" or "three ways you might have experienced prejudice or stigma." Time is given, and once the three issues have been chosen and discussed, then the teams are asked to go back into their subgroups and choose the one that is most relevant to them in the here and now. Often, I ask the groups to name themselves by a chosen color, so I can identify each subgroup, easily. At this point the teams are given two instructions: make a sculpt (a *tableaux vivant*) of your chosen theme that you will present to the whole group and give it a secret caption (a title that no one else but the subgroup knows). Each team presents their sculpt in the center of the room, while the other participants walk around and free associate, out loud, about the frozen silent sculpt they are witnessing. They say whatever comes into their head that they associate to the physicalized theme. Then, the group states their secret caption. In this fashion, each team has a turn. At the end, there is a vote (only one vote by each participant) by the whole group on which theme they want to work with. The secret caption may become the title of that theme (This was the same process used in the caregivers' workshop described in Chapter 5).

The perspective of sociometry, as developed by Moreno, is very important to this work. "Put simply, sociometry is the assessment of social choices and a set of intervention tools designed to facilitate social change" (Garcia & Buchanan in Johnson & Emunah, 2009, p. 397). This quote highlights the social activist intention of sociometry. In a more philosophical vein, Moreno writes, "The principle which set sociometry in motion is the twin concept of spontaneity and creativity, not as abstractions but as a function in actual human beings and in their relationships" (1953/1993, p. 16). Sociometry is a measurement of those relationships between the members of a group. As pointed out by Buchanan, "However, sociometry as used by the field of psychodrama also means the assessment of groups and a set of intervention tools to enhance positive group dynamics" (2016, p. 72). Tools, like the action spectrogram, described in previous chapters, help to locate what the group wants to focus on and how individuals relate, emotionally and psychologically, to such an issue, but they also help build the coherence of the group.

Once the theme has been chosen, the subgroup who created the sculpt for this theme reconstructs their tableau, and from this we begin to build a sociodrama around this theme.

My work in ethnodramatherapy, at this point, is very akin to Moreno's sociodrama method.

I want the first step to be collective and not based on one person's lived experience. This is the essential difference between psychodrama and sociodrama. The group chooses a fictional plot and roles, as they build an imaginary scenario to explore the issue they have chosen to work on.

As Sternberg and Garcia describe, "The members of a sociodrama group will work with a situation in which they would like to gain greater understanding" (Sternberg & Garcia in Johnson & Emunah, 2009, p. 424). Starting from a collective, hypothetical perspective provides distance and safety, especially when the issue may be highly charged for group members.

The Themes Chosen in the Four Workshops

In the workshops in China, we had to go slower than usual, because of translation, and to make sure that each step of the way was clearly understood. There is such trust and intimacy in choosing a theme, collectively, that great sensitivity and awareness, is needed, at this point, to make sure that all voices are heard, and everyone understands exactly what is being agreed to.

In the four workshops, each group chose a unique theme, connected to its own chemistry and what was "cooking" in the group on that particular day. As I will identify each group by their chosen theme in the following pages, I will state, here, the essential title that the group gave to the issue they finally decided to work with, after undergoing the sociometric exercise described above. I list these themes in the order of the time when the workshop happened.

#1 "The Oppression of Women in Contemporary China"
#2 "The Impact of the One-Child Policy"
#3 "Pressures on the Family in regard to Education"
#4 "Women's Sexuality in China, Today"

Methods Employed in the Four Workshops

A sample of the most significant methods used to evoke personal material around the central theme will be delineated. These will include drama therapy techniques, expressive arts media and interviews done by a participant on the chosen issue of their group, with someone outside the group. The personal expression emerging out of this process became material for the improvised ethnodrama.

The Women's Oppression in China Group

In preparing to explore the theme, we had done an action spectrogram (See Chapter 4, p. 114) on "older cultural ideas of men's and women's place in the world." It focused somewhat more on the female perspective, as there was only one male in the group. Out of this emerged an improvisation in which the women went into poses based on value judgments of certain qualities: age, appearance, profession, social status, etc. The single male then went around and imaginarily stamped them with a monetary value. This was a real concretization of the theme of oppression. It was later used in the performance.

A Playback Theatre Scene

In a playback theatre process, one woman told a story of when she was 20 years old and was a new worker in a factory. She came to know that she was being underpaid in comparison to the male workers. She was hurt and angry. She tried to get a friend to help her protest, but she was afraid to. The boss (played by a female participant with a strong theatre/dance background) was portrayed as being an arrogant and oblivious man. The only male participant played his obsequious lackey. This added a lot of humor to the scene. Finally, the big boss just laughingly dismissed the young woman, and she was left in tears. This true story was later rehearsed and became a scene in the play.

A Scene Emerges from a Psychodrama

One of participants volunteered to do a psychodrama about some problems she was having communicating with her husband. This transformed into a moment from her childhood, when she witnessed her father verbally abusing her mother. A walk and talk was done with the Protagonist and myself, as the Director. The Protagonist was asked if she would like go back to that time when she was a six-year-old and experienced this family violence. We made that contract. The Protagonist played herself as a child. The Direc-tor asked the Protagonist to cast Auxiliaries for the mother and father, and she did so. Re-enacting the scene led to tears of catharsis. I asked if the Protagonist would like to do a "future projection," where she could talk to both her father and mother as an adult. She agreed. Again, this brought up a lot of emotion. There was a powerful "sharing," with all group members participating. Afterwards, the Protagonist and the group agreed to use this a scene in our ethnodrama, as it was so dynamic and relevant. The Protagonist asked if another actor could play her role. I thought this was a good idea to give her some distance when she would see it as a theatrical scene. This is a good example of translating the emotional authenticity that is present in a psychodrama into a theatrical moment in ethnodrama, as long as the Protag-onist consents to this.

An Interview Is Used as a Monologue

Another way dynamic and authentic moments are established for the im-provised performance is through the interview process. In the same way as I have described in previous chapters, I gave the workshop participants a brief introduction on how to do an ethnographic interview using open-ended questions. The questions were to be based on our theme of "Oppression of

Women." Each participant was asked to do an interview with someone outside the class, asking questions about this topic. One of the female group members interviewed her aunt who told a harrowing story of being forced by the government's One-Child policy to have an IUD (interuterine device) implanted after she already had her one allowed child. Because the IUD had remained in her body for 27 years, it took a horrifically painful operation, one that lasted for hours, to remove it. Here is an excerpt of the transcribed interview, presented as a monologue and translated from the Chinese:

> During that period, the primary goal of the Chinese government was controlling the number of people: therefore, they asked all women to wear the IUD. In the countryside, the women were carried by wooden wheelbarrows like pigs being sent to be slaughtered. It was impossible to reject the surgery … From 1981 to 1988, the authorities forced every woman who might get pregnant to have an IUD. If you did not do it, you would be accused forever. After the surgery (for the removal of the IUD), I still remember the doctor said, "It is impossible that she is still alive after suffering this process."
>
> (Anonymous, July 2018)

The participant delivering this speech in the performance was a talented actress. It clearly, emotionally and forcefully made the point concerning the experience of women's oppression in China.

'Half the Sky': A New Title for the Improvised Play

As we concluded the rehearsal period, one of the women brought up an image from a famous Chinese proverb of how "Women Hold Up Half the Sky." It resonated emotionally with the whole group. As Spraker wrote in an essay of the same name "What it evokes is a picture of women fully bringing their unique gifts to the task, bringing their ways of holding up the sky" (Spraker, 2008, p. 1). Although our focus was mainly about the oppression of women in contemporary China, it was certainly also about them finding their voice and their empowerment. I was personally touched by this image. The group decided to reword the title as "Half the Sky – Exploration of the Modern Chinese Woman." This title went on the final scenario.

The One-Child Policy Group

The next workshop group, four months later, actually chose "The Emotional and Psychological Impact of the One-Child Policy" as its theme. This was a whole new group with different people and a new translator. How and why did they choose this topic to explore?

In terms of the sociometric exercise previously described, the group was given a gentle catalyst: find a personal challenge that is deeply related to contemporary Chinese society that you share with two other group members. Out of the subgroups, several themes emerged. The one that took hold was "Stress of the Single Child." Many group members revealed experience related to this subject. We discussed what this term meant to everyone. Then, we improvised a sociodrama based on one person's story of "a stressful day," although all members contributed images and ideas to this improvised drama around stresses that come from being a "single child." This is exactly the format for creating a sociodrama where all share their ideas on the topic, so it becomes a collective creation (Sternberg & Garcia, 1994).

A Sociodrama Becomes a Scene in the Play

This was an example of the direct transfer of a sociodramatic scene into an ethnodrama performance. It began with the lines of the original storyteller, "I am a single child. I am also a single mother with a single child. Sometimes, my days are very stressful. Like, today, my mother had a stroke!" Immediately sirens blare and an ambulance (two actors carrying the grandmother) hastens to the emergency room where they find the two attending doctors embroiled in a heated argument. The grandmother complains about everything. Then, the single mom gets a call from her child's teacher – problems at school. Then, the single mother's boyfriend arrives and says he is breaking up with her to move to Canada. We wanted to take the concept of a "stressful day" to the limit, so the audience would laugh. At that point, the single mother narrator says, "So, you think this is funny!? You think this is crazy!? This is my life as a single child …" This was the opening scene of our ethnodrama on the "One-Child Policy."

Organic Emergence of a Big Theme: "The One-Child Policy"

I, of course, had heard about this important historical episode in Chinese society, but I really did not know much about it. So, I had to follow the lead of the workshop participants. It was obviously a highly charged theme for them. As Zhang relates, "the legacy of the one-child policy, which has affected millions of people for over 30 years, continues to be of great interest" (2017, p. 142). From the 1970s, Chairman Mao had demanded greater population control for China. By 1979, the one-child policy was founded and birth control planning was enforced (Zhang, 2017, pp. 142–144). In our ethnodrama, we had the central government policy read aloud by one of the participants in the performance. This policy was especially cruel and harmful to females. As one author states, "As male children are particularly valued for cultural and historical reasons, sex-selective abortion is commonly practiced as a way to ensure that the sole pregnancy is male" (Howden & Zhou, 2014, p. 354). Another writer makes it crystal clear that there was a prevalence of female infanticide specifically due to the one-child policy (Banister, 2004). All of this led to an intense exploration in our group as to how this policy had impacted individual lives.

A Powerful Psychodrama Takes the Group Deeper into the Theme

The sociodrama scene reflected the dynamic impact of the government's "One-Child Policy" on peoples' lives, even a generation later. It begged the question: in what other ways did this government rule affect individuals and their families? Many experiences of such were shared by participants, and many of these became scenes or monologues in the performance. One of the most powerful was a psychodramatic enactment based on a woman's experience of a miscarriage. Having a miscarriage is a sad event for any couple, but when you are *only allowed to have one child*, it is especially emotionally and psychologically poignant. As Howden and Zhou cite, "Families are exposed to emotional hardship if their only child passes away" (2014, p. 36). In the personal story of her miscarriage, the Protagonist essentially wanted to say "goodbye" to this child she had lost. We made a contract to do that, she cast an Auxiliary as her husband, and we reviewed several historical scenes in her life. She felt guilty as she was too busy working during her pregnancy. After the miscarriage, she did not feel her husband really understood her pain. Finally, we did a "surplus reality" scene where she was able to say goodbye to this baby that was never born. Tears of catharsis emerged, and the group tenderly held her in the "sharing" and closing ritual. An abbreviated version of all of this became a scene in the play.

The Group Creates an Astonishing Ritual

Like a molecular chain reaction, peoples' sharing and improvisations begin to deeply affect each other. A pool of empathy begins to form in the group, much like the concept of Armand Volkas' *culture of empathy* in his "Healing the Wounds of History" method (Volkas in Johnson & Emunah, 2009, p. 148). After the conclusion of this psychodrama, one of the members came up with the idea for a ritual which would be performed to honor all of the female infants that were killed as a direct result of the "One-Child Policy." She had the idea for a solemn march to a circle formation with everyone holding a lit red candle. A set of tiny Tibetan hand cymbals (*Tingsha*) would move the march along. It was simple and elegant. I thought the idea was great, but I wanted to make sure the whole group supported it. They did. So, the only question left was: Where do we get 50 red candles in one day (this was the number the ritual's creator said she wanted)? The answer came quickly – amazon.com. And, indeed, the candles arrived, the next day!

A Personal Story as a Monologue

Out of the emotional interconnections, the pool of empathy and the group's spontaneity, other powerful contributions emerged. One participant who was very moved by the collective stories she was hearing decided to write down her own story. In a sense, she interviewed herself, around a very emotionally charged personal narrative. It was performed by another actor. I relate it, here, verbatim, as it was translated from the Chinese.

> According to my mother's account, I was regarded to be a boy before I was born, so that they took extra care of me and were particularly worried about my being miscarried. This kind of narration makes me feel sick and angry. It is clear that the birth of girls is made even more bleak by the one-child policy. Because your birth will let all people around you feel heavy. When they saw a mother give birth to a girl they feel it is a disaster and came to tears. When I was born, it is said my father cried, not because of joy, but because of helplessness and pain. Then, less than a month later, I was sent away. Psychologically, such separation at an early age will cast a shadow on a child's psyche. One year (as an adult), I went home for the Spring Festival, listening to our driver, he said that a lot of girls were sent away after they were born. Some were thrown away in the mountains or by the roadside, and no one knows if they were starved to death, frozen to death or eaten by wild dogs. This was my fate and that for many girls in those years.
>
> (Anonymous, December 2018)

The EDT process, with its many drama therapy techniques and Synaesthetic Spontaneity, can create a nexus for a formidable exploration of a theme and a deep sharing of related experiences.

The Priority of Education in the Chinese Family Group

How did we get to this particular theme? As usual, I opened this new group with warm-ups to get acquainted, relaxed, and to build trust in the **playspace**, a term developed by David Read Johnson (Johnson in Johnson & Emunah,

2009, p. 93–94). One of my favorite immediate and fun warm-ups that I learned from a psychiatric nurse at a conference in London is the "Mexican Hat Dance." Partners take each other by both hands, standing face to face. I begin to sing the melody of the number. When I shout "switch," then people change partners. This goes on until all are spent. It evokes great spontaneity and laughter. This group had so much fun with it that, later on, we decided to open the performance with it!

As we did the sociometric process of theme-location, many ideas came up around education and its very high cost in contemporary China; also, its great importance to the family and the resultant pressures on the family. The group wanted to mainly focus, then, on the pressures of prioritizing the child's education at all costs.

A Playback Scene on the Theme

A scene was developed around a true story of a woman whose daughter was accepted into a very elite school. The role of the principal, the mother, the daughter and the father were filled by the playback actors. The principal of the school telephones the mother concerning the child's acceptance and the costs of her program. The mother goes into a soliloquy on how excited and thrilled she is, but she is worried about how her husband will react to the steep fees. He returns home from his workday. The mother plies him with pleasurable comforts of food and drink and a soft pillow on his chair. Finally, she presents the exciting news, but when she mentions the cost, her husband goes through the roof. They argue. In the end, she convinces him to borrow on their mortgage to provide their child with this excellent education. The group expressed a lot of laugher and anxiety around this scene. It reflected the enormous pressures many Chinese people experience. Using some poetic license, this playback scene was adapted for a scene in the play, as it so perfectly portrayed the pressures in the contemporary family around education.

Scene Developed from a Psychodrama Process

A scene on a subtheme of "Education begins at Home" emerged out of a psychodrama. It was a very painful moment from one participant's childhood. A walk and talk was used to set the contract. In the scene, she is four years old, and her mother screams at her for jumping in a mud puddle with her new boots on. The Protagonist reversed roles to show the Auxiliary how the mother screamed.[2] It was big and very harsh, out of control. To concretize

---

2 This is a very common use of "role reversal" in psychodrama: to role train the Auxiliary on how to play their role.

the re-enactment of this memory, I had the Protagonist get down on the floor while the Auxiliary playing the mother was asked to stand on a chair and amplify that critical voice in her yelling at her daughter. Later, we did a "future projection," with the adult daughter confronting the mother. Finally, the Protagonist role reversed with the mother and gave an apology to the daughter/herself. Tears were released. The group had a very deep sharing around the impact of parents' harsh criticism and how it can stymie a child's natural curiosity and desire to learn. In the psychodrama, the mother was given a line by the Protagonist, "Why did I have such a stupid daughter?" As we developed it for a scene in the play, three actors as Chorus repeated this line to the little girl. It was very effective, dramatically.

Post-Performance Forum

This scene above, and other scenes like it in the play, provoked a very interesting dialogue with the audience in the forum after the performance that concluded this six-day workshop. As part of the purpose of EDT is to create social change, the mirror function of theatre, here, revealed a very sensitive issue for many Chinese families, and audience members were keen to discuss it and search for solutions. The units of the improvised performance provided many nuanced reflections on the theme of "Education in Contemporary China," from a battle between a father and his adolescent son around the overuse of a cellphone to a gentle grandfather offering to pay for his granddaughter's education; from a child wounded by the harsh criticism of her mother to the re-enactment of a joyous high school graduation party, with the whole cast as family, friends and neighbors. This pastiche of the group's real experiences around the issue definitely catalyzed the audience to think about the theme. As with each of the four workshops' post-performance forums, at least a few moments of public reflection were given to an important topic in contemporary Chinese society.

The Women's Sexuality Group

The last of the four groups was made up of all women and women of very different ages and backgrounds. I honestly did not know what to expect and was quite surprised by the theme that emerged from the group. However, my job as director is to listen closely to the yearnings and urges of the group and to impartially and sensitively guide them where they want to go.

Out of the sociometric process came many ideas that related to sexuality: "longing," "touch," "early sexual experiences," "sex education," "extra-marital sex," "sexual harassment," etc. One subgroup created a caption for their final sculpture: "The Human Sexuality Thing." The group as a whole chose to create a sociodrama on the topic: "Sexuality in Senior Citizens."

The Scene that Evolved from a Sociodramatic Enactment

One of the participants had worked in a nursing home and so the whole idea of sexuality in the lives of senior citizens was discussed. Eventually, we established a fictional scenario based on an 82-year-old male nursing home resident who tries to seduce a young and naïve female volunteer. He was the archetypal "dirty old man" who tries to grab the young lady's derrière when she turned her back to him. The roles cast were Mr. Wong, the old man, the young volunteer, and a nurse and a social worker, both employees of the nursing home. A collective scenario was constructed, with a great deal of use of the "Freeze" technique, where all action is frozen and the director can ask questions directly to other members of the group, such as "What do you think might happen, here?," etc. There was a mood of glee in building this scene as the whole group found it very amusing. This was the first or second meeting of the group and everyone was feeling very playful. The resultant scenario went like this: After the first incident the young volunteer went to the nurse and complained; the nurse showed her where the emergency bell in the room was and said to ring her if this happened again. Sure enough, same behavior on the next visit. The volunteer rings the bell, the nurse comes and reprimands Mr. Wong. Next visit, same thing, so the nurse calls the social worker who comes down and talks with Mr. Wong: "There will be no more volunteer if you continue this way!" But Mr. Wong is incorrigible. The third incident and the pretty young volunteer is told she can no longer visit Mr. Wong. This scene that started as a sociodrama became the fifth unit in the actual performed scenario. It was done in a very comedic style.

A Poignant Scene from a Psychodrama

As we explored the central theme, many personal stories of sex and sexuality were revealed. Listening to a middle-aged women's story about an affair she had with a co-worker, I asked if she would like to use psychodrama to investigate what this all really meant to her. We made a contract for what the drama would focus on through a walk and talk. There had been a lot of pressure in her family. Her husband had a fight with her father. She was feeling quite distraught. She went to a hotel bar after work with a couple of male colleagues, and she ended up spending the night in the hotel with one of them. Finally, the scene boiled down to the two lovers in the hotel room. The whole thing sounded pretty clichéd, but after exploring this last scene through a psychodramatic enactment with role reversals, doubling and a soliloquy, it turned out to be one of the most meaningful events of the Protagonist's life – a curious turning point for her. The love-making was tender and gentle. She said goodbye with thanks to her one-time lover and actually never saw him again. Later on, she told her husband about it. He forgave her and they remained together. The Protagonist was alright with her story becoming a scene in the play. In the performance it was constructed as quasi-playback theatre: the Protagonist became the narrator, told her story, cast the roles. She announced this scene as an example of "sex happens outside of marriage, too." At the end she describes how sweet the sex was and what a beautiful orgasm she had. We staged the sex as a shadow play behind a translucent half-curtain. The orgasm was represented by a single arm going up in the air (à la the scene of the young lovers in the car in the movie *Titanic*). The scene had humor, romance and pathos, and the audience was touched by it.

A Moving Monologue Based on a Childhood Memory

The whole improvised ethnodrama that evolved from the workshops was like a kaleidoscope of various takes on sex and sexuality, from childhood experiences of sexuality to accidentally watching a Hong Kong porno film on TV; from a boyfriend who said he "would never marry a bisexual!" to a monologue based on an interview with a bisexual male; from a talk on sex and spirituality to a "vagina monologue." We covered a whole spectrum of personal experiences. I had shown the group some video segment's from CAHD's 2014 ethnodrama, "The Amazing Adventure of Relationships" (described in Chapter 4). I believe the group responded by realizing they had a great deal of freedom in exploring their theme.

One of the older women told a very tragic story. In her town, when she was a girl, she witnessed an adolescent boy expose himself and saw his penis. The boy was arrested and put in prison for a very long time. Although this had happened a quarter-century before, she had always felt sadness when she thought of this incident. It was such a cruel punishment for a teenager's foolish act that had no intended malevolence. Was he just showing off? After she completed telling the tale, she asked the audience: "Would this have happened if we had better sex education in China?"

Poetry, Art and Dance in the EDT Six-Day Process

In each of the four workshops, there was at least one day where we explored using arts media other than drama to express thoughts and feelings on the chosen theme. The "Women's Sexuality Group," in particular, wove art, poetry, song and dance into their performance. For instance, after the story above was first told, I used the "Group Poem" method (Emunah, 1994, p. 237) to close the group. Each person added a line on a piece of paper that was folded so the next contributor could not see the line written before theirs. The theme for the poem was summing up what the group now felt about sex and sexuality at the end of our workshops. It was incredibly powerful.

A decision was made to put it into Chinese calligraphy on a large piece of paper in order to "ritualize" its presentation for the audience. It was used in the performance. Sadly, it got lost in the wake of an exciting evening with a larger-than-usual audience in attendance.

Another participant had made a colorful drawing on a large piece of paper. It was on the theme of "Sex and Spirituality." She held it up for the audience to see when she gave her talk on this topic. Another performer did the same with her artwork on her "love for her vagina." Another group member, a highly skilled dancer, had created a dance on "a woman's capacity to fully accept her body," with music that she specifically chose for her choreography. All of these selections that came from the workshop process grew out of our framework for Synaesthetic Spontaneity.

Finally, we created a song for the opening of the show. I wrote the English lyrics, and they were translated into Chinese, so the group could sing them. They went like this:

Sex, Sex,
Sex is like a circus!

Sex, Sex,
Does it make you nervous?

Sex, Sex,
Yes, it can disturb us!

Sex, Sex,
But, it has a purpose!

Sex!!!

The play began with a group sculpt that came from one of the subgroup's sociometric processes and quintessentially embodied our theme. The rest of the group moved around it and said associated words, out loud. Then, the cast formed a straight line from stage left to stage right. One of our members, who was a very talented gymnast, did complete flips in the air, on a diagonal, from one side of the "stage" to the other. After the applause, the cast sang the song above, and then, a narrator began: "Our play is about sex and sex spans all of the human life cycle. Here is an example with seniors." And we did the scene with Mr. Wong and the young volunteer in the nursing home.

For probably the obvious reason, this ethnodrama attracted the largest audience we had ever had for one of these performances that were the conclusion of the Six-Day EDT workshops in China. People were really interested to discuss sex. So, after the curtain call, the cast and I came out and we had a serious 90-minute discussion with the audience on this topic.

How the Scenario Is Created

The "scripts" for these performances were scenarios in the old tradition of the *commedia dell'arte*, "the actors worked from a plot outline, on the basis of which they improvised dialogue and action" (Brockett, 1968, p. 150). This was the basic format and all the materials came out of improvisation. However, it was not the plotline of a story, but rather the plotline of a theme. At the center of everything was the theme. All the units of action were constellated around this. As a director, I often like to speak about these units as "the pieces of the puzzle." The scenario is the sequence of things to be enacted or performed.

As the group moves through the first five days of the workshops, the pieces begin to emerge spontaneously out of all the exercises. If they feel right to the group, they are selected and reviewed. As the ultimate goal is an improvised performance that will represent the group's five days of research on the topic, the ethnodramatherapist works in collaboration with the group to produce the scenario. The construction of the scenario begins after the third day, although ideas for contents will often begin after the first meeting. Often, the sociodrama becomes the first scene in the play. Sometimes, material from warm-ups even get selected as contents. This was the case with the "Mexican Hat Dance" and, as described above, the sociometric sculpt for the opening of the "Women's Sexuality" performance.

Informant validation takes place in a more informal and spontaneous manner in the Six-Day model. As the scenario gets created, all participants must agree that the material selected authentically relates to the chosen theme.

By the end of the fifth day a real rehearsal process is put in place. The materials that are in the scenario, must be brought to the most "performable" state possible in the time left. The dress rehearsal, which is the main event on the sixth day, is the time when the group fully owns its performance. This is the final moment of informant validation of the performance. If any member of the group feels uncomfortable or dissatisfied with a specific unit, it could be removed at this point. However, I cannot remember an incident of this happening. The period is so intense – we likely only have a half-day before the audience comes in! – that people have already worked out if they feel comfortable with the material or not. The one thing I do recall is people who have been a Protagonist in a psychodrama that had now become a scene, asking for someone else to play their role. This would usually happen before the "dress rehearsal."

By this point, the scenario has also been printed out, so that each actor can have a copy to refer to as the performance unfolds. With such a short rehearsal time, this is an absolute necessity. There are no stage manager's warnings. This is the only way the cast can literally stay on the same page. Here is an example of such a scenario (Figure 7.3, p. 212).

How Rehearsals are Conducted

As spontaneity and improvisation are the major frames for the whole process, the question is how to keep the content alive, fresh and dynamic for the actual performance. The drama therapy techniques, as well as improvisational exercises are the ways to accomplish this goal, so that the performance, itself, is a kind of improvisation (Kaufman et al., 2018; Lindheim, 2011).

Repetition is the French word for rehearsal. Like its English correlate, it implies the push towards virtuosity, like singing every note perfectly in Opera, or reciting every iambic pentameter, accurately, as in Shakespeare. This is not the case at all for rehearsal in the Six-Day EDT process. Firstly, there is not enough time and few of the actors are professionals; most are amateurs, and some are even neophytes. This is not the mastery of a script, but rather learning the basic outline (scenario) and keeping the "pieces of the puzzle" intact, so they hold together as one entity in the performance. The performers still have to know their parts, but not to the point of perfection.

As many have created their own pieces, they can rehearse them on their own in preparation for the last two days of rehearsals. There is not a problem

Scenario 剧本

1. opening ritual 开幕仪式
2. Scene of stress 压力的场景
          line 柳的台词
   -ambulance 救护车
   -2 doctor's fighting 2 个医生在吵架
   -Boss calls 老板打来电话
   -Grandma 祖母
   -teacher calls 老师打来电话
   - Boyfriend's farewell 男朋友的告别
   -all scream and freeze 尖叫并定格
3.   monologue   的独白
4.   All in line:title 所有人排成一排 ： 标题
5.   government policy announce   的政府政策通告
6.   line   的台词
7.   monologue   的独白
8.   monologue with artwork 杨的独白，带上艺术作品
9.   story with Fluids   的故事，流动雕塑
10.   story with   as a boy and   and   as parents
          的故事，   扮演男孩，   和   扮演父母
11.   artworks with song by   的作品，杨唱歌
12.   Dr. He Divorce solution scene
          何博士的场景 离婚解决方案
13.   doing   story   说   的故事
14.   poem   的诗
15.   artwork   的艺术作品
16.   poem with   on drum   的诗，   打鼓
17.   scene with husband and candle (candle lit)   和丈夫的场景，丈夫蜡烛
给   蜡烛点上
18.The ritual circle with candles 蜡烛仪式
19.   song 柳的歌
20.Fireworks 烟花
Each with statement and gesture 陈述加手势

Curtain call 闭幕

Figure 7.3   Model Scenario for EDT Workshop on the "One-Child Policy" (permission from Dr. Li Weixiao)

with reading a monologue from an interview that is still on paper. The same for poetry that has been written. If the actor tells a story that is portrayed in a drawing, they can just hold the original drawing up for the audience to see.

Individual dances that have been set to selected music will be rehearsed from the CD that will also be used in the performance. The evening of the performance the entire scenario may also be written on a blackboard or a white board, so the cast can refer to it. The whole idea is to keep the informal and improvisational spirit that has been part of the six-day workshop process.

Basic Formula of the Six-Day EDT Process

There are four main areas to consider in reviewing the basic formula of the Six-Day EDT process, as has been established through the Chinese workshops: (1) Creating an Ensemble; (2) Locating a Dynamic Theme in the Group; (3) Collecting Material Based on Authentic Personal Experience; and (4) Holding the Group as a Group Therapist.

Creating an Ensemble

One could also call this establishing coherence for a group therapy process. It amounts to the same thing, with the exception that the group is making a commitment to devise an improvised performance as a final outcome. The task of the director/therapist is to build a safe and playful space where the participants feel free to share their authentic selves. This is a high order, but, in fact, this is the pre-requisite for any drama therapy group (Emunah, 1994; Johnson in Johnson & Emunah, 2009; Jones, 1996). Safety is created by implementing many exercises that create trust. It is through these practices, some of them already described, that group trust can be established, very quickly. Along with this, a contract of agreements is created by the group in the first session. The ingredients include an agreement for confidentiality and a commitment to respect each other and the space. Also included, are the freedom to say "no" to any exercise that a participant does not want to engage in and a framework for asking questions at any time. Other than these, anything else the participant would like an agreement for, such as breaktimes, bathroom breaks, etc., are established. Then, the full schedule of the six days is given to all. The ground for the sociometric work is set. The group is ready to plunge into the playspace.

Locating a Dynamic Theme

The sociometric work of subgroup discussions and sculpts has been described in previous sections. However, it is crucial to emphasize that this segment of the process is a *sine qua non*.

Finding a genuine theme that resonates with all the participants is the major step to moving forward with the process. The sociometric work creates the crucible of networks, conscious and unconscious, that evoke the central theme. The group is finding, itself, in this moment. What is it really all about? Who are we? The chosen theme will profoundly reflect who this group is and how the individuals in it connect. Usually, this gestalt will be clearly embodied in the first sociodrama.

Collecting Authentic Personal Material

All the media and processes implemented in the first few days of the process, after the central theme is established, are aimed at collecting the content for the improvised ethnodrama. Drama therapy, art-making, interviews and all and every form for artistic expression are utilized to capture authentic narratives and images related to the theme. This is all done in the frame of Synaesthetic Spontaneity, where movement, visual art, storytelling and poetry engage the group members in sensual forms of self-expression that will become the body of the work. It is all meant to be highly processual, although the end product will be a *performance*. I have often quoted Renée Emunah on this point, in terms of drama therapy: "The therapeutic impact of performance is different from, and often greater than, process-oriented drama therapy (1994, p. 251). The intensity of the Six-Day EDT workshop model resonates with this perspective.

Holding the Group Like a Good Group Psychotherapist

One of the four roles in EDT (see Figure 3.1) is that of "Therapist" and this fully applies in the Six-Day format, as well. The director/therapist needs to be present for each individual who is going through the intense initiatory experience that this process can represent. I have often looked upon therapeutic theatre as a kind of ritual initiation around identity, i.e., constructing a new identity in the performance process (Snow in Johnson & Emunah, 2009; Snow in Gersie, 1996). I believe this also holds true for this model. Opportunities should be created for the director/therapist to have individual sessions with the participants, if these are required to help work through psychological issues that come up in the process or to relieve stress caused by engaging in self-exploration. The director/therapist is there to "hold the space" and keep it safe and healthy for all group members. The job is that of a guide, holding together the therapy, aesthetic, research and social activist functions, as in all EDT, but in a much shorter and smaller framework.

Final Thoughts on the Six-Day Model

The Power of Spontaneity

The power of being in the moment and creating from the moment is confirmed by many authors (Kaufman et al., 2018; Lindheim, 2011; Moreno, 1946; Spolin,1963). The goal, then, of the process is not virtuosity, but spontaneous authentic self-expression. This is how I view the Six-Day EDT Workshop model. It is all done in the framework of Synaesthetic Spontaneity. Each day of the workshop evokes unique self-narratives through the media of all the arts, with drama being the paradigmatic modality. A poem on a relevant childhood experience, a dance based on an emotional encounter with a loved one, an artwork around one's experience of one's own body, a song that reviews a meaningful lived moment – every instance of self-expression in the workshops can be incorporated into the final improvised ethnodrama. They give it life, presence and authenticity. They culminate in a living reflection of the group's process.

The Pros and Cons of Time Limitation

In a model of EDT, shrunk down to six days or less, there is no possibility of completely furnishing out a production with all the elements of set, lighting, costume design, intricate staging and choreography, and a perfected flow of dramatic units. This can be approached in a six-month or longer process, but not in a week or less. Relinquishing this loss of the attempt at a perfected aesthetic, a different view must be taken of performance. This would be closer to how Schechner has defined the term: "performance is the art that is open, unfinished, decentered, liminal. Performance is a paradigm of process" (1986, p. 8). The process is the key. Working with "process-oriented" drama therapy, we can spontaneously explore individual self-expression in relation to the chosen theme. We can enhance this with the use of other arts media. We can locate these expressions in the moment and aim to keep them in the moment, right through to the time of performance. This has been the case for many EDT workshops that I have done in a day or half-day model at conferences in Los Angeles, New York, Philadelphia and Montreal, as well as in workshops in Israel and Sri Lanka. Even in a very brief time, the process of EDT can give the participant a profound personal experience and an introduction to how the method works.

Formulating a Training Model

The six-day model that I developed for the workshops in China became an inspiration to formulate a "training program" for EDT. At the end of the six-day workshops in China, some students asked how they could receive further training. Recognizing what a dynamic introductory training the six-day program offered to these participants, I began to ask myself: "What would be needed for a student to become truly competent as a director of EDT – to be qualified as a full-fledged, skilled and ethical ethnodramatherapist? I began to conceive of a training sequence that would fully qualify a trainee.

The basic formula I conceived of was as follows: (1) a student would take the six-day workshop, twice, and then, under my supervision, direct a six-day ethnodramatherapy process that culminated in a brief improvised ethnodrama. At this point, they would be certified as an "Assistant Director-in-Training." (2) Next, they would need to develop and realize a six-week EDT project which I would supervise. The successful completion of this project would qualify them as "Assistant Director of EDT." (3) Finally, they would need to create a six-month EDT project under my supervision and take an exam to earn the title of "Director of EDT."

The goal in developing this training program is to make it rigorous enough that the practitioner is skilled and confident in applying the method, understands how to facilitate the method in an ethical manner and has knowledge of all the theories behind EDT. The model gives the participants a full introduction to the theories and techniques, and in-depth experience of practice of EDT. It is somewhat based on the model of psychodrama certification which also requires many hours of practicum, plus a final exam.

At this point, the design for this training is still being worked out. I am considering developing an Ethnodramatherapy Training Institute in Montreal. I presently have two Assistant Directors-in-Training who, when they fulfill the whole certification process, will likely become trainers themselves. The idea is definitely to be able to also travel to sites to give trainings as I have already done in Sri Lanka, Israel and China. All is in the planning stage at this point. However, there seems to be interest in and desire for such a training program, so it is highly likely that it will be implemented in the near future.[3]

---

3 Inquiries into training in EDT may be done through contacting the author at stephen.snow@concordia.ca. This training program is just being established in 2021. However, it is based on the formulation of the process described in this book, especially the Six-Day model.

References

Banister, J. (2004). Shortage of girls in China today. *Journal of Population Research,* *21*(1), 19–45.

Brockett, O. G. (1968). *History of the theatre.* Allyn & Bacon.

Buchanan, D. R. (2016). Practical application of step-in sociometry: Increasing sociometric intelligence via self-disclosure and connection. *Journal of Psychodrama, Sociometry, and Group Psychotherapy,* 64(1), 71–78.

Emunah, R. (1994). *Drama therapy: Process, technique, and performance.* Brunner-Mazel Publishers.

Garcia, A., & Buchanan, D.R. (2009). Psychodrama. In D. R. Johnson & R. Emunah (Eds.), *Current approaches in drama therapy* (2nd ed., pp. 393–423). C. C. Thomas Publisher.

Howden, D., & Zhou, Y. (2014). China's one-child policy: Some unintended consequences. *Economic Affairs,* *31*(3), 353–369.

Johnson, D. R. (2009). Developmental transformations: Towards the body as presence. In D. R. Johnson & R. Emunah (Eds.), *Current approaches in drama therapy* (2nd ed., pp. 89–116). C. C. Thomas Publisher.

Jones, P. (1996). *Drama as therapy, theatre as living.* Routledge.

Kaufman, M., McAdams, B. P, Fondakowski, L, Pierotti, G., Paris, A, Simpkins, K. Maize, J., & Barrow, S. (2018). *Moment work: Tectonic Theatre Project's process of devising theatre.* Vintage Books.

Lindheim, J. (2011). *Trusting the moment: Unlocking your creativity and imagination. A handbook for individual and group work.* Satya House Publications.

Moreno, J. L. (1946). *Psychodrama, First Volume.* Beacon House.

_____. (1993). *Who shall survive?: Foundations of sociometry, group therapy and sociodrama.* American Society of Group Psychotherapy and Psychodrama (Original work published 1953).

_____. (2019). *Autobiography of a genius.* (E. Schreiber, S. Kelley, & S. Giacomucci, Eds.),The North-West Psychodrama Association.

Schechner, R. (1986). Victor Turner's last adventure. In V. Turner (author and editor), *The anthropology of performance* (pp. 7–20). PAJ Publications.

Snow, S. (1996). Focusing on mythic imagery in brief dramatherapy with psychotic individuals. In A. Gersie, *Dramatic approaches to brief therapy* (pp. 216–235). Jessica Kingsley Publishers.

_____. (2009). Ritual/Theatre/Therapy. In D. R. Johnson & R. Emunah (Eds.), *Current approaches in drama therapy* (2nd ed., pp. 117–144). C. C. Thomas Publisher.

Spolin, V. (1963). *Improvisation for the theatre: A handbook of teaching and directing techniques*. Northwestern University Press.

_____. (1986). *Theatre games for the classroom: A teacher's handbook*. Northwestern University Press.

Spraker, B. J. (2008). Women hold up half the sky. Antioch University, 1–9. Retrieved from www.antioch.edu/seattle/wp-content/uploads/sites/5/2017/02/Women-Hold-up-Half-the-Sky.pdf.

Sternberg, P., & Garcia, A. (1994). *Sociodrama: Who's in Your Shoes?* Praeger.

_____. (2009). Sociodrama. In D. R. Johnson & R. Emunah (Eds.). *Current approaches in drama therapy* (2nd ed., pp. 424–444). C. C. Thomas Publisher.

Volkas, A. (2009). Healing the wounds of history: Drama therapy in collective trauma and intercultural conflict resolution. In D. R. Johnson & R. Emunah (Eds.). *Current approaches in drama therapy* (2nd ed., pp. 145–171). C. C. Thomas Publisher.

Zang, J. (2017). The evolution of China's one-child policy and its effects on family outcomes. *Journal of Economic Perspectives, 31*(1), 141–160.

Part III
Ethics and Philosophies

8

Ethical Challenges in Ethnodramatherapy

This chapter is emphatic in the demand for ethical responsibility in presentation and that the rights of researchers and performers can not usurp the rights of audience members and whomever may be impacted indirectly by effects related to the performance.

(Morgan, Mienczakowski & Smith, 2001)

Ethical Challenges in This Field

Why Are Ethics So Important to This Work?

As Paul and Elder suggest at the beginning of their booklet, *Ethical Reasoning*, the general public mostly confuses ethics with social values, religion, morality and the law; they state: "Most people do not see ethics as a domain unto itself, *a set of concepts and principles that guide us in determining what behavior helps or harms sentient creatures* (italics mine, 2003, p. i). I like this little definition as it brings it all down to earth and has a full environmental resonance as well. Our job as *ethical* human beings is to do *no harm* to other living creatures. Of course, this is an immensely complex challenge on multiple levels. In the frame of the human service professions, this concept regulates the practitioners' actions towards their clients. In this way, a professional code of ethics aims to protect the clients against harm and enhance their well-being.

Ethics are crucial to the process of ethnodramatherapy because of its multiple framework. It is due to this multidisciplinary approach that ethical dilemmas often emerge. Dickinson and Bailey give a good succinct definition for this concept, "An *ethical dilemma* is a situation in which the therapist has to make a difficult choice that goes against an ethical principle" (2021, p. 177). This definition relates directly to the therapy function in EDT. In the case of drama therapy, we have a professional code of

DOI: 10.4324/9781003083818-11

ethics to follow. As researchers, we are bound by the ethics certificate of the institution that is sponsoring our work. However, there often are no ethical codes in theatre or in social activism. As will be seen in this chapter, ethical dilemmas frequently arise when two or more of the four functions of EDT come into conflict. Focused in one role, the ethnodramatherapist may be blind to ethical challenges occurring for another role. It is for this reason that a protocol for ethics needs to be established for *all* participants at the very beginning of an EDT project. I am in agreement with the authors above that: "A strong understanding of how to use ethical guidelines strengthens future practitioners' abilities to reflect on their own work, provides clear ground rules and boundaries to follow in complex and volatile situations and brings a clear-eyed responsibility to practice" (Bailey & Dickinson, 2018, p. 227).[1]

Mienczakowski's Team Address Ethics in Ethnodrama

Jim Mienczakowski, who created ethnodrama as a form of performance ethnography, along with his colleagues Stephen Morgan and Lynn Smith, seriously address the issue of "ethical responsibility" in their 2001 article, "Extreme dilemmas in performance ethnography: unleashed emotionality of performance in critical areas of suicide, abuse, and madness" (Morgan et al. 2001). As described in earlier chapters, Mienczakowski and his colleagues took on challenging subjects from the very beginning: schizophrenia, substance abuse, rape and brain damage. He and his team acknowledge the potential for harm in ethnodramatic productions:

> But since we hold an encompassing framework of social criticism, seeking to impact favorably upon social circumstances for marginalized persons with whom we cite allegiance, then we must take seriously the notion that these events and thereby these projects may have caused some harm.
> (Morgan et al., 2001, pp. 170–171)

They specifically look at the negative effects of mirroring suicidal experience dramatically. In one instance, a play that contained a scene portraying a suicide seems to have catalyzed an actual suicide by a person associated with the performance group. This experience and other drastic responses to

---

1 The writing of these two drama therapists on ethics (Bailey & Dickinson, 2018; Dickinson & Bailey, 2021) are very useful for therapists and applied theatre practitioners. I highly recommend them for future practitioners of EDT. Also, the NADTA Code of Ethical Principles can be found at www.nadta.org/about-nadta/code-of-ethics.html.

their ethnodramas forced Mienczakowski and his colleagues to review the profound responsibility that ethnodramatists have towards their audiences. They conclude: "Unlike other versions of research reports, dramatic presentations can be emotionally loaded for audiences and participants as any gun" (Morgan et al., 2001, p. 176).

In examining the ethical responsibilities involved in the ethnodramatherapy process, I believe it is very important to search out, first, how many others have analyzed the multiple dimensions of ethical challenges that arise in their *ethnodrama* work.

The International Ethnodrama Community Reviews Their Ethical Challenges

Johnny Saldana, a professor of theatre and a major proponent of ethnodrama in the USA, undertook a very significant self-exploration in regard to his own work. In his 1998 article, "Ethical issues in an ethnographic performance text: The 'dramatic impact' of the 'juicy stuff,'" he considers a possible ethical failure on his part in his very first ethnodrama, *Maybe Someday if I'm Famous*. In his script, he followed the development of a young man, Barry, in his theatre training, from childhood through adolescence. Saldana also directed the production in which he had the real Barry play the role of himself. He cites this as a directorial technique with a clear purpose: "Withholding his true identity until the end of the text was a playwriting choice for dramatic impact, and a directorial tactic to engage audience members' reflexivity throughout the performance" (1998, p. 189). However, this caused some ethical concerns in those involved with the post-performance forum where Barry was present. Were these artistic choices harmful to the informant/performer or the audience members? Saldana purports, "If discussion had progressed with 'the real Barry' in a covert role, deception would have been operative, with the results potentially embarrassing for the participant and the audience" (1998, p. 189). This seems like a pretty minor infraction of ethics and, in fact, Mienczakowski, in his response to Saldana's article absolves him of his "guilty conscience" around his confessed ethical *faux pas* (Mienczakowski, 1999). This does, however, bring up the paramount importance of *choices* made by the creators of an ethnodrama. Making responsible choices in this work is a major theme of the dialogue on this topic in the international ethnodrama community.

Saldana goes on to address an even more sensitive issue. There were some highly intense issues in Barry's family – the " juicy stuff" – that Saldana knew would have had a strong dramatic impact on an audience, but he refrained from incorporating them into the script/performance as "had I included this material … the results would have been a breach of researcher ethics to protect them and respect their privacy" (1998, p. 191).

I admire Saldana's conscientiousness, and his writings on ethical issues are a great service to this research/creation community. He really helps to define the parameters of ethical responsibility in the ethnodramatist's work:

> first responsibility is the people he or she interviewed and observed. The second responsibility is to one's self as a researcher and artist, maintaining personal integrity and standards of excellence. The audience, our third responsibility, then witnesses what the first two parties have collaborated on and becomes a group of new collaborators in the ethnotheatrical event.
>
> (2011, p. 43)

Two other international researchers who have contributed greatly to the ethics discussion are Judith Ackroyd, from Regent's College, London, and John O'Toole, from the University of Melbourne. They have significantly investigated the role of ethics in ethnodrama in their book on this topic (2010). They especially emphasize "the inevitable tensions between art-making and the gathering and reporting of research" (2010, p. 33). A big question is raised: as the *performance* is a research report of the data gathered, how much latitude does the ethnodramatist have, *creatively* and *artistically*? This is a question that must be addressed by anyone who undertakes this work. Like Saldana, they acknowledge the potential tension between the artistic needs of a production and being ethically responsible to the interviews collected from informants as part of the ethnographic research. As they write, "A division opens up here between artistry and instrumentality, between aesthetic considerations and the need for the original stories to be appropriately honoured" (2010, p. 54).

I have certainly experienced this tension in my own ethnodramatherapy productions, when a strong desire to create artistic dramatic expression wants to override the concrete expression collected from the informant. Most of the time, I do my best to adhere to Mienczakowski's well-articulated perspective: "My personal view is that ethnographies, and in particular ethnodramas, are most useful when informant voices are articulated and heard in open and continuous collaboration with the informants themselves" (1999, p. 98).

Ackroyd and O'Toole (2010) present other potential pitfalls in the ethno-drama process, when conflicts arise between the research, educational and artistic functions. With a strong focus on the educational goals of ethno-drama, they recognize "the inevitable tensions which this creates between aesthetic, educational and research dynamics" (p. 17). They present many valuable case examples of ethnodrama productions in which these tensions were made manifest.

Perhaps no one has paid more attention to the minute particulars of ethical challenges in performed research than Canadian Kathy Bishop. In her 2014 article, "Six perspectives in search of an ethical solution: Utilizing a moral imperative with a multiple ethics paradigm to guide research-based theatre/ applied theatre," she seeks an holistic way to answer all the potential ethic's questions that may emerge in producing theatrical performance that is based on research. Her stated goal is to get researchers: "to think about ethical issues in a comprehensive manner to support their own ethical practice and further discussions towards new ethical paradigms in the field" (2014, p. 64). To accomplish this task, she created a survey interview for six major figures in this field, including two ethnodramatists – Mienczakowski and Saldana. In searching to establish a "moral imperative," i.e., a general framework for evaluating ethics, in the domain of performed research, she locates four es-sential frames: justice, critique, care and profession. Like Kant's "Categorical Imperative," her umbrella framing in her "moral imperative" will provide "a moral compass, or a wa y by which a human being understands what is mor-ally right, and behaves accordingly" (Boone, 2017, p. 94), in this case in relation to research-based performance. However, this is not as simple as it sounds.

Bishop presents a multidimensional perspective to analyze her fourfold framework. First, *justice* indicates that the same rules apply to everyone – whether a theatre researcher or a biochemist, the institutional governance of ethics must be the same. This would relate to university and agency re-search boards, whose ethical regulations must be adhered to, as has been discussed in Chapters 2–6, herein. Secondly, Bishop, reviews the frame of *critique*, by which she means the exposing of the inequities in systems. She writes: "the ethic of critique – in contrast with justice – targets inconsist-encies inherent in laws and policies. It challenges the status quo and ques-tions oppression and social inequities" (2014, p. 68). The third frame, *care*, is equivalent to Saldana's three dimensions of responsibility: the research participants, one's self as researcher/artist and the audience. They all need to be cared for. The fourth category is *profession*. To help define this frame,

Bishop uses a succinct and cogent quote from her interview with Kathleen Gallagher in regard to *profession*: "It's moral imperative, if there is one, might be: Don't let artistic questions cloud the ethical dimensions/relationships of the work AND don't let ethical assumptions obscure the drive towards robust artistic work" (2014, p. 70). This is similar to Saldana's "maintaining personal integrity and standards of excellence." It is about being a genuine professional as a researcher/creator.

Bishop has also looked into the *political* dimension and power dynamics that may occur in a theatre-based research project. She writes: "when practitioners go into particular sites to do intimate applied theatre work, they must seek to also understand what is happening on a broader political level and how a project can be (mis)represented, (mis)interpreted and/or (mis)used" (2014, p. 68). Following Bishop's lead, Canadian scholars and drama therapists Jessica Bleuer and I have explored how power dynamics can catalyze ethical challenges in ethnodramatherapy processes. We state: "Other ways in which power dynamics may be influencing the emotional safety of everyone involved in the project must also be considered" (Snow & Bleuer, in Johnson & Emunah, 2020, p. 270).

In the end, Bishop's efforts to create a comprehensive framework for making ethical choices in research-based performance projects contributes a useful and effective way to consider the difficult challenges that present themselves in this kind of work. The whole quest is to do the right thing and feel good about it. She concludes:

> The root of my belief is that ethics start with the person who perceives the ethical issues. Therefore, to engage ethically in the work, choosing with good character is critical. In order to do so, practitioners need to consistently engage in reflective practices and have the opportunity to "to *talk* about … ethics and share stories of ethical dilemmas."
>
> (2014, p. 73)

Ethical Tensions Multiply in Ethnodramatherapy

Tensions from the Quadrated Perspective

As ethnodramatherapy adds the therapeutic function to those of research and art-making, as well as a commitment to social activism (see Figure 1.4), the potential ethical conflicts multiply in the EDT process. Reviewing Figure 1.4, what I call the "Diamond of Ethnodramatherapy," we see the whole field in play. Tensions can move in at least four different directions. The goal is to realize all four functions in a healthy and ethical manner, keeping them all in balance. However, many ethical dilemmas do emerge in the tensions between these four functions.

As already expressed by Mienczakowski (in Morgan et al., 2001), Saldana (1998), Ackroyd and O'Toole (2010) and Bishop (2014), many tensions are manifested between the main functions or frames in ethnodrama. The tensions are the result of conflicts between one category and another.

All of these conflicts are also present in EDT. For instance, the essential conflict between research and aesthetic values is a constant issue. As Gallagher has pointed out, the big question is how to not sacrifice one for the other. As the director of many EDT projects, I can say that this has often been a real tightrope walk for me. How to give each function equal attention and value is perhaps the most common conundrum in the EDT process. Research and aesthetics must not override the extremely important therapeutic function, nor should that function supersede the goals of social activism. Mienczakowski recognized a potential conflict between the value of accuracy in research and the therapeutic potential for informants, "Although this scene may amply demonstrate the effectiveness of the accurate portrayal of experience … one must question the impact of this validation in terms of the recuperative processes of our informants" (in Morgan et al., 2001, p. 169). In EDT, with its added therapeutic concerns, the medical ethics maxim "Do no harm" becomes an essential measure of the success of a project.

Making Ethical Choices

Making ethical choices may be even more complex in the context of EDT, especially with all the shades of grey betwixt and between the four functions. For instance, the difficult choice to omit powerful material because it is in the best interest of the informant can create a major ethical dilemma. As in Saldana's experience, the fundamental rule should be "to protect and respect the informant." However, this can be a real strain on the concepts and goals of the writer/director. Because, like ethnodrama, EDT is a collective and collaborative process, there can be real differences of opinion between the ethnodramatherapist and her research participants. It may even be necessary to stop the production at some point. Morgan, Mienczakowski and Smith give an example of a production, when "the entire project stalled as participants were unable to democratically agree as to the validity and ethics in all sections of the text" (2001, p. 166). Although, I have not had this particular experience, after 15 years of developing ethnodramas in the specific framework of EDT, I can attest to many incidents of ethical challenges arising from the collision of its four functions. They often emerge spontaneously and quite unexpectedly, as the research protocols, the therapeutic goals, the artistic perspective and the social activist intentions collide. In the next section, I will delineate a few occasions when these types of conflicts erupted.

Specific Ethical Challenges in Our EDT Productions

Official Ethics Reviews as Prevention

As described in Chapters 2–6, the scrutiny that occurs in being reviewed by an official Human Research Ethics Committee (HREC), which examines in detail the potential risks to participants in your proposed project, can be enormously helpful. It is the first step towards prevention of making bad choices and creating an infraction of ethics. I can not overemphasize how important this has been to my own learning process in regard to ethics and how necessary it is for this work. Any future practitioner of EDT should learn the ropes of passing an ethics review. This is why I have spent some pains to delineate our own development of the Summary Protocol Forms (SPF) for our EDT projects in the early chapters of this book.

However, being human and fallible, breaches of ethics do occur. In this section, I aim to be as honest as possible in revealing the ethical quandaries that we have faced over the past 15 years, in developing and implementing EDT. Some of these have been very subtle, and some have been gross errors in judgement. I hope this will serve to enlighten future practitioners as to how and why these instances happened and how they can be avoided.

Are the Informants Being Taken Advantage of in Any Way?

In our 2006–2008 project, "It's a Wonderful World," we were working with a vulnerable population of adults with a wide variety of developmental disabilities. Part Three of the SPF dealt with "Ethical Concerns." The first item to be reviewed was "**Informed Consent**." Our co-researchers had intellectual and cognitive challenges that might impede their ability to understand every aspect of the research, so the HREC demanded that we write our consent forms in language that they could comprehend (see Chapter 2). The second question dealt with "**Deception**." The SPF states: "Deception may include the following: deliberate presentation of false information; suppression of material information; selection of information designed to mislead; and selective disclosure" (Concordia University SPF Form, 2003, p. 7). We put down that "There is no deception use in this study." However, in retrospect, there may have been a very subtle form of deception. Dr. Nisha Sajnani, who was a Ph.D.-level research assistant for the project and, later, wrote her dissertation, using our production as a case example, has pointed out that, in so fully supporting the informants' performance and having professional theatre artists do the set, lights and music, we may have been forcing on the audience a false image of the participants. She writes: "though the *overt* message celebrated through such performances is one of the empowerment of the marginalized group, the *covert* message (i.e., that they are not capable) is held in the shadows, as a conversation that cannot be held simultaneously, and that therefore goes unexamined or challenged" (2010, pp. 70–71).

The professional members of the research team had struggled with this issue. We asked ourselves: What would it look like if the informant/performers were given complete autonomy? If they ran the lights and played all the music? Sajnani's critique acknowledged an ethical conflict in our process between the research goal of portraying the authentic life experience of participants and aiming to produce a highly aesthetic theatre performance, i.e., researcher versus theatre artist. In hedging on the side of aesthetics, had we deceived the audience and taken advantage of the participants? And we wanted it to be a therapeutic and positive experience for the latter. If the audience did not enjoy the performance, would this have a negative effect on the performers? This is a perennial question in all forms of therapeutic theatre. In this case, it highlights the potential conflict between aesthetics and therapeutic goals. If the performers are presenting an inauthentic image of themselves, how could this be therapeutic for them?

In the end, I feel Sajnani's question is very valuable and points us in the direction of needing to evaluate the limits of informant/performers as well as the intentions of the professional members of the research team. It represents a challenge to go further in stretching the possibilities of self-expression for participants (it could be very interesting to see adults with developmental disabilities completely in charge of music for a production) and in being more forthright as to the nature of support provided by the other members of the research team.[2]

Was this a breach of ethics of any kind? If it was, it was very minor, but very worthwhile to put under the microscope for honest self-reflection. In general, we had taken great precaution in this production in answering all

2 If the reader would like to see the actual performance of "It's A Wonderful World," just go to www. psychotherapy.net and type in Snow.

the HREC's questions concerning "Risk Factors" (questions 4 and 5 on the SPF for the participants). We did our very best to prevent potential ethical problems. In fact, our SPF was commended as an example of conscientious pre-planning (Connolly & Reid, 2007). However, there is always room for error and the possibility of breaching an ethics protocol.

Am I Competent to Apply These Methods with This Population?

In our 2012 ethnodramatherapy project with female adolescents in Youth Protection, a similar critique was made by an M.A.-level research assistant; it also relates to important ethical considerations. Art therapy graduate student Claudia Corradetti was both working on our research team and doing her clinical internship at the center where the project took place. She has developed considerable background working with this population, so I felt her thoughts on this matter really needed to be carefully reviewed. In discussing the project, eight years later, she writes:

> There were significant trust issues, in particular for youth who have experienced early developmental trauma – so more clarity was needed from the beginning about what the project entailed, and this would allow for us to maintain a sturdier frame. For such a group, consistency, predictability, and sturdiness is so essential; and would have allowed for a deeper process to unfold. We needed to listen better to the participants and have them be more in control of the process.
> (C. Corradetti, personal communication, May 2, 2020)

Corradetti is correct. It was extremely difficult to establish trust with these young women due to their psychological wounding and the traumatic experiences in their personal histories. Trust was a central issue for all of them. As Corradetti says, they needed "consistency, predictability and sturdiness." We tried to provide that through our weekly sessions in art therapy and drama therapy over half a year. However, it was an enormous challenge.

The question presented, above, "How to give them more control?" is quintessential. I think a big part of the problem was that I did not have the skill, as the director of the project, to create a pathway for their greater autonomy. Again, my roles as principal investigator, therapy supervisor and theatre director were in conflict. I only had minimal experience with this specific population and this lack of in-depth experience may have created a negative dynamic. As described in Chapter 3, the female adolescents seemed to have a very negative transference towards me as an older, white, male authority figure.

Had I breached the principles of my own professional Code of Ethics (NADTA, 2019) by not being competent enough to provide proper safety and containment for these young women? I had recruited an art therapy supervisor who was highly skilled with this population to be a co-researcher, but I was the leader of the team. Ultimately, the framing of all aspects of the project was my responsibility. Was my function as theatre director too strong and my role as therapist too weak here? I was on a very steep learning curve in this process, and the conflict between my roles, and my weakness in the therapist role, may have contributed to a breach in ethics, although I believe the participants were not harmed by the project. Mostly, they seemed to have quite a positive experience (see Chapter 3).

This case example points to the need for the ethnodramatherapist to be qualified in all four roles of the EDT process and to balance them in an ethical manner. Alternatively, as will be discussed in Chapter 10, a qualified individual needs to be located to take a role for which the ethnodramatherapist is not qualified. All four functions of EDT – research, therapeutic, aesthetic and social activist – require a high level of skill and, sometimes, this is too much to ask of one person.

Are All Researchers in the PAR Framework Being Fully Empowered?

In our 2014 project that focused on romance, intimacy and sexuality in the lives of adults with developmental disabilities, the "Risk Factors" were around vulnerability and exploitation. We answered all the questions to the satisfaction of Concordia University's HREC. However, as we were fully implementing a participatory action research approach for this project, did we really create a level playing field, so that all the co-researchers could equally participate? This question has ethical ramifications as instances of excluding co-researchers from the PAR process could possibly represent a breach of research ethics. The ideal in PAR is for *all* co-researchers to participate in *all* the research activities. As Chevalier and Buckles state, "The change agent and the client group thus carry out all phases of the research process jointly. The analysis and interpretation of data and observed behaviour is no longer the prerogative of the expert alone" (2019, p. 20). Again, this reflects Sajnani's critique around limitations in the "client group" and Bleuer and my examination of power dynamics – who has the power? The professional members of our research team – "the change agent" – wanted to change public attitudes about sexuality in the lives of adults with developmental disabilities. However, the client group did not have the capacity to analyze results from our post-performance questionnaires, thus they were excluded from "the analysis of the data." Could we have tried harder to involve them in this aspect of the research? Was their exclusion from this discussion a minor breach of ethics?

We were also presented with an ironic twist in regard to equal participation. At the 2017 NADTA conference, a group of our research team members gave an afternoon workshop on this project, entitled, "Whose Sex Life is it, Anyway? An Ethnodramatic Exploration with Adults with DD/ID." Towards the end of the event, Dr. Jason Butler, the Director of the Drama Therapy Program at Lesley University, asked a very provocative question, along the lines of: "You asked them (the "client group") to reveal and describe their sex lives to you (the professional staff of therapists and theatre artists), did you do the same for them?" I have to admit the panel members were a bit nonplussed. Why had we never considered this? Perhaps, we should have had a team member with a developmental disability on this panel. It would have been very interesting to see how they might have responded to this question. This instance brings up the whole issue of how to optimally create a genuinely level playing field in PAR research. Our research was not a game of strip poker; however, self-disclosure by all co-researchers might have been a more honest approach. On the other hand, would this, then, have been an infraction of clinical ethics for us, as therapists, to talk about our own sex lives? The balancing of roles and functions in EDT is a complex business!

Is the Director Asking the Performers to Do Something Unethical?

I had an extremely difficult incident happen to me in this framework, when I was directing the *Pro Bono Playback Theatre Company* in 2014–2015. This work was a prelude to the EDT project as described in Chapter 5. Personally, this was one of the most painful moments I have ever experienced as a theatre director in any theatrical format, therapeutic theatre or otherwise. As mentioned, the performers felt it was a breach of ethics to perform the role of a mentally ill person. In the story, the Teller had recounted meeting an old school friend on the streets of a big city, ten years after their friendship during high school. His old friend had become seriously mentally ill and was raving in the middle of the streets. The Teller described him as having schizophrenia. He said, at first, he was embarrassed to talk with his old friend and walked away, But, then he felt guilty and decided to return and engage his former friend in a conversation. The Teller described this as being awkward and also embarrassing. He could not re-connect to the person he once knew so well. He ended up feeling very badly and saddened by this encounter.

In the playback, the actors played the two young men in this strange encounter. It was painful to watch, but seemed reasonably accurate in regard to the Teller's description. Then, after the performance, a complaint was made by the actors that it did not feel ethical to portray this mentally ill person. As the director, I held a firm stance that *this was playback theatre, of which the first principle is that you aim to truthfully portray the Teller's story this*. And, this was the Teller's story, not his friend's. How could these young actors not see the difference! I felt hurt and betrayed. I thought we had established a deep bond of trust in our company, but now it was fragmenting due to questioning the ethics of our work together. In the end, I would say it was a conflict of opinions about what is ethical in playback theatre practice. I did not feel I was asking the actors to do anything unethical, but some of them did. We needed to sit down and process this moment, but it did not happen. I regret that, very much. And, I also remained hurt that some of the actors quit the company, so abruptly. The lesson learned, here, is that ethical issues need to be deeply discussed by all involved, so all sides can fully express their points of view and find a way to work through the conflicts. A project like this is always a process and, fortunately, in this case (as described in Chapter 5), a valuable new way of doing playback, integrating psychodramatic techniques, evolved out of this process.

The Dangers of the "Juicy Stuff"

In the "Caregiver Project" (2015–2017), the greatest ethical concern was in exploiting the informants in regard to their deeply personal and often painful stories. This brings up Saldana's whole question around keeping the "Juicy Stuff," without infringing on the research ethics to "protect and respect" our informants. This is what creates the difficult choices.

Of course, we had informed consent for the use of all the transcribed interview material that was transformed into monologues and scenes (see Chapter 5). However, there were certain informant stories the use of which felt like being on the borderline of trespassing into an infraction of the research ethics to "protect and respect." One of these was Natalie's story of her traumatic experience when her son, who has been diagnosed with paranoid schizophrenia, tried to kill her. This story is the kind of material that Saldana refers to as having high "dramatic impact." In the production, we staged it as a dance with the son, circling beneath Natalie's window, threatening to burn down the house with his mother inside. At the end, the actress playing Natalie did a verbatim monologue of how she had to call the police and have her son incarcerated in a mental institution. It was both a true story and highly theatrical. Was it the right choice to use it in our performance/research report?

The use of a story like the above may begin to approach what is now called "trauma porn," i.e. "the exploitive sharing of the darkest, creepiest, most jarring parts of our trauma, specifically for the purpose of shocking others" (Zipursky, 2018, p. 1). Although this particular project did not engage a therapeutic function, as the informants were not the performers, was it harmful psychologically for the real "Natalie" to relive this experience as an audience member? In our productions I can think of several stories like this one where the question must be asked: Is this a potential breach of research or clinical ethics?

I will answer the best I can for this specific case. I think a framework of safety was provided for the real "Natalie," with whom I developed a strong personal connection. She validated both the script and the performance of this personal material. She had been supported through AMI-Québec. She had been completely informed about the precise use of the material and signed a consent for its presentation in the performance. I met with her, a year later, and did a videotaped interview with her for a documentary on the "Caregiver Project." She was very articulate in analyzing this experience and about her relationship with her son. In the end, I believe in this case we kept on the right side of ethics. However, ethical considerations should always be explored for this kind of personal material.

Three Infractions of Clinical Ethics on My Part

I am certainly not proud of these three instances that came in the heat of rehearsal and theatrical production of our *Nobody's Perfect* project, in 2018, but they all happened, and I think it is most important to be truthful about this kind of ethical mistake to prevent future occurrences and to understand the potential for this kind of collision of roles in the EDT process.

They all, to my mind, represent the extreme tension that can emerge between the role of theatre artist and that of drama therapist. This has been a zone of great vulnerability for me, as a person who has passion and skill in both domains. The first example I will cite came at the height of the rehearsal process for our ethnodrama, "Nobody's Perfect". I have described it in some detail in Chapter 6. So, let me just say here that the role of theatre director, at this point, had just about completely taken over my focus. We were in the last week of rehearsal and only going to have a couple of days on our real stage. The use of time was urgent and critical. One of the "client group members," whom I will call "Barry," began acting out by banging his head on the wall in the hallway. I was trying desperately to concentrate on staging a scene that needed to be polished. Barry kept it up. One of the research assistants went to support Barry. But Barry continued his noisome interruption, and I just blew up. I yelled at Barry and said he would have to leave the space, immediately. In truth, this was the last straw. Barry had been uncooperative since day one and we tried every way possible to engage him. It was a fool's errand, as Barry really did not want to be part of this process. Later, I understood the problem was that his parents wanted him in this project. He had never really consented to be part of it. He resisted from the beginning. We should have seen this and allowed him his real choice. In fact, when I told him to leave and, later, that he would not be part of the performance, he seemed enormously relieved. This incident spotlights the important issue of how "Informed Consent" is attained.

I am not saying this to defend my action, only to give some context of how a bad choice, or several bad choices, were made. What I did by yelling at a client was totally inappropriate and a breach of my professional ethics as a drama therapist. It has made me very aware of how, especially in the final phase of rehearsal, the tension between the roles of therapist and artist can be in the extreme.

Another possible breach of ethics in the "Nobody's Perfect" project was a decision I made to use a specific drama therapy technique in the rehearsal process. I had been using psychodrama techniques throughout the process to evoke authentic narratives from all the informants. We were enacting many personal stories related to mental health and mental illness. For the most part, this seemed to be a positive and effective approach (see Chapter 7 to review several successful examples of the use of psychodrama in the ethnodramatherapy process). However, I made a mistake in using this methodology in trying to evoke the "Juicy Stuff" in one participant. His specific disability probably made it a contraindicated approach.

I will call him "Mack." In the psychodrama, I had taken Mack back to the time when, as a ten-year-old boy, he had allegedly been beaten by a staff member on the ward of a psychiatric hospital. It was a difficult memory for him, but it was accompanied by more pleasant memories when he was discharged from the hospital and given a pencil box at his new school. The way he had cherished the pencil box was very touching. This all seemed like great material for the play. But was it good for Mack? Regressing to that painful childhood memory seemed to catalyze an agitation in him. It was reported by his caregiver that he was perseverating about his incident at home. The **perseveration** became so bad that she removed him from the program at CAHD the following year.

What was my responsibility here? I believed I was a competent drama therapist using psychodramatic techniques in an appropriate manner, so that there would be a therapeutic benefit for the client. What I did not perceive, and probably should have, was that Mack's intellectual and cognitive disability did not allow him to process the psychodrama experience in a healthy way. He got stuck in it and perseverated, talking about it all the time. His reaction seemed to be destructive to himself and to his relationship with his caregiver. I may have broken the NADTA code regarding "Competence" here, as I should have known that he would not effectively process it and gain some distance from his early emotional experience. His tendency to perseverate was noted in his chart at CAHD. This was a real clinical error on my part. Reflecting on these two case examples, I see I should have been more cautious and careful. With Barry, I should have tuned into his discomfort with the process much earlier and found a way for him to exit with dignity. I should not have allowed my frustration with his nonparticipation to build to an explosion during the final week of rehearsals. It was unhealthy for both of us. It was bad clinical practice. With Mack, I should have been much more cautious about utilizing a technique that might have a negative effect on him and not been so eager to find "Juicy Material" for our ethnodrama. These were both hard lessons. From these experiences, I believe I have learned to be aware of the dangers of the clinical frame during the heightened tensions of theatre-making. The clinical hat must stay on one's head even in the hurricane of the final days of creating a performance. In the final sections, I will present few ideas on how to prevent such incidents from occurring through self-awareness and clinical vigilance.

I would say this next incident was more of a *faux pas* than a breach of ethics. However, it still contains an important lesson for myself and future practitioners to take to heart. It may well also fall under the rubric of "haste maketh waste."

The interview is at the very core of the EDT process. It establishes powerfully authentic material to be used in the play. As Dickinson and Bailey write,

> Ethnodrama is created from interviews. Ethnodramatists need to evaluate their transcripts to be sure they are accurate and allow the interviewee an

opportunity to clarify any aspect of what was said or request that certain information not be included.

(2021, p. 190)

In the incident I am reporting, here, I had done an interview with a young woman about her experience of being placed in a psychiatric hospital under her psychiatrist's authority. She told the whole story and gave her consent to use it in the play. However, as we were under great time pressure in the production, I did not give her the script to read. Because of this, it turned out that I completely misinterpreted an important moment in the scene of her mother visiting her and having to say "goodbye" when visiting hours were up. As an ethnodramatist, a script writer, listening to the recorded interview, I heard a single line that stood out for me as I felt it captured this moving moment when her mother was in tears before she left, but, for the interviewee, it was actually something very different – a specific phrase her mother said as she left. Of course, her interpretation should have been honored!

This had a humorous ending. I asked the same individual to do an interview for a documentary I was making about that same EDT project. I wanted her to discuss how she felt seeing her story performed. That was when I learned I had completely misinterpreted that moment and some other aspects of the way she felt at that time. She said she was shocked when she saw the way the actress performed it on stage. In her words, it took "a very different direction."[3] She was not angry. She laughed and was just surprised that we portrayed that moment, so differently than she experienced it. This indelibly imprinted on my brain: *Always show the transcribed interview and how it is to be used in the play to the interviewee.*

Primum Non Nocere

First, Do No Harm!

Like Morgan, Mienczakowski and Smith, I want my writing to be a cautionary tale on ethics for my own self-reflection and for those who would like to practice EDT. As they state in their article on "Extreme Dilemmas in Performance Ethnography," "the primary intention is to wave a cautionary flag indicating perilous waters ahead, while also attempting to construct cogent approaches toward solutions" (2001, p. 170). All of us would do well to take

---

3 This videotaped interview can be seen in the documentary, *Nobody's Perfect*, online, through the CAHD website at www.concordia.ca/finearts/research/cahd.html in the Research section under Ethnodrama Mental Health Education Series: video documentary.

the principal precept of bioethics to heart – *Primum non nocere* – First, do no harm! This phrase is attributed to Hippocrates and a derivative of it has been part of the Hippocratic Oath taken by physicians for centuries (*Primum non nocere*, 2020). Like the work of physicians, our practices in ethnodrama and ethnodramatherapy can have benefits as well as negative consequences. We do well to be very vigilant in preventing the latter.

With the inclusion of the therapeutic function in EDT, practitioners must be very aware of how conflicts with negative consequences may emerge from the tensions between therapy and art-making, therapy and research, and therapy and social activism. We need to be conscientious and self-reflective. We need to recognize potential conflicts and nip them in the bud before they flower into ethnical disasters. We need to promote dialogue between practitioners on the ethics of practice. Practitioners need to be trained on how to present well-prepared proposals to Human Research Ethics Committees, so that prevention – Do No Harm! – will be at the forefront of their work. Tensions between the functions are real, but with careful planning and sensitivity, solutions can be developed for the many knotty challenges for those who wish to practice EDT.

Ethics are of utmost importance in this work. It is important to maintain an ethical perspective at all times: "ethics is about right versus wrong – both in terms of defining those extremes and how to act on the side of 'right'" (Boone, 2017, p. 16). And we have guides to help us. As a professional drama therapist (RDT), I am committed to follow the NADTA Code of Ethics, and I do my best to do that. If I fail, which obviously I have at times, I must admit my mistakes and address them with proper knowledge and supervision. As a 35-year veteran of therapeutic theatre, who in the last 15 years has integrated his knowledge of drama therapy and performance ethnography, I find I agree wholeheartedly with my colleagues at New York University's *As Performance* program, "Aesthetics and ethical considerations in therapeutic theatre require ongoing examination and study" (Hodermarska et al., 2015, p. 173).

We need to keep an open ear to all potential breaches of ethics. We need to attune our body and emotions to identify danger zones where harmful moments might occur. We need to practice a mindfulness in staying aware of what is going on in the moment and what might be of detriment to any of the participants in the project – to catch the red flags before anything harmful can occur. Finally, we need to foster an open space for dialogue and discussion around any topics of ethical concern that may arise in the group. I totally agree with Bishop that we, as applied theatre researchers, ethnodramatists and ethnodramatherapists, must "consistently engage in reflective practices" (2014, p. 73). When we screw up, we must admit it and really look at why this happened, so as ongoing practitioners of our methods, we can continually move towards *best practice* in the ethics related to our unique professional work.

References

Ackroyd, J., & O'Toole, J. (2010). *Performing research: Tensions, triumphs and trade-offs of ethnodrama*. Trentham Books.

Bailey, S., & Dickinson, P. (2018). Teaching beyond the traditional: Generating ethics and social justice in applied theatre curriculum. In A. Fliotus & G. S. Medford (Eds.), *New directions in teaching theatre arts* (pp. 225–248). Palgrave Macmillan.

Bishop, K. (2014). Six perspectives in search of an ethical solution: Utilizing a moral imperative with a multiple ethics paradigm to guide research-based theatre/applied theatre. *The Journal of Applied Theatre and Performance, 19*(1), 64–75.

Boone, B. (2017). *Ethics 101: From altruism and utilitarianism to bioethics and political ethics: An exploration of the concepts of right and wrong*. Adams media.

Chevalier, J. M., & Buckles, D. J. (2019). *Participatory action research: Theory and methods of engaged inquiry* (2nd ed.). Routledge.

Concordia University Summary Protocol Form, Rev. 10 (December 2003). Concordia University.

Connolly, K., & Reid, A. (2007). Ethics review for qualitative inquiry: Adopting a value-based, facilitative approach. *Qualitative Inquiry, 13*(7), 1031–1047.

Dickinson, P., & Bailey, S. (2021). Ethics. In P. Dickinson & S. Bailey, *The drama therapy decision tree: Connecting drama therapy interventions to treatment* (pp.175–202). Intellect.

Hodermarska, M., Landy, R., Dintino, C., Mowers, D., & Sajnani, N. (2015). As *Performance*: Ethical considerations for therapeutic theatre. *The Drama Therapy Review, 1*(2), 173–186.

Mienczakowski, J. (1999). Emerging forms: Comments upon Johnny Saldana's "Ethical issues in an ethnographic performance text: The 'dramatic impact' of 'juicy stuff.'" *Research in Drama Education, 4*(1), 97–100.

Morgan, S., Mienczakowski, J., & Smith, L. (2001). Extreme dilemmas in performance ethnography: Unleashed emotionality of performance in critical areas of suicide, abuse and madness. In K. R. Gilbert (Ed.), *The emotional nature of qualitative research* (pp. 163–178). CRC Press.

North American Drama Therapy Association (2019). *NADTA Code, Ethical Principles*. www.nadta.org/about-nadta/code-of-ethics.html.

Paul, R., & Elder, L. (2003). *The miniature guide to understanding the foundations of ethical reasoning: Based on critical thinking concepts & principles*. The Foundation for Critical Thinking.

Primum non nocere. (2020, October 30). In Wikipedia. https//:en.wikipedia.org/wiki/Primum-non-nocere#Origin.

Saldana, J. (1998). Ethical issues in an ethnographic performance text: The "dramatic impact" of "juicy stuff." *Research in Drama Education, 3*(2), 181–196.

_____. (2011). *Ethnodrama: Research from page to stage*. Left Coast Press.

Snow, S., & Bleuer, J. (2020). In D. R. Johnson & R. Emunah (Eds.), *Current approaches in drama therapy* (3rd ed., pp. 250–283). C. C. Thomas Publisher.

Zipursky, A. (2018). When they want trauma porn instead of your truth: How we tell stories of child sex abuse and incest. *Healing Honestly*, January 12. Retrieved from https:/healing honestly.com/ pop-culture/when-they-want-trauma-porn-instead-your truth.

9
Essential Philosophies Underlying Ethnodramatherapy

This interdisciplinary perspective can provide the theoretical foundation for graduate study in drama therapy. Principles of drama therapy and appropriate research methodologies can be developed from these interrelated perspectives. But the process of delineating principles and research methods must be carefully conceived and subject to much discussion and experimentation. Students need to realize the difficulties inherent in studying a new field that is essentially a hybrid.

(Robert Landy, 1982)

Introduction

There are several major philosophical concepts that support the practice of ethnodramatherapy. These grand ideas, like Plato's famous Cave Allegory or Kant's Categorical Imperative, are meant in some way to illuminate the truth of human existence. They belong to that realm of philosophy which Aristotle delineates as "the knowledge of the truth" (ca. 350 BC/1963). However, they are also the intellectual scaffold upon which EDT has been constructed. Four of these big concepts, derived from such philosophical traditions, will be reviewed in this chapter: The Philosophy of Phenomenology, The Philosophy of Emancipation, The Philosophy of Social Progress and Moreno's Philosophy of Spontaneity–Creativity. Perhaps, the grandest of these is "The Philosophy of Emancipation." In his dissertation (1995a), Mienczakowski has recapitulated the history of the concept of emancipation, from Immanuel Kant to Jürgen Habermas. It has been extremely important for me to review and understand this concept as it forms a guiding principle for ethnodrama and, therefore, for ethnodramatherapy as well. It establishes the basis for a two-pronged perspective in the potential for human freedom: the psychological and the social. Mienczakowski's work is so significant, here, as he discovered a unique way to approach emancipatory experience in both these domains. The first realm might be epitomized in William Blake's well-known

DOI: 10.4324/9781003083818-12

line from his poem "London": "The mind-forged manacles I hear" (Blake, 1975, p. 112). On the psychological level, the task of emancipation is to awaken the individual to his or her own blindness (unconsciousness). The second domain could be summed up in Max Weber's famous idea: "man is an animal suspended in the webs of significance he himself has spun" (Geertz, 1973, p. 5). The webs of course are the tissues of culture and society that disallow the potential for human freedom. Habermas and Moreno, as will be seen, have many thoughts on how to support social groups breaking through these manacles and webs; of course, from very different philosophical stances, but still with the same goal, which is also the goal of EDT.

In this chapter these large philosophical schemata will be distilled into the methods that make them practicable. This chapter is meant to be of benefit to the student or professional who would like to put EDT into practice and, at the same time, have a good understanding of the theories that underlie it. It might be wise for students of EDT to heed Landy's advice in the epigraph above, and consider and embrace the complexities involved in a hybrid methodology that integrates four different fields (Figure 1.4). The philosophies described herein are all foundational to the theories that guide the practice of EDT. As Aristotle recognized, they are ideas that are meant to be put into practice. As the great philosopher states, "Truth is the aim of a contemplative study, action that of a practical study; for even if practical men do study the state of a thing, they do not study its cause for its own sake, but for some immediate and relative purpose" (ca. 350 BC/1963, p. 56). These philosophical concepts have such a purpose; they are eventually distilled into clinical and research methodologies, supporting the two-pronged approach established by Mienczakowski and further developed by myself. This transformation is eminently visible in the following review of phenomenology which begins as a philosophy that is later translated into research methods in both psychology and ethnography.

The Philosophy of Phenomenology

Phenomenology as Philosophy

> Phenomenology counts as one of the dominant traditions in 20th-century philosophy … a proper grasp of phenomenology is, consequently, important not only for its own sake, but also because it remains a *sine qua non* for an understanding of subsequent developments in 20th-century theorizing.
>
> (Zahavi, 2019, p. 1)

The founder of phenomenology was the philosopher Edmund Husserl (1859–1938), who, as Betensky points out, "tried to reduce the perception of phenomena to their essence" (1995, p. 3). This is a very simple articulation of a very complex intellectual process and, when taken up by other philosophers such as Heidegger, Merleau-Ponty and Sartre, to name just a few, becomes a very complex, variegated system of ideas.

In his book, *Phenomenological Research Methods*, Clark Moustakas attempts to succinctly summarize Husserl's concept of "transcendental phenomenology." He writes:

> transcendental phenomenology is a scientific study of the appearance of things, of phenomena just as we see them and as they appear to us in consciousness. Any phenomenon represents a suitable starting point for phenomenological reflection. The very appearance of something makes it a phenomenon. The challenge is to explicate the phenomenon in terms of its constituents and possible meanings, thus discerning the features of consciousness and arriving at an understanding of the essences of the experience.
>
> (1994, p. 49)

Most writers on phenomenology seem to agree that there are four major aspects of the procedure involved in practicing it: intentionality, intersubjectivity, empathy and the Epoche. Betensky cogently defines intentionality as meaning that "I am intent upon the thing that I am looking at. By means of my intent look, I make that thing appear to my consciousness more clearly than before I was intent on looking at it" (1995, p. 6). Moustakas deftly describes intersubjectivity as "the Other is within me and I am within the Other. My existence and the Other's existence are copresent in intentional communion" (1994, p. 37). Zahavi clarifies the use of the term, empathy, in phenomenology as "a basic, perceptually based form of other-understanding, one that other more complex and indirect forms of interpersonal understanding presuppose and rely on" (2019, p. 92). Another take on the concept of empathy in phenomenology is presented by Maso,

> Experiencing the experiences of others is called 'empathy' … This is the way in which, in a phenomenological approach, we are not only able to consider others as humans like ourselves … but also to acquire an understanding of the experiences "behind" their perceptible expressions.
>
> (Maso in Atkinson et al., 2007, p. 139)

As Moustakas states, "Evidence for phenomenological research is derived from first-person reports of life experiences" (1994, p. 84). Husserl wanted the reporting of such experience to be as free from suppositions as possible. To make this viable, he invented the technique of the Epoche. This is a method that forces the researcher to reflect upon her own potential biases. As Moustakas puts it, "In the Epoche, we set aside our prejudgments, biases, and preconceived ideas about things. We 'invalidate,' 'inhibit,' and 'disqualify' all commitments with reference to previous knowledge and experience" (1994, p. 85).

The job of the phenomenological investigator is to produce the purest possible reflection on another human being's experience. This approach is valuable in both psychology and ethnography, where profoundly personal and culturally saturated experiences are the focus of the researcher.

Psychological Phenomenology

Amedeo Giorgi, an experimental psychologist, discovered the work of Husserl and with that a new approach to research that was relevant to his own desire to "study the whole person" (2012).

Afterwards, he developed his method of "Descriptive Phenomenology," to explore the lived experience of people. As he writes in reference to his study of Husserl, "Phenomenology does not dictate to phenomena but rather it wants to understand how the phenomena present themselves to consciousness and the elucidation of this process is a descriptive task" (2012, p. 6).

Georgi built upon Husserl's concept of "psychological phenomenological reduction." In his own approach, Georgi reviews the description of a lived experience; then re-reads it and breaks it down into "meaning units"; and finally utilizes the technique of "free imaginative variation," which helps to establish the way in which "the essential structure is then used to help clarify and interpret the raw data of the research" (2012, p. 6). Again, this is actualizing Husserl's goal of producing the most authentic report on a given human experience that is possible.

This is very like the process Mienczakowski used in his first two ethnodrama projects, exploring the experiences of persons having schizophrenia and those with substance abuse issues, respectively: "The phenomenological reduction of themes further includes an analysis of the functions represented by actions performed by respondents in the clinical setting" (1995a, p. 163). This is also similar to our EDT projects (see Chapters 2–6), in evoking the themes and in locating the essential details of informants' lived experiences. Giorgi elaborates:

> The method is descriptive because the researcher posits that there is a specific expression that will satisfy the problem with which he is confronted (a good psychological description of the participant's lifeworld expression) but he does not yet know what that is … He or she begins the

process of imaginative variation, examining various possible expressions, and then the researcher comes across a description that fits precisely the intentional act her or she was seeking to fulfill. The fulfilling expression then is precisely described.

(2012, p. 8)

This sounds very much like the producing of a "thick description," the ideal of the documentation of personal and cultural experiences as proposed by Geertz (1973) and Moustakas (1994) and valued as the content of the research report in both ethnodrama and EDT.

Phenomenological Ethnography

Phenomenology has also been applied to the field of ethnography. In Chapter 5, I made the case for EDT making use of a form of ethnography that is essentially phenomenological. I quoted Katz and Csordas, "Phenomenology is a natural perspective for ethnographic research that would probe beneath the locally warranted definitions of a local culture to grasp the active foundations of its everyday reconstruction" (2003, pp. 284–285). In other words, as with all phenomenological investigations, we want an in-depth understanding of the lifeworld of the group being studied. In my research, the focus was the lived experience of family caregivers for loved ones with a mental illness.

In ethnography, we are aiming to discover the web of interconnecting thoughts and behaviors that define the "culture" of the group. In EDT research, we focus on a way of looking at the world that is specific to a group that has had very similar life experiences, like adolescent females in Youth Protection. What are the ideas and attitudes held in common by this particular group of individuals? However, as Maso reflects, "phenomenological ethnographers assume that there are individual differences as well as different ways of looking between each other and within a group" (Maso in Atkinson et al., 2007, p. 144).

As delineated in Chapters 2 to 6, the ethnographic interview is the crucial tool for entering the lifeworld of informants. "Using the ethnographic interviewing technique as a means of data collection the researcher aims to explicate the ways that people understand and account for their day-to-day situations" (Maggs-Rapport, 2000, p. 220). It is through this method that we are able to grasp the "lived experience" of the persons we wish to understand. Van Manen, especially, investigated and theorized about the phenomenon of "lived experience." He sees this as the heart of the phenomenological approach:

> Lived experience is the starting point and end point of phenomenological research. The aim of phenomenology is to transform lived experience into a textual expression of its essence – in such a way that the effect

of the text is at once a reflexive re-living and a reflective appropriation of something meaningful: a notion by which a reader is powerfully animated in his or her own lived experience.

(2016, p. 36)

Just replace the word "reader," in the statement above, with "audience member" and you will see clearly how the mirror function of theatre can be harnessed in a similar way in order to render a phenomenological report that can catalyze a visceral empathy between the audience of an EDT performance and the informant's text. This would seem to confirm Norman Denzin's hypothesis that "The performance text is the single, most powerful way for ethnography to recover yet interrogate the meanings of lived experience" (1997, pp. 94–95).

The Philosophy of Emancipation

The Concept

The terms "emancipation" or "emancipatory" are used over 100 times in Mienczakowski's dissertation (1995a), where he formulates his essential definition of ethnodrama. Obviously, the notion of emancipation is a core concept for his work. At one point, he simply asks, "emancipation from what?" (1995a, p. 95). This is perhaps the crucial question. Mienczakowski answers himself in the following way,

> I construe this as representing emancipation as a democratically founded process in which oppression is not defined for health consumers but by them, and the action sought in order to achieve emancipation need not be political but is pragmatically dependent upon health consumer needs.
> (1995a, p. 107)

The whole philosophical tradition of "Emancipation" is brought to bear, here, on Mienczakowski's microcosmic domain of research. He spends a great deal of time defining the meaning of "oppression" and in explicating the means by which it can be overcome both for the individual and the group in which he or she lives. In doing so, he acknowledges his debt to the development of **critical theory** and the philosophical tradition from which it emerges. As he cites "critical theory with its interest in emancipatory practices is central to the thesis" (1995a, p. 1).

As ethnodramatherapy is derived from ethnodrama, it also embraces this crucial concept and shares the essential goal of producing emancipatory experiences for both individual informants and the social system which they inhabit. In Mienczakowski's early work, these were health care systems and, for the most part in my own work, I have continued this focus. For both, the most dynamic underlying and guiding principle is the concept of "emancipation." I will take time, in this section, to carefully deconstruct its meaning.

The Philosophical Tradition of Emancipatory Ideals and Ideas

In his review of the philosophical tradition related to emancipatory ideals and ideas, Mienczakowski explores the evolution of thinking on the topic, from Immanuel Kant to Jürgen Habermas. He cites Kant's views on oppression as root source of the concept of critical theory, "in Kantian terms, oppression is derived through individuals unwittingly remaining uncritical of the established structures and power relationships governing their lives, enlightenment, therefore, partially consists of the development of powers of critical thinking" (1995a, p. 15). In his book, *Knowledge and Human Interests* (1971), Habermas also reviews this philosophical tradition beginning with Kant. He analyses "Hegel's Critique of Kant" and "Marx's Metacritique of Hegel," evidencing the continuous advancement of thought on emancipation and, finally, establishing his own theory of emancipation. Mienczakowski makes great use of Habermas' work. As he writes, "Habermasian critical theory holds appeal precisely because it continues to speak in the name of emancipation" (1995a, p. 62).

In the 1960s, Jürgen Habermas, a German philosopher and sociologist, located new ways of locating and defining critical knowledge (Aristotle's search for "truth"), based on new ideas that differentiated his approach from positivism in science and the humanities ("Jürgen Habermas," 2020). In a review of a recent lecture he gave at the age of 90, entitled "The Unfinished Project of Enlightenment: Jürgen Habermas at 90," the author describes how "it was fitting that one of the greatest moral thinkers would close more than a half century of public intellectual life with a return to his roots, with yet another reflection on Kant, Hegel, and Marx" (Mendieta, 2019, p. 3). Habermas is so important as he spent most of his life investigating the philosophical issues directly related to emancipation and developed a communicative action method for producing it.

The second thinker on emancipation who has most influenced Mienczakowski is the Italian sociologist and journalist Francesco Alberoni, whose concept of the "Nascent State" (Alberoni, 1984) is crucial to Mienczakowski's own arguments about emancipation.

Mienczakowski's Original and Dynamic Synthesis of Habermas and Alberoni

What Mienczakowski integrated, in solving the problem addressed in his Ph.D. thesis, was: "Habermas' notion of human communicative consensus as the fundamental grounds for seeking emancipation and Alberoni's conception of enlightenment within the nascent state" (1995a, p. 93). I see this as a brilliant and original synthesis that must be understood to realize the emancipatory potential in ethnodrama and, therefore, subsequently, in EDT. It is this synthesis, along with the invention of Informant Validation, that marks Mienczakowski's very significant contribution to the field of performance ethnography.

The two major conceptual approaches that Habermas has given towards the accomplishment of emancipation are "communicative consensus" and the "**ideal speech situation.**" Mienczakowski has incorporated these into his own method. These two constructs are formulated in Habermas' great work, *The Theory of Communicative Action: Reason and the Rationalization of Society* (1986). They constitute a democratic move towards social justice through dialogue. This is perhaps best summarized by the translator of Habermas' book, Thomas McCarthy, in his "Translator's Introduction: "it is, in fact, to the experience of achieving mutual understanding in communication that is free from coercion that Habermas looks in developing his idea of rationality" (1986, p. xii). Habermas diligently focuses on the process of producing "uncoerced communicative consensus," which McCarthy goes on to describe as "communicatively *achieved* agreement" (1986, p. xxxix). Habermas elucidates this process in his own words:

> I shall speak of *communicative* action whenever the actions of agents involved are coordinated not through egocentric calculations of success, but through acts of reaching understanding. In communicative action participants are not primarily oriented to their individual successes; they pursue their individual goals under the condition that they can harmonize their plans of action on the basis of common situation definitions.
>
> (1986, pp. 285–286)

And, this kind of unified, concerted effort towards "understanding" has to take place at just the "right" and prepared for moment; what Habermas designates as "the ideal speech situation." This is the moment when the most possible emancipatory effects can be actualized and sustained. As Mienczakowski observes, "Emancipation, in Habermas' terms, must be relegated to an ideal which is approached through strategies aimed at dealing with institutions and conditions that continually preclude the creation of an ideal speech situation, but strive to achieve them" (1995a, p. 74). It is in this context, that Mienczakowski frequently speaks of "limited" and "latent" emancipatory potential in his work.

To these major constructs, Mienczakowski insightfully adds the concept of the "Nascent State," developed by Alberoni. In his book, *Movement and Institution*, Alberoni defines this terminology:

> It is, therefore, a transitional state, and it appears when there is a failure of those forces which constitute social solidarity. In such a case, solidarity is reconstructed beginning from certain points in the social system having quite specific properties. Broadly speaking, the nascent state is a proposal for reconstruction made by one part of the social system.
>
> (1986, p. 20)

This is clearly a concept of social change. This why it is so valuable to a program seeking emancipatory outcomes. It can be interpreted as a social process, but it can also be viewed as a psychological process (as shortly, it will be seen has been done by Moreno). It is the change in a group's perspective of itself. When does it occur that the group is ready for this? Let's consider an instance like Mienczakowski's group in Detox becoming aware of how the enormous stigmatization of alcoholism affects their treatment, both clinically and personally; or the adults with developmental disabilities in my research (Chapter 2) who begin to see the role that stigmatization plays in their lives and begin developing the impulse to advocate for themselves against this force of oppression. It is a new awareness in the group, but also a new consciousness for individuals in the group. As Mienczakowski states in light of his incorporation of Alberoni's concept into his ethnodramatic process: "both enlightenment and emancipation are defined by personal and individual need and not by the global prerequisites of any given political project" (1995a, p. 37). It is this consideration of *individual* needs that eventually leads Mienczakowski to intimate a therapeutic potential for his method and which I have further developed in defining a full therapeutic function for ethnodramatherapy.

The Two-Pronged Research Focus in EDT

Mienczakowski's dynamic synthesis of Habermas and Alberoni paves the way for my own establishment of a dual research focus in EDT. As he writes in connection to integrating Alberoni's ideas with those of Habermas, "Combined with Habermas' practical basis for emancipation, it reveals the potential to pursue emancipation on an individuated level" (1995a, p. 38). This inspired me to create a clinical research program for EDT. As described in previous chapters, individual therapeutic goals were set for each of the informants in our projects. Our aim was to provide evidence of therapeutic changes that occurred for participants during the process. This may be the weakest component of the EDT method, so far, as we are still searching for a way to effectively produce such clinical evidence (see Chapter 10). However, we have strived to achieve such proof of "emancipation on an individuated level" since the beginning.

Research in EDT is two-pronged as we are always investigating both the emancipatory (educational) value of performed research for the audience as well as the emancipatory (therapeutic) effects on the informant/performers. Based on Mienczakowski's idea that an ethnodrama can engage "therapeutic strategies leading to individual change" (Mienczakowski, Smith & Sinclair, 1996, p. 445), I have developed a complete process of therapy, utilizing clinical methods from creative arts therapies, drama therapy and psychodrama, that is a major component of EDT. Along with the implementation of these clinical practices, we also have aimed to produce both qualitative and quantitative evidence that demonstrates the therapeutic effectiveness of EDT (see Chapters 2–6).

Our second research frame is structured so that we can measure the educational efficacy of the performance/research report. We regularly administer pre- and post-performance questionnaires to our audiences. This educational focus is quite like Mienczakowski's, where he has borrowed Freire's notion of how emancipatory pedagogy can create *Conscientizacao* in the students (audience members) (Freire, 1974). As Mienczakowski expresses it, his method is meant to "impact upon the lives of the subjects of the study by forcing confrontation with the real problems of their existence; engaging in processes of conscientiation" (1995a, pp. 46–47). This latter is in consideration of the informants; however, it can also be applied to the audience who are moved and changed by the informants' performance text. This is a function of the emancipatory potential of education. As with Mienczakowski, whose work seeks "ascertaining emancipation as a recognizable outcome or product of ethno-drama" (1995a, p. 250), in EDT, we also want to prove the effectiveness of our process in changing peoples' attitudes and behaviors.

The Philosophy of Social Progress Based on Collaborative Research with Members of the Community Being Researched

Participatory Action Research

This long title above is, of course, simply saying "Participatory Action Research (PAR)." It is a vital component of EDT. But, how is it a philosophy?

First of all, PAR can be seen as a reaction against the philosophical stance of Positivism, which considers only information derived from sensory experience, using the scientific method, as valid knowledge, or "knowledge of truth," as articulated in Aristotle's model of philosophy. This reaction was especially heated in the German-speaking countries in the first half of the 20th-century. There was a strong movement towards building a new "social" science that did not subscribe to the views of Positivism. As Fuchs proposes, "Once the narrow positivistic interpretation of the social scientific concept of 'experience' is broken … it seems quite possible to count means of political and social practice as research techniques and everyday communication processes as social research" (McTaggart, 1997, p. 46). What a powerful statement of how the doors were opening to a new way of investigating social phenomena, which, of course, includes "lived experience," the central focus of phenomenology.

One of the major voices in the early PAR movement was German ex-patriot Kurt Lewin who "first used the expression in his 1946 paper "Action Research and Minority Problems" (Chevalier & Buckles, 2019, p. 19). He and his colleagues transformed research by embedding social action into the process. Thus, the name "Action Research." Another German thinker who comes on the scene in the 1950s is Jürgen Habermas. Along with Freire and others, he influences the development of a form of PAR known as the "Critical–Emancipatory" school. As Chevalier and Buckles write, "Practitioners inspired by the works of Habermas … have also stressed the socially critical mission of PAR. They make a compelling case for the infusion of critical theory into PAR, motivated by 'a deep concern to overcome social injustice'" (2019, p. 49).

As delineated in Chapters 2–6, EDT utilizes PAR as a way to bring in members of the community being studied as co-researchers on the projects. This democratizes the process and enhances the potential for emancipatory experience. This reflects the notion that "The principal modality of action research is tacitly 'participative and democratic, working with participants and towards knowledge in action'" (Chevalier & Buckles, 2019, p. 24). Although perhaps imperfectly implemented, especially in the early projects, the fundamental philosophy of PAR has been fully embraced by our EDT approach.

Mienczakowski and his team had previously espoused "Participatory Experiential and Compelling Action Research" for their own projects in the mid-1990s (Mienczakowski & Morgan, 2001). In our 2007–2018 research with participants with developmental disabilities at The Centre for the Arts in Human Development (see Table 2.1), we began to locate ways to specifically adapt PAR for that population. It also seemed like a very useful approach in terms of creating a sense of self-advocacy in our participants. This concurs with the findings of Cock and Cockram (1995) in regard to using PAR with individuals with developmental and intellectual disabilities. These authors state that "participatory research may have usefulness through the medium of advocacy efforts, particularly those of self-advocacy and self-help … Participatory processes and methodologies are intrinsically empowering and thus directly relevant to the struggles of these groups" (pp. 33–34). We certainly witnessed the empowering effect on our informant co-researchers at CAHD. In fact, from this research study we developed a documentary entitled "Empowering Adults with Developmental Disabilities."[1]

As with each of the philosophical frameworks discussed in this chapter, ultimately the grand philosophical schemata are boiled down to methods to be put into practice. In the case of PAR, the large ideas and ideals of social action and social justice are distilled into ways of adapting PAR processes to the specific group in the community that is the focus of the research study. It is important, I believe, for the students of EDT to have awareness of both the big concepts and the practices derived from them in order to fully comprehend the praxis of EDT. PAR is an essential component of EDT and another tool for actualizing the humanistic values instilled in the philosophy of "Emancipation."

Moreno's Philosophy of Spontaneity–Creativity and His Method of Sociometry

Much of the previous discussion of philosophical ideas in this chapter is derived from concepts already explored in the works of Mienczakowski. I am highly indebted to him for his exegesis of these important philosophical and methodological perspectives. They have significantly shaped my own development of EDT. It is at this point that I truly add something new – the philosophical ideas of J.L. Moreno regarding Spontaneity–Creativity and his theory and practice of sociometry. As the reader will see, these latter have become foundational constructs in EDT.

Moreno is most well-known for his creation of psychodrama. I have been studying psychodrama, off and on, for nearly 40 years. I have been very fortunate to have studied with some of the great masters of this tradition. However, it is only quite recently that I have come to understand the profound significance of sociometry to the philosophy of Spontaneity–Creativity that

---

1 This documentary is available through **psychotherapy.net**. Simply type in "Snow" and you can see a sample section or rent the streaming of the whole documentary.

Moreno created. A few years back, I attended a psychodrama conference in New York City. The opening address was given by Dr. Robert Siroka, a major disciple of Moreno. With a kind of impersonation of Moreno (deceased at that time), Siroka proclaimed, "I get them in with psychodrama, but what I want to teach them is *Sociometry*!" Since then, I have learned what a powerful approach sociometry is to the service of social and psychological emancipation and how deeply it is rooted in Moreno's grand vision for a therapy to serve the world-at-large: "A truly therapeutic procedure cannot have less an objective than the whole of mankind" (Moreno, 1953/1993, p. 3).

Mienczakowski does mention Moreno once in his dissertation where he reviews how "Within the spheres of psychodrama (Moreno, 1977; Ruscombe-King, 1983) and emancipatory theatre (Boal, 1979) the main focus of performance practice is to engage in therapy through critical self-reflection" (1995a, p. 53). I have taken this nascent reflection on the therapeutic potential in ethnodrama and developed it into a full-fledged therapeutic program in EDT. This therapeutic framework is profoundly indebted to Moreno's thinking.

Moreno's "Philosophy" of Spontaneity–Creativity

How is Moreno's theorization around Spontaneity–Creativity a philosophy? One has only to read a little of Moreno's writing on this topic to understand what a deep, all-pervasive world view he has established. It is a paradigm of how the world works in terms of human development and interaction. Garcia and Buchanan (2009) in their analysis of Moreno's "Canon of Creativity," cite a core principle, "In Morenean philosophy anxiety is caused by the breach between the First and Second Universe. Moreno referred to anxiety as cosmic hunger to maintain identity with the entire universe" (p. 400). These two major psychodramatists are relating this construct to Moreno's grand conception of spontaneity in the child (First Universe) who doesn't see a separation between herself and the world. The psychological development of this separation (The Second Universe) is the beginning of alienation and potential pathology (anxiety). As adults we lose our spontaneity and its retrieval is the purpose of psychodrama as a therapeutic tool.

The grand conception of spontaneity in Moreno's work, in fact, begins to take on a theological tone. In discussing how spontaneity and creativity never come perfectly together in human experience, he writes, "God is an exceptional case because in God all spontaneity has become creativity. He is the one case in which spontaneity and creativity are identical" (1953/1993, p. 11). It is important to see that Moreno had deified spontaneity as identical with the Prime Mover of the universe.

In *Psychodrama, First Volume*, Moreno states, "It is evident that a spontaneous creative process is the matrix and the initial stage of any cultural conserve – whether a form of religion, a work of art or a technological invention" (1946, p. 109). Ontologically, Moreno sees spontaneity at the core of all human experience and culture. It is the source of cultural creations like the three named above. The problem is that people get stuck in these **culture conserves** and at some point, they become "Mind-forged Manacles" that block future creativity; they become the social webs that deny the potential for human freedom. This concept may be one of the most important in Moreno's philosophy. It predicates the requirement for "Spontaneity Training" that is at the core of Moreno's methods. As he cites, "Spontaneity 'training' is therefore the most auspicious skill to be taught to therapists in all our institutions of learning and it is his task to teach his clients how to be more spontaneous without becoming excessive" (1953/1993, p. 14).

Moreno has literally written volumes on his paradigm of Spontaneity–Creativity (to get some perspective on this, see the bibliography of Moreno at the Countway Medical Library at Harvard University[2]). It is a philosophy in the sense of the definition of such in the *Oxford Dictionary of English*: "The study of the fundamental nature of knowledge, reality and existence" (2005, p. 1323). In Moreno's conception, it is the very basis of human existence and is the cause of both evolution and devolution. His methods are aimed to promote social evolution through the emancipation of the individuals from the imprisoning grasp of the culture conserves; to promote greater creative thinking on both the social and individual level.

How is Sociometry Born out of the Spontaneity–Creativity Paradigm?

Moreno clearly answers this question. He tells us "The cornerstones of sociometric conceptualization are the universal concepts of spontaneity and creativity. Sociometry has taken these concepts from the metaphysical and philosophical level and brought them to empirical test by means of the sociometric method" (1953/1993, p. 11). The twin concepts of spontaneity and creativity are the matrix for the method. Again, this is another example of the distillation of method from philosophy. Some of the techniques of

---

2 See full collection of Moreno's writings at www.morenomuseum.org/en/content/harvard-library-jacob-l-moreno-papers-1906-1911-1977.

sociometry have been discussed in previous chapters; however, here, I want to give a quintessential formulation of sociometry and its great value to EDT.

Sociometry as the word implies, is the measurement of relations in a group of people, whether society as a whole on the macro level or the small therapy group on the micro level. However, the idea of measurement – 'empirical test' as stated above – barely touches the surface of what Moreno means by this term. Sociometry is ultimately a means of healing the group and the individuals within it, with the goal of moving from dysfunction to healthy functioning, based on deep mutual understanding between group members. This can work on the macro level and the micro level. On the macro level, according to Moreno's thinking, "With the cooperation of 'all' the people we should be able to create a social order worthy of the highest aspirations of our times. This is the meaning of revolutionary, dynamic sociometry" (1953/1993, p. 29). This is the "political" framework for Moreno's method. On the micro level, this means achieving the most positive outcome for the group therapy process. EDT can be regarded, in this light, as a group therapy practice. In Habermasian terms, sociometry is applied to create the greatest potential for the "ideal speech situation."

It is through Moreno's many ways of measuring "social networks" and his techniques for creating positive models for the same that EDT can find immense value in sociometry. Psychodrama and sociodrama are both tools for establishing deep *communicative action* and *ideal speech situations* in the small groups that are the focus of any given EDT project. Finally, it is important to note that, within his work in sociometry, Moreno himself created a form of ethnodrama.

Moreno's Version of Ethnodrama

At the very beginning of his great tome, *Who Shall Survive?*, Moreno makes an important statement of what will be included in his study of sociometry theory and practice, "Among the sociatric approaches, particular attention will be given to group psychotherapy, psychodrama, sociodrama and *ethnodrama*" (Italics mine, 1953/1993, p. xxii). This is the first time I had ever observed the term, ethnodrama, in his writings. However, searching through the whole 325-page volume, I have not been able to find another use of it. So, what was ethnodrama for Moreno?

Moreno uses the adjective *sociatric* to frame his statement. This term is derived from the noun, *sociatry*, which means the treatment of group or social pathology. "Sociatry treats the pathological syndromes of normal society, of inter-related individuals and of inter-related groups" (Moreno, 1953/1993, p. 90). So, we know we are dealing with a group phenomena and social process. But what form does this take? Obviously, we get a clue from the first half of the terminology – *ethno*. We are dealing with cultural phenomena. Continuing my research on Moreno's particular usage of the term, I discovered a couple of articles by anthropologists, from the 1950s and the 1960s, respectively, as well as a more recent article on "Race Relations" in Brazil by two Brazilian psychodramatists.

The individual who actually first coined the term, *ethnodrama*, seems to have been anthropologist Joseph Bram. After observing psychodrama sessions at Moreno's New York Institute in the early 1950s, he realized the value of this approach to anthropological research. He writes:

> In this connection, I suggested to Dr. Moreno that psychodrama, when used in this context, should perhaps be identified under a separate name, such as ethnodrama. Dr. Moreno approved the idea and authorized me to bring my students from New York University to his Psychodrama Theatre for experimental sessions. In the meantime, I continued attending weekly sessions at the Institute and also took advantage of the Beacon Workshop for Training in Psychodrama.
>
> (1953, p. 255)

So, Bram, an anthropologist, became immersed in psychodrama and found a way to integrate it into his own cultural investigations. This is confirmed a decade later by another anthropologist, Jerry M. Rosenberg, who states that "Dr. J. Bram has suggested using this method as 'a tool for cross-cultural study of human behavior,' and has contributed the useful neologism 'ethnodrama'"(1962, p. 237). Rosenberg goes on to point out the value of this new method: "ethnodrama offers dramatic prospects for acquiring insights into a culture … Dr. Bram has already indicated progress in a research-project 'regarding the value-system and the personality' of an ethnic group in New York City"(1962, p. 243). And all this, more than 30 years before Mienczakowski used the term ethnodrama!

In my detective work on this issue, I have been able to locate one more article that employs the word ethnodrama as part of its research study. This case is particularly interesting as it deals with a clearly sociatric problem: tensions between the races in Brazil and, so, fits very well into Moreno's conception of a dynamic sociometry and how sociometric networks "have the function of shaping social tradition and public opinion" (Moreno, 1953/1993, p. 25). The study was exploring the tradition of racism in a specific cultural context.

In their 2016 article, the researchers specifically cite Moreno's "method for dealing with ethnic problems, called Ethnodrama, which he defines as 'a synthesis of psychodrama with the research of ethnic problems, conflicts of ethnic groups'" (Malaquias, Nonoyo & Cesarino, 2016, p. 92). I feel very fortunate to have found an English translation of this article that came out of a psychodrama conference in Brazil. I feel like EDT would have a great deal of sympatico with this Brazilian team's focus on ethnic conflict as the topic for an ethnodrama.

I believe that further research into how Moreno shaped his own concept of ethnodrama will be most valuable to the further development of EDT and how psychodrama, sociodrama and sociometry can be best integrated into this method.

Summary

We have reviewed some very grand philosophical concepts in this chapter. Perhaps what is most important is how these intellectual frameworks support and justify the actual praxis of EDT. Phenomenology, especially in its psychological and ethnographic iterations, is a crucial underlying perspective to EDT practice. The Critical–Emancipatory school of participatory action research embraces a philosophy of social change and social activism that are major components in EDT's agenda. Embedded in the whole evolutionary philosophical system is emancipatory critical theory. Sociometry with its accompanying techniques of psychodrama, sociodrama, and Moreno's version of ethnodrama, echo these approaches in their intention to actualize human freedom which is the paramount goal of EDT.

There are many interconnections, both theoretically and methodologically, between these various schools of thought. One significant example is the concept of "Nascent State" that is articulated by both Alberoni and Moreno. For Alberoni it represents a particular transitional moment in social structure when the status quo must be replaced by something new. For Moreno, it is part of the creative process, the moment when new ideas, images and forms are born; when they are still fragile and not solidified as a "culture conserve; when they still contain the spontaneity out of which they grew. The concept can be applied to both the social and individual goal of change that is at the heart of EDT. This connection will be further analyzed in Chapter 10.

What I have added to Mienczakowski's ethnodramatic approach is a dynamic therapeutic function which utilizes both drama therapy and psychodrama.

I am extremely indebted to Moreno for his conceptualization of sociometry. As I further include more sociometric theory and practice in my own work, I concur with Moreno's grand vision of the therapeutic procedure with evolutionary potential for all of humankind. I hope this will be at the center of the practice of EDT, as we seek to actualize emancipation for individuals and the groups that they live in. In the end, I have aimed to follow Aristotle's pronouncement, studying all of these philosophies and correspondent practices, with the "immediate and relevant purpose" of defining an effective synthesis – ethnodramatherapy.

References

Alberoni, F. (1984). *Institution and movement* (P. C. A. Delmoro, Trans.). Columbia University Press.

Aristotle. (1963). *The philosophy of Aristotle* (J. L. Creed & A. E. Wardman, Trans.). The New American Library (Original work published in 350 BCE).

Betensky, M. (1995). *What do you see? Phenomenology of therapeutic art expression.* Jessica Kingsley Publishers.

Blake, W. (1975). *The portable Blake* (A. Kazin, Ed.). The Viking Press.

Bram, J. (1953). The application of psychodrama to research in social anthropology. *The New York State Academy of Sciences, 15*(7): 253–257.

Chevalier, J. M., & Buckles, D. J. (2019). *Participatory action research: Theory and methods of engaged inquiry* (2nd ed.). Routledge.

Cock, E., & Cockram, J. (1995). The participatory research paradigm and intellectual disability. *BILD Publications, 8*(1), 25–37.

Denzin, N. K. (1997). *Interpretive ethnography: Ethnographic practices in the 21st Century.* Sage Publications.

Freire, P. (1974). *Education for critical consciousness.* Bloomsbury Academic.

Garcia, N., & Buchanan, D. R. (2009). Psychodrama. In D. R. Johnson & R. Emunah (Eds.), *Current approaches in drama therapy* (2nd ed., pp. 393–423). C. C. Thomas Publisher.

Geertz, C. (1973). *The interpretation of cultures.* Basic Books.

Giorgi, A. (2012). The descriptive phenomenological psychological method. *Journal of Phenomenological Psychology, 43*, 2–12.

Habermas, J. (1971). *Knowledge and human interests.* Beacon Press.

_____. (1986). *The theory of communicative action: Reason and the rationalization of society*. Polity Press.

Jürgen Habermas. (2020, December 29) In Wikipedia. https://en.wikipedia.org/wiki/J%C3%BCrgen_Habermas

Katz, J., & Csordas, T. J. (2003). Phenomenological ethnography in sociology and anthropology. *Ethnography, 4*(3), 275–288.

Landy, R. (1982). Training the drama therapist: A four-part model. *The Arts in Psychotherapy, 9*, 91–99.

Maggs-Rapport, F. (2000). Combining methodological approaches in research: Ethnography and interpretive phenomenology. *Journal of Advanced Nursing, 31*(1), 219–225.

Malaquisas, M. C., Nonoya, D. S., & Cesarino, A. C. (2016). Psychodrama and race relations. *Revista Brasileira de Psicodrama, 24*(2), 91–100.

Maso, I. (2007). Phenomenology and ethnography. In P. Atkinson, A. Coffey, S. Delamont, J. Lofland & L. Lofland (Eds.), *Handbook of ethnography* (pp. 136–144). Sage Publications.

McTaggart, R. (Ed.). (1997). *Participatory action research: International contexts and consequences*. State University of New York Press.

Mendieta, E. (2019). The unfinished project of enlightenment; Jürgen Haberman at 90. *Los Angeles Review of Books*, 1–12. https://lareviewofbooks.org/article.unfinished-project-Enlightenment-jurgen-habermas-90/.

Mienczakowski, J. (1995a). *The application of critical ethno-drama to health settings*. [Unpublished doctoral dissertation]. Griffith University, Australia.

Mienczakowski, J., & Morgan, S. (2001). Ethnodrama: Constructing participatory action, experiential and compelling action research through performance. In P. Reason & H. Bradbury (Eds.), *Handbook of action research: Participative inquiry and practice*. Sage Publications.

Mienczakowski, J., Smith, R., & Sinclair, M. (1996). On the road to catharsis: A theoretical framework of change. *Qualitative Inquiry, 2*(4), 439–462.

Moreno, J. L. (1946). *Psychodrama, First Volume*. Beacon House.

_____. (1993). *Who shall survive?: Foundations of sociometry, group therapy and sociodrama*. American Society of Group Psychotherapy and Psychodrama. (Original work published 1953).

Moustakas, C. (1994). *Phenomenological research methods*. Sage Publications.

Oxford Dictionary of English. (2005). (2nd ed. Revised). Oxford University Press.

Rosenberg, J. (1962). Ethnodrama as a research method in anthropology. *Group Psychotherapy*, *15*(3), 236–243.

van Manen, M. (2016). *Researching lived experience: Human science for an action sensitive pedagogy* (2nd ed). Routledge.

Zahavi, D. (2019). *Phenomenology: The basics*. Routledge.

Part IV
Integration and Future Possibilities

10

Integrating Research, Therapy, Theatre and Social Activism into One Method

Expression Necessary to Evolution.
(Attributed to Charles Wesley Emerson, Founder of Emerson
College of Oratory, 1880)

Introduction: Moving Forward or Evolution

These words, "Expression Necessary to Evolution" were emblazoned on my consciousness when I was a freshman at Emerson College in 1964. They are the motto of my college. Over the years, I have often thought of them in different contexts and this deep thought, "Expression is necessary to evolution," has carried multiple meanings for me. In the context of couples counselling, it means that moment when unspoken emotions of resentment and anger are *expressed*, and a couple can move forwards to develop their relationship. For a writer, it means that moment when she finds her true voice and can continue to evolve as an artist, *expressing* her unique individuality. In terms of human evolution, it is the *expression* of those new ideas – new breakthroughs in consciousness – that move us forward as a species. In this chapter, I am going to apply it to the emancipatory potential of ethnodramatherapy and discuss it in relation to human evolution.

When I matriculated at Emerson College in the mid-1960s, it still had one foot in the 19th century. To this day, one of my favorite memories is the wonderful old actor, Will Geer, giving a reading of Walt Whitman's poetry in our carriage house theatre behind 130 Beacon Street. The school had evolved from Boston Conservatory of Elocution, Oratory and Dramatic Art in the 1880s. Even in the 1960s, one had to study Voice and Articulation, Public Speaking and the Oral Interpretation of Literature. This intense focus on Voice and Speech was derived from the passion for the arts of Oratory, Rhetoric, Voice Culture and the Oral Interpretation of Literature of

DOI: 10.4324/9781003083818-14

the school's founder, Charles Wesley Emerson, for whom the college was eventually named. He is an interesting mid-19th-century figure. A distant cousin of Ralph Waldo Emerson, he was a Unitarian minister, earned an MD from the University of Pennsylvania, and was profoundly engaged in the study of Voice and Speech ("Charles Wesley Emerson," 2020). Around the turn of the century, he published a booklet entitled *Evolution of Expression* (1905/1964). It is in this short work that Charles Wesley Emerson articulates his ideas about evolution and its relation to "expression."

By "expression," he meant the full force of the voice to catalyze feeling, thought, spirituality and "enlightenment" in the person. His two major vehicles were Oratory and the Oral interpretation of Literature. Early in the short treatise, he writes:

> These principles of natural evolution have been applied by the writer to the study of oratory ... [the orator] can not escape the necessity of cultivating his powers by the same process of evolution which the race needed centuries to pass through.
>
> (1905/1964, p. 7)

Born in 1837, Charles Wesley must have been coming of age not long after Darwin published his *Origin of the Species* 1847. His writing is steeped in evolutionary thought, colored with a touch of New England Transcendentalism and a dash of Swedenborg. A little later on in the tract, he quotes his famous cousin, "The individual repeats in himself the history of the race" (1905/1964, p. 9). This, of course, is a paraphrase of the well-known "principle of recapitulation," popular in that era, which states that "ontogeny repeats phylogeny" (Simpson & Beck, 1965, p. 240). Charles Wesley was searching for a way for his original thinking on the dynamics of Speech and Voice to be related to the new perspectives on human evolution in his times. As a theologian, he saw his work on oral expression as a way to inspire "the soul." His concluding statement in the booklet, reveals his spiritual outlook on the powers of Voice and Speech:

> When the speaker has become a free channel for truth, a transparent medium for high thought, then his forms of expression no longer call attention to themselves, but lend themselves in perfect service. The everlasting thirst of the soul is to be free.
>
> (1905/1964, p. 42)

I hope the reader will indulge me in this little reminiscence and a brief detour into 19th-century thought. I think it is important to understand the original intellectual background of this phrase, "Expression Necessary to Evolution," before I apply it to a wider and more contemporary framework.

Charles Wesley Emerson's maxim was couched in Victorian idealism, poetic vision and 19th-century evolutionary thinking. Times change. This is the nature of evolution. We build on the great thinkers that come before us. We correct their mistakes, aiming to produce a more lucid, enlightening and truthful portrait of life. We move forward.

As an example of times changing, let me report a brief experience that really changed my personal perspective on a social issue and opened me up to want to use EDT for a new theme.

A Personal Expression with Social Consequence

In 2020, the president of Emerson College was an African American scholar and educator, Dr. M. Lee Pelton. He holds a Ph.D. from Harvard University and has been both dean and college president at several other institutions. He is a dynamic administrator who has vigorously pushed Emerson into the 21st-century. However, on May 31, 2020, he wrote to the community as a Black man in deep pain. Here are his own words:

> I didn't sleep Friday night. Instead, I spent the night, like a moth drawn to a flame, looking again and again at the video of George Floyd's murder at the hands of a Minneapolis white police officer. It was a legalized lynching. I also intently watched the fiery protests in American cities. America is on fire, I thought. Even in the face of a viral pandemic that had closed down much of human society, it could not stop a black man from being murdered in public view […] I watched the video over and over again well into the morning hours because I was mesmerized by the casualness with which the Minneapolis police officer Derek Chauvin murdered George Floyd. Chauvin dug his knee into his neck for almost nine minutes, even as Floyd repeatedly said, "I can't breathe. I can't breathe." As he called on his Mama before he took his last breath, Chauvin continued to talk, he looked as if he didn't have a care in the world. He didn't stop until Floyd was unresponsive.
>
> George Floyd was invisible. And it was his invisibility, a brutal white power structure and Chauvin's dehumanization of him that killed him.
>
> Floyd has a history. And so do I.
>
> I was born in a house that had no indoor plumbing until I was six years old. Until they died, my mother and both of my grandmothers cleaned houses for middle class and rich white folks. My father was a laborer until he got a good paying job working at the City of Wichita, Kansas, where I was born and raised.
>
> In my lifetime, I have been called the n-word by white people in every state and every city that I have ever lived in.

I have been pulled over driving while black more times than I can remember. I have been spit on by a white parking lot attendant. I was stopped 20 feet from my house by two white police officers in their cruiser, the searing heat of their spot lights on the back of my neck, guns drawn on either side of my car because I looked like a black man who was alleged to have stolen something from a convenience store. When I was living on the West Coast, I was pulled over twice in a single night by police officers because, according to each, I didn't turn on my turn signal the proper feet before a stop sign. As President of Willamette University, two teenage boys drove up on the sidewalk to block my path home because I looked like someone who was suspected of stealing from neighborhood homes. When I asked what that person looked like they described someone more than twenty years younger than me. While visiting my cousins in Conway, Arkansas in the '70s, I suffered the deep humiliation of having to go to the back alley of a local restaurant to order food. I was twenty years old. I was angry at the overt racism and at my cousins for enduring such indignities almost a decade after the passages of the two Civil Rights Acts of the mid-'60s [...]

What happened to George Floyd is not new. It is as old as 250 years of slavery and the Jim Crow laws that sought to marginalize and shut out black Americans from American society.

As my wise friend reminded me, quoting James Baldwin, "Any real change implies the breaking of the world as one has always known it, the loss of all that gave one an identity, the end of safety."

Black folks are sick and tired of being sick and tired.

So, I have no words of comfort today because they would be inauthentic. They would absolve so many from coming to terms with their own silent complicity in the world in which we live.

As I wrote to someone today, "This is not a black problem, but a structural issue built on white supremacy and centuries of racism. It's your problem. And until you understand that, we are doomed to relive this week's tragic events over and over again. What changes will you make in your own life? Begin with answering that question and maybe, just maybe we will get somewhere."

The most important question is: What are **you** going to do?
(Alumni Monthly News Letter: Special Edition, June 15, 2020)[1]

---

1 To read Dr. Pelton's complete letter go to https://today.emerson.edu/2020/06/01/letter-to-the-emerson-community-may-31-2020/.

I was profoundly moved by Dr. Pelton's letter. Along with the events of those days in May/June 2020, his deep, sincere, personal expression of his own emotions touched me in a way that motivated and inspired me. I was about to turn 75-years-old. I knew, then and there, I wanted to spend rest of my life finding effective ways to work on eradicating systemic racism. I want to use the method I have developed, EDT, to create empathy and emancipatory potential in relation to this deeply engrained social issue. "Expression Necessary to Evolution" took on a whole new meaning for me.

"Expression Necessary to Evolution" in a Wider Frame

Charles Wesley Emerson was inspired by the exciting new thinking on evolution in his day. He saw the power of speech communication as effecting the evolutionary process. His emphasis on speech to create change in human culture will, hopefully, become more relevant when I shortly connect it to Habermas' emancipatory concept of "The Ideal Speech Situation."

The power of speech and language changed the whole course of human evolution. As the Israeli historian Yuval Noah Harari writes: "The appearance of new ways of thinking and communicating, between 70,000 and 30,000 years ago, constitutes the Cognitive Revolution. What caused it?" (2014, p. 21). This nodal point in the history of human evolution was clearly related to the emergence of speech and language. Harari goes on to say, "The most common answer is that our language is amazingly supple. We can connect a limited number of sounds and signs to produce an infinite number of sentences, each with a distinct meaning" (2014, p. 22). The advent of language is what distinguishes humankind from the rest of the animal world, especially in terms of the human evolutionary trajectory. The power to cooperate on massive scales is the result of our language communication skills. It is our astounding speech/language function of "expression" that predicates all the advances in human cultures or what the palaeontologist Teilhard de Chardin calls the "hominization" of the planet (1965). De Chardin also points to the development of our speech/language capacity as a kind of spiritual principle. He states, "The impetus of the world, glimpsed in the great drive of consciousness, can only have its ultimate source in some *inner* principle, which alone can explain its irreversible advance towards higher psychisms" (1965, p. 149). In my interpretation, he is saying it is the power of internal thought, or consciousness, that is responsible for the intensive evolution of humans and that progress in human society happens through its expression in speech/language. Is this so far from Charles Wesley Emerson's dictum? For de Chardin, the process is stated in his formula: "geogenesis to biogenesis to psychogenesis." However, it is now, from our 30,000-year-old utilization of speech, that, in our present phase of "psychogenesis," we can advance the evolution of the species. And this is in the framework of what de Chardin designates as the "**Noosphere**." It is that space of emancipatory potential, like Charles Wesley Emerson's "The everlasting thirst of the soul to be free …," where humanity as a whole has the potential to function on the highest level of communication, sharing and empathy. De Chardin calls this "the progressive, phyletic spiritualisation in human civilisation of all the forces contained in the animal world" (1965, p. 180). And he attributes this immense emancipatory potential to "categorical expression in consciousness and through the voice of the species" (1965, p. 306). Another way of saying, "Expression Necessary to Evolution."

Social Evolution via Public Voice Ethnography

Coming right back to the manifold challenges of humanity today, I want to look on a very grounded level as to how the theory of expression effectively catalyzing evolution can be put to work. As described in previous chapters, the value of EDT, as "Public Voice Ethnography," can bring about change on a social level as a form of social activism. As a form of group therapy, EDT can also effect change in the individual, catalyzing growth and healing. Expression is a very significant construct in the study of how change occurs in psychotherapy. As Armstrong and her colleagues have written: "emotional expression is necessary for therapeutic change to occur … Emotional expression is beneficial to clients when combined with emotional processing" (Armstrong et al., 2015, p. 149). When we are able to speak with and/or act out our lived experience of emotional pain with a therapist, we can foster personal growth. Later, I will pursue this important theme of individual psychological development through deep self-expression and how to measure its therapeutic effectiveness. Presently, I want to focus on the aspect of collective, social evolution.

As said, I was deeply moved by the analysis of "Racism in America" by Dr. Lee Pelton in his powerful self-revelatory letter. It made me want to work on this issue through the EDT process, aiming to create the "Ideal Speech Situation," as formulated by Habermas, in order to actualize a transformative conversation about race.

Following Mienczakowski's earliest theorizing about the emancipatory potential of ethnodrama, it is clear that he sees the construction of the "Ideal Speech Situation" as key. He devotes ten pages of his dissertation to defining this concept (1995a, pp. 40–49). He largely follows the analysis of Habermas' translator, Thomas McCarthy, who articulates "The conditions of the Ideal Speech Situation" and further elucidates the meaning of this construct: "The conditions of the ideal speech situation must insure not only unlimited discussion but also discussion which is free from all constraints of domination, whether the source be conscious strategic behavior or communication barriers secured through ideology or neurosis" (1973, pp. 145–146). What is implied, here, is a context of fundamental respect without any pressures to dominate the other party in the dialogue; rather, an openness and willingness to listen to the other party's point of view. Mienczakowski sees this as "another method of assessing consciousness" (1995a, p. 41). Both Mienczakowski and McCarthy are excellent interpreters of Habermas, but perhaps it is best to let this "master thinker" speak for himself. In his book, *Moral Consciousness and Communicative Action*, Habermas delineates his concept of the "ideal situation":

> The agreement made possible by discourse depends on two things. The individual's inalienable right to say yes or no and his overcoming of his egocentric viewpoint. Without the individual's uninfringeable freedom to respond "yes" or "no" to criticizable validity claims, consent is merely factual rather than truly universal. Conversely, without empathic sensitivity by each person to everyone else, no solution deserving universal consent will result from the deliberation.
>
> (1990, p. 202)

In EDT, such a situation is the result of opening a dialogue among audience members who have witnessed a research-based theatre performance that deals with a controversial social issue. The post-performance forum is designed to bring about a consensus, in order to strategize together, on how to create social action to solve the problem. The "Ideal Speech Situation" provides a framework for building a consensus on changing ideas, attitudes, policies and perspectives and putting a new program into action. Thus, it is a key factor in creating change in ethnodrama, and, subsequently, EDT.

The Shape and Content of the Post-Performance Forum

However, it is never a perfect situation. Over the past 15 years, we have aimed to create post-performance forums that provide the audience with as much safety as possible, and with a framework for open discussion. We often start with a written questionnaire that guarantees full confidentiality through a coding system. These responses are later analyzed to provide us with information on the educational value of the experience of witnessing the play (see Chapters 5 and 6). After this we go into an open Q & A discussion with the audience. Often, I have asked experts on the topic to be part of a panel. For instance, in the June 2018 performance of "Through the Eyes of Caregivers," I invited two psychiatrists, a high school student who is an advocate for the de-stigmatization of mental illness, a family caregiver and the executive director of an agency for mental health advocacy. There were many carers and mental health professionals in the audience. Serious comments and questions were presented on how and why "the system of mental health services" needs to be changed.[2] Perhaps, we should have had a government mental health administrator there as well. The provisional "Ideal Speech Situation" must be shaped to evoke new ideas on how to best change a system and how to establish actions to realize these ideas. And, of course, there must be follow-up to see that the proposed actions are implemented. Mostly, this latter activity has been beyond the scope of our EDT projects.

In the situation, itself, in that moment when performers, audience members and professional experts meet, a nexus for change is created, however imperfect. It is a manifestation of what Habermas recognizes as an "ideal community of communication" (1990, p. 202), where freedom of expression and respect for each other's point of view are inherent in the communicative process. In discussing the influence of Habermas on his own work, Mienczakowski states, "My take on the ideal grounds for human communicative competence aspect, therefore, has been that ethnodrama provides an avenue for collective, emancipatory dialogue" (J. Mienczakowski, personal communication, March 30, 2021). This modest and limited appraisal for the potential of the "Ideal Speech Situation" is also the case for EDT.

Integration Model #1: Wearing All Four Hats at Once

My Personal Integration

Combining my 35 years' experience in drama therapy and therapeutic theatre with my training in performance ethnography represents a genuine personal integration for me. As described in Chapter 1, I have had significant trainings in theatre, performance studies, performance theory and performance ethnography, as well as drama therapy and psychodrama. Putting all of this together in the past 15 years has been my personal journey of integration.

---

2 This post-performance forum session can be viewed in the documentary, *For Those Who Care*, to be released in 2022. Please contact the author at stephen.snow@concordia.ca for further information.

It has allowed me to wear "four hats at once," with all the challenges and complications that can involve. The "four hats," here, are an analogue for the four roles of the ethnodramatherapist: drama therapist, researcher, theatre artist and social activist (see Figure 3.1). The latter has been the most recently developed role, or it can be seen as a return to a role that was very alive for me as a young man in the 1960s and 1970s.

A Re-Awakened Social Activist

The social activist role has been re-awakened in me because of three historical factors (1) a toxic presidency in the USA that became a threat to democracy; (2) the stark reality of the global climate crisis; and (3) the irrefutable identification of systemic racism in America that emerged in 2020. As said, I was profoundly moved by the raw and lucid letter of Dr. Lee Pelton, responding to the televised murder of George Floyd on May 25, 2020. I think, like for myself, many people took this naked revelation of the systemic racism in our world as a clarion call for collective action.

I have said "re-awakened," as in my twenties I was very involved in the anti-Vietnam war movement. I was committed to the focus on social justice in the Civil Rights movement. In graduate school, in my thirties, I was engaged in the anti-Nuclear Proliferation movement. I always felt a deep connection with the environmental movement, but more in a philosophical way than in an activist role. By my mid-forties, I was so involved in developing a Centre for the Arts in Human Development and a graduate program in drama therapy, I found time for little else. It took up all of my energy. My focus was in the arts as tools for personal healing – the creative arts therapies – which had become my career. I looked for transformation on a personal and spiritual level through Jungian analysis and meditation.

However, being a professor for three decades and constantly hearing the voices of the younger generations, I was made aware of contemporary issues of gender prejudice, racial inequality and other social issues. I was not unsympathetic to the call for social change. I just was not an activist. It took my engagement in ethnodrama to begin to rekindle the flame of social activism in me. It was the development of EDT that refocused my attention on how to develop programs to catalyze social change. There were parallels to my experience in other senior members of the drama therapy community. David Read Johnson, in his introduction to the recently released *Current Approaches in Drama Therapy* (3rd ed.), describes a new emergence of social consciousness that has occurred in the field of drama therapy in North America:

This transformation is primarily driven by a greater awareness and deeper commitment of younger generations to the state of the world. The greater attention to psychological, cultural, systemic and historical trauma has also had an influence. Several of the pioneers who initially developed clinically-oriented approaches have found ways of extending their work into social justice areas…

(2020, pp. 18–19)

Johnson mentions ethnodramatherapy as one of the methods that focus on social justice. I am proud to be named as part of this group of "re-awakened" senior drama therapists. I feel truly motivated, at this point in my life, to use my integrated method to work on issues such as systemic racism and the ecological crisis. Whatever wisdom in drama therapy I have garnered over the past 35 years, I want to put it, now, towards social change, especially in these two areas.

The Challenges of Wearing Four Hats at Once

The model of EDT I have created, going back to 2005, has always had me wearing all four hats. I was the principal investigator (research), the supervising drama therapist (therapy), the theatre director (theatre), and with the inclusion of the participatory action research framework, I was the guide (social activist), leading the process towards realizing the end goals of social change. Over a decade, I got used to this balancing act and, I would say there were, in fact, some great values to this unitary approach. The primary one was the unity of vision that could be sustained by one person overseeing all four functions of EDT. It is the same rationale for having only one director in theatre. The potentials for harm are also the same: the emergence of authoritarianism and the misuse and abuse of power by one person who controls everything. It could also be said the ethical quandaries in EDT are perhaps amplified by the one-person-in-charge model (see Chapter 8). The four functions (see Figure 1.4) can very easily come into conflict, most especially, the theatre artist with the therapist, the researcher with the therapist, and the researcher with the theatre artist. These moments of conflict can be intense and painful. I can bear witness to this with the case examples of such that I have written about in Chapter 8, where I felt the excruciating discomfort between the conflicting roles of therapist and theatre director in specific moments. These instances could perhaps provide arguments for having different individuals in the different roles. At least, then, the conflicts could be resolved between separate persons and not only within the one person in charge of everything. It's a big question and one that I will take up, shortly.

Some Specific Challenges for the Ethnographer

Ethnography like anthropology has come into some disrepute in recent years. I addressed this briefly in Chapter 1 (Trouillot, 1991). There is a kind of animosity towards these fields from the younger generation who see resonances of colonialism, racism and prejudice, especially in white North Americans and European "authorities" investigating the cultural realities of non-white cultures. "Who has the right to speak for another culture that is not one's own?" This is the big question. I was trained in ethnography as part of my doctoral work in performance studies (Snow, 1993). I have taken pride in and enjoyed my work in other cultures. So, these negative attitudes towards ethnography have been painful for me. I certainly agree with some of the thinking around anti-colonialism and anti-white supremacy, but I believe very strongly that ethnography still has its place as a valid social science. The researcher in EDT is mostly a phenomenological ethnographer. For myself, I wish to use the performance ethnography methods in EDT to support the correction of social injustices, and I believe they can do that.

So, for a few years, now, I have been searching for new issues that would be worthwhile to explore in EDT. In August 2015, I went to see a New York City International Fringe Festival theatre piece, entitled "Exact Change: Changing Your Gender Isn't as Hard as Changing Your Mind." It was written and performed by Christine Howey, a person who had transitioned from male to female, earlier in her life. It was a formidable self-revelatory performance about her life's experience, her painful identity crises, periods of suicidal ideation, and the relief of finally living in her "true body." She was seventy years old when she performed it. I was deeply moved by the piece. In the very last part of the production, Christine, via a screened PowerPoint, presented the horrific statistics on suicide, abuse and murder of transgender persons. It was shattering. I was moved to want to create an EDT process for "the correction of social injustice" that I saw depicted at the end of the play. I felt very motivated, but the big question was, "Can I find a group of transgender people to work with me?" "How would I go about doing this?" I began to research the topic. I read the National Geographic Special Edition on the "Gender Revolution" (2017). I began to meet with transgender individuals to gauge the feasibility of such a project. I reviewed newspaper stories like that of Canadian actor Elaine Page changing her name to Elliot and asking to be addressed as "him/his" (Rosenberg, December 5, 2020, p. B7). I approached some of my students who identified as "transgender." I did the normal preliminary work that any ethnographer would do. In the end, I got the culminating response, "Who are you to direct a project on us? You are not one of us!"

This was a huge challenge to me in the role of ethnographic researcher. It brought up many questions for me. It brought up the whole concept and practice of **cultural humility** (see definition in Glossary). I had really wanted to make use of my ethnographic skills to create an authentic portrait of the lived experience of transgender persons. I wanted to make a public audience more aware of the social injustices they face. Hadn't I already done this for adults with developmental disabilities and female adolescents in Youth Protection? However, I was being told, "You are not one of us, so you can not create an authentic portrait of our lives!" I was being challenged to the core of my ethnographic bones! I thought, "Wouldn't *informant validation* empower them and put the control in their hands?" "Was I being a *colonialist* wanting to invade *their* world?" "Was my interest in their lives more prurient than scientific?" I really wanted to do this project, and I probably should have stuck to my original motivation, having been so moved by Christine Howey's story. In the end, I let it go, under the rationalization, "This is not the right place and time for me to do this."

This experience brought up another big question for me, "Am I really limited in the roles I can play – in the number of hats I can wear – in EDT? I had formulated the method out of my own life's experiences as an integrated approach with one leader. I had done this for more than 15 years, but was there a better way? After the disappointment of letting go of the potential transgender project, I really began to think this through.

Integration Model #2: Sharing the Four Hats with Individual Team Members

Another Point of View

The idea was dawning on me that it might be better to share the main roles amongst different members of a team where, perhaps, four individuals would take one role, each. In fact, during a 6-hour workshop on EDT at the North American Drama Therapy Association, in Philadelphia, in 2019, a seasoned drama therapist, Carlos Rodriguez Perez, suggested just such a model. For that day, I had two young assistants, sometimes taking over the roles of therapist or theatre director. So, Carlos' point struck home. Why not create a team where one person is the researcher, one the therapist, a third, the theatre artist, and a fourth, the guide for social activism. Why had I not thought of this before? It seemed so obvious.

A New Model for EDT Emerges

Because I had been so immersed for 15 years in doing EDT a certain way, largely as portrayed in Chapters 2–7, I had not conceived of a team approach where roles could be divided into four. Perhaps, it was also my egocentric ownership of the method that I have been in the process of creating during all that time that prevented me from seeing an obvious possibility. At this point, however, in 2019, it began to make sense. Now, I was ready to plunge into such a hypothetical model. I could see developing a team approach along the lines of participatory action research. Such a cooperative approach has been articulated by Chevalier and Buckles: "We espouse the idea of partnering creatively, towards the *interfacing* of views, goals, skill sets and forms of knowledge and experience that can be brought to bear and evolve through action research" (2019, p. 27). In this model, each major function of EDT would be guided by a team leader who would be responsible for realizing the methods and goals of their assigned function, even while working with all the team as co-researchers in accordance with the PAR perspective.

By 2019, I had already started to do some of this creative partnering by co-authoring the chapter on "Ethnodramatherapy" for *Current Approaches in Drama Therapy* (3rd ed.) with a younger colleague. In co-authoring this chapter with Jessica Bleuer, I was able to have the advantage of Jessica's substantial knowledge of the "critical social consciousness frame" and, together, we adapted this dynamic framework to the EDT process. As she states in the chapter's section on "Best Practices in Critical Ethnodramatherapy", "the *critical social consciousness frame* reminds us of our interdependence, and that unequal power dynamics left unacknowledged will ultimately undermine social justice as well as therapeutic potential" (2020, p. 269). In other words, the process of the team will be a model for implementing a democratic social process in the community through EDT. It is an idealistic perspective in regard to human cooperation and communication, and quite like the concept of Habermas' "Ideal Speech Situation," where there is empathy and sensitivity and no pressures to dominate, either "through ideology or neurosis." This was a very significant contribution to the further development of EDT theory and practice, and I feel indebted to my younger colleagues who have assisted in this task.[3] My eyes have been opened to a more collaborative,

3 Both Jessica Bleuer and Simon Driver, the second assistant at the 2019 NADTA conference, have been instrumental in the development of EDT. They are in training with me to become EDT directors. I am delighted to have these two talented drama therapy teachers and practitioners engaged in the further development of EDT.

interdependent way of doing EDT. I still have some doubts about this highly collegial approach, as it has yet to be tested, but my basic feeling is that it could be, and may well be, the optimal way of doing EDT.

New Complexities with Ethics

A more collaborative, collegial approach also brings with it some new, complex ethical issues. There would now be four sets of eyes reviewing ethical challenges emerging in the process. Team members would need to come together and become acquainted with each others' values and principles. This would necessitate the kind of open and honest interpersonal communication mentioned above. An agreement would need to be made on which code of ethics is to be followed for the project at hand. The NADTA Code of Ethics (2019) would be useful as a central model. But, would a psychological or ethnographic researcher want to follow another code? Again, earnest dialogue and discussion would be a *sine qua non*. Review of potential ethical violations, and *how* to discuss them when they do occur, would need to be addressed, so that the interdisciplinary team could avoid defensive, non-productive communication where members don't really listen to each other. A framework of empathic listening should be invoked from the beginning. A preparatory perspective for prevention of miscommunication or negative communication would be most valuable, especially in regard to the inevitable dialogue on ethical issues that will arise. All the vicissitudes of working together as a team would have to be faced and dealt with.

The Pros and Cons of the Two Models

As already mentioned, the great value of the single individual guiding all the functions – the "Wearing the Four Hats at Once" approach – is the potential for unity of vision and purpose in a project. This is often a consideration in theatre productions, where the adage "Too Many Chefs Spoil the Soup" has been experienced with real consequences such as a production just disintegrating through personality conflicts and no singular vision. With the "One Chief-in-Charge" model, one solitary vision can be realized through the intelligence, sensitivity and leadership skills of a single guide. However, this is dependent on enormous trust-building with the entire team and excellent communication skills on the part of everyone involved.

On the other hand – the "Share the Hats Amongst the Team" model – can harness the positive spin that "More Heads Are Better than One." The advantage of the multiple team leader approach would seem to be in effecting a mirror of a democratic dialogue process that works towards social justice. It invokes a process of interdependence, like the model of the "Ideal Speech Situation," where dialogue must be profoundly honest and open. Again, this is dependent on enormous trust-building and excellent communication skills on the part of everyone involved.

So, it is clearly not a case of Dictatorship versus Democracy with these two models, but of adjustments to genuine communication amongst the team, either with one person or with four. I have not fully experienced the latter, but I have had intimations of it in my work over the past 15 years. I have seen this when I had to come to terms with my own weaknesses in a specific area and became dependent on others to fill these roles. For example, I was never really trained in quantitative research methods and have very little skill with them. I had to reach out to Dr. Miranda D'Amico and Dr. Norman Segalowitz for help in this domain. These two colleagues of mine at Concordia University, in Education and Psychology, respectively, were able to provide their skills in statistical analysis, so we were able, consequently, to develop evidence for the effectiveness of our educational purpose in EDT (See Chapters 5 and 6, especially). This experience suggests to me that a fully collaborative team approach is possible, and with effective leadership in each of EDT's four functions, a real synergy is possible that could enhance the EDT process.

Conclusion

Effecting Social Change

Ethnodramatherapy is an integrated method aimed at effecting positive social change around a chosen social issue. It requires deep, authentic expression from those who have lived this issue and have become informant/co-researcher/performers in the EDT group process. As a phenomenological approach, it can create a vivid portrait of this lived experience and move an audience to change attitudes towards the issue through experiencing it in the powerful mirror of theatrical performance. This performance, in fact, constitutes the group's research report. The forum following the performance offers the audience, the performers and the researchers an opportunity to dialogue on the issue, come to consensus about necessary action and strategize on practical ways to embody an action plan. With the many urgent issues facing society, today – systemic racism, climate change, poverty, sexual and gender violence – EDT is a tool that can be harnessed to catalyze social evolution through its dynamic mode of theatrical expression.

Effecting Individual Change

As a form of group psychotherapy, EDT is meant to create psychological change in the individual participants in the group. Through various techniques of drama therapy, psychodrama and other creative arts therapies, participants are supported to engage in deep, personal, emotional expression within a therapeutic framework. This is a clear exemplification of the maxim, "Expression Necessary for Evolution"; although, in this case, the "Evolution" is the psychological development of an individual human being.

One of the great challenges for the EDT Method, actually for the whole field of drama therapy, has been to accurately measure the effectiveness of the therapeutic process. As Armstrong and her colleagues state, "It has not been demonstrated beyond anecdotal evidence that those processes are, in fact, effective" (2016, p. 28). This has been one of the most disappointing areas of research in EDT: to provide evidence that the parallel therapeutic process genuinely gives the participants an experience of positive therapeutic change. However, new methods for measuring therapeutic efficacy are beginning to evolve in the field of drama therapy. The NADTA has recently put a link on its website that specifically deals with this area.[4] Entitled, "Measures for Drama Therapy Research," this link offers invaluable information on how to use quantitative scales to establish effectiveness of the drama therapy process and provide statistical evidence for the same. One of these scales represented in this compendium is the Outcome Questionnaire (OQ-45.2), created by Lambert and Burlingame (Lambert et al., 1996). I had planned to use this scale on a major prospective project, "Utilizing the Ethnodramatherapy Method to Create a Model for both Group Therapy and Dynamic Mental Health Education for Canadian University Students." Unfortunately, I did not receive the funding from the Canadian Institutes of Health Research for this three-year project. However, this is definitely the direction I would take with any future research projects in EDT. I would hire skilled quantitative

---

4 www.nadta.org/what-is-drama-therapy/research/measures.html. I highly recommend this link to any reader interested in the quantitative measurement of the therapy process.

researchers to administer scales like the OQ-45.2 and analyze results of the application of the scale at the beginning, middle and end of the project. The aim would be to finally produce some strong evidence that the EDT group therapy component is effective and, in fact, generates real therapeutic experiences for participants.

Effectively Employing the Art of Theatre

Effectively employing the art of theatre in the service of emancipatory experience for the audience is at the heart of EDT. And by this, I mean fully engaging in the artistic practice of theatre and using its powerful tools to provide a profound experience for the audience, i.e., taking the role of theatre artist seriously. It is honoring the great art of theatre's immense capacity for effective communication. It is harnessing all the dramatic media – lights, sound, music, singing, dance, scenic design, puppets, masks, poetry, storytelling and acting – in the service of providing catharsis and insight to the audience. As a form of artistic expression, both in virtuosity and in spontaneity, the mirroring function of theatre has been a vehicle for change throughout human history. It is another mode of "Expression Necessary to Evolution."

Effectively Implementing Phenomenological Ethnography

Mienczakowski created a new form of performance ethnography. I have embraced his method and wanted to make it even stronger by adding a therapeutic experience for the informants. I saw the nascent ideas for therapy in his writings and teased them out to become a full-fledged component of my own synthesized method. I know that not all groups will want to work with me or with this method. However, some will. Creating "the group" to be engaged in exploring their own lived experience around a significant social issue is perhaps the greatest challenge in EDT. Trust is a *sine qua non*. As a director of a project, it is getting the group to trust you and each other that is the quintessential challenge. Using Moreno's method of sociometry and the many trust-building exercises in drama therapy are ways to establish trust in the group and assist them in feeling safe enough to share their lived experience around the central theme. Locating and framing the "Ideal Speech Situation" as the performance/research report is presented to the audience allows the ethnography to find its public voice and be a vehicle for change. On the local level, in its own social context, such as in health service environments, the communicative action of EDT can effect changes in attitudes of politicians, administrators and health service professionals. The central goal of the method is to use its powerful tools of expression to promote the healthy evolution of human systems. It potentially validates the assertion: "Expression Necessary to Evolution."

References

Armstrong, C. R., Tanaka, S., Reoch, L., Bronstein, L., Honce, J. Rosenberg, M., & Powell, M. A. (2015). Emotional arousal in two drama therapy core processes: Dramatic embodiment and dramatic projection. *Drama Therapy Review, 1*(2), 147–160.

Armstrong, C. R., Rosenberg, M., Powell, M. A., Honce, J., Bronstein, L. Gingras, G., & Han, E. (2016). A step toward empirical evidence: Operationalizing and uncovering drama therapy change processes. *The Arts in Psychotherapy, 49,* 27–33.

Charles Wesley Emerson. (2020, December 23). In Wikipedia. https://en.wikipedia.org/wiki/Charles_Wesley_Emerson

Chevalier, J. M., & Buckles, D. J. (2019). *Participatory action research: Theory and methods of engaged inquiry* (2nd ed.). Routledge.

de Chardin, T. (1965). *The phenomenon of man.* Harper Torchbooks.

Emerson, C. W. (1964). *Evolution of expression.* Emerson College Press. (Original work published in 1905).

Habermas, J. (1990). *Moral consciousness and communicative action* (C. Lenhardt & S. W. Nicholsen, Trans.). MIT Press.

Harari, Y. N. (2014). *Sapiens: A brief history of humankind.* McClelland & Stewart.

Johnson, D. R. (2020). Development of the modern profession of drama therapy in North America. In D. R. Johnson & R. Emunah (Eds.), *Current approaches in drama therapy* (3rd ed., pp. 5–21). C.C. Thomas Publisher.

Lambert, M. J., Burlingame, G. M., Umphress, V., Hansen, N. B., Vermeersch, D. A., Clouse, G. et al., (1996). The reliability and validity of the outcome questionnaire. *Clinical Psychology and Psychotherapy, 3*(4), 249–258.

McCarthy, T. A. (1973). A theory of communicative competence. *Philosophy of the Social Sciences, 3,* 135–156.

Mienczakowski, J. (1995a). *The application of critical ethno-drama to health settings* [Unpublished doctoral dissertation]. Griffith University, Australia.

National Geographic (2017, January). *Special issue: Gender revolution.*

North American Drama Therapy Association (2019). *NADTA Code, Ethical Principles*. Retrieved from www.nadta.org/about-nadta/code-of-ethics.html.

Pelton, L. (2020, June 15). Message from President Pelton: America is on fire. *Alumni Monthly Newsletter; Special Edition*. Emerson College, Boston, Massachusetts.

Rosenberg, A. (2020, December 5). Page of disruption. *The Montreal Gazette*, B7.

Simpson, G. G, & Beck, W. S. (1965). *Life: An introduction to biology* (2nd ed.). Harcourt, Brace & World.

Snow, S. (1993). *Performing the pilgrims: A study of ethnohistorical role-playing at Plimoth Plantation*. University Press of Mississippi.

Snow, S., & Bleuer, J. (2020). Ethnodramatherapy. In D. R. Johnson & R. Emunah (Eds.), *Current approaches in drama therapy* (3rd ed., pp. 250–283). C. C. Thomas Publisher.

Trouillot, M. R. (1991). Anthropology and the savage plot: The poetics and politics of others. In *Recapturing anthropology: Working in the present* (pp. 17–44). School of American Research Press.

Glossary

This glossary is by no means exhaustive of every term in the four major domains that are the focus of this book: research, therapy, theatre and social activism. However, it seemed like it would be valuable in such an interdisciplinary framework to provide definitions that may not be well known to practitioners in different disciplines. For instance, a theatre artist may not be familiar with diagnoses like ADHD or bipolar disorder. On the other hand, a drama therapist may have never heard of Habermas' "ideal speech situation," or "performance ethnography." The attempt is to spread a wide enough net that the basic concepts from each discipline can be made available to all readers. To save space, citations for some references have been set in an abbreviated code as follows: **M-W.com** represents Merriam-Webster. (n.d.). In *Merriam-Webster.com dictionary*; **DSM-V** signifies American Psychiatric Association. (2013). *Diagnostic and statistical manual of mental disorders* (5th ed.); APA-DPsy means American Psychological Association. (n.d.). In APA *dictionary of psychology*. **Wikipedia** is simply identified as such. If specific authors have been used to define or clarify a specific term, they will be cited individually in the Reference List.

ADHD attention-deficit/hyperactivity disorder: "a behavioral syndrome characterized by the persistent presence of six or more symptoms involving (a) inattention (e.g., failure to complete tasks or listen carefully, difficulty in concentrating, distractibility) or (b) impulsivity or hyperactivity (e.g., blurting out answers; impatience; restlessness; fidgeting; difficulty in organizing work, taking turns, or staying seated; excessive talking; running about; climbing on things." (APA-DPsy)

Applied Theatre "is an umbrella term for the use of theatrical practices and creativity that take participants and audience members further than mainstream theatre, that is often in response to conventional people with real life stories. The work also often happens in non-conventional theatre spaces and social settings e.g. schools, prisons, streets and alternative educational provisions." ("Applied Theatre," Wikipedia, 2021)

Art Therapy is the use of art media, images and creative art processes in conjunction with patient/client/participant responses to the created art production as reflections of an individual's development, abilities, personality, interests, concerns and conflicts. Art therapy can help reconcile emotional conflicts, develop self-awareness, enhance social skills, facilitate problem solving and behavior management and improve self-esteem (see also American Art Therapy Association at www.arttherapy.org).

Asperger's syndrome: "an autism spectrum disorder that is characterized by impaired social interaction, by repetitive patterns of behavior and restricted interests, by normal language and cognitive development but poor conversational skills and difficulty with nonverbal communication, and often by above average performance in a narrow field against a general background of impaired functioning." (M-W.com)

Assessment is the process of gathering information to make decisions; the integration of a variety of data through such means as paper and pencil tests, case studies, behavioral observations and tests assessing psychological attributes.

Autism Spectrum Disorder: "any of a group of developmental disorders (such as autism and Asperger's syndrome) marked by impairments in the ability to communicate and interact socially and by the presence of repetitive behaviors or restricted interests." (M-W.com)

Auxiliary is the title for the members of a psychodrama group who step into the roles in the Protagonist's drama. They are chosen most often by the Protagonist, but sometimes a Director will assign an Auxiliary as specific role. In this format, many members of the group will have an embodied role-playing experience in the group therapy process of psychodrama.

Bipolar Disorder: "any of several psychological disorders of mood characterized usually by alternating episodes of depression and mania – called also *manic depression, manic-depressive illness*" (M-W.com)

Borderline personality disorder: "a personality disorder that is marked by unstable, intense emotions and mood with symptoms including instability in interpersonal relationships and self-image, fear of abandonment, and impulsive or unpredictable behavior and that has an onset during adolescence or early adulthood." (M-W.com)

Catharsis is a term used in both theatre and psychotherapy. It is the word that Aristotle used to describe the psychological experience of the audience when they go through a powerful purgation of emotions while witnessing a Greek tragedy. Moreno saw it as the experience of a release of pent-up emotion in the Protagonist, when they re-experience deep emotions or trauma from earlier in their lives in a psychodrama. It is a complex psychological phenomenon (see Scheff, 1979).

Cerebral palsy: "a disability resulting from damage to the brain before, during, or shortly after birth and outwardly manifested by muscular incoordination and speech disturbances." (M-W.com)

Creative Arts Therapies is the branch of mental health practice that uses the arts as a means of psychotherapy, rehabilitation and personal development. According to the National Coalition of Creative Arts Therapy Associations (NCCATA) in the USA, the six representative modalities are art therapy, music therapy, dance movement therapy, drama therapy, poetry therapy and psychodrama (see also www.nccata.org).

Critical Theory "is an approach to social philosophy that focuses on reflective assessment and critique of society and culture in order to reveal and challenge power structures. With origins in sociology and literary criticism, it argues that social problems are influenced and created more by societal structures and cultural assumptions than by individual and psychological factors" ("Critical Theory," Wikipedia, 2021).

Cronbach's alpha is a measure of the internal reliability or consistency of a set of scale items. A questionnaire with a strong Cronbach's alpha, around .70 or greater, means that its items have been responded to as a group in a consistent way.

Cultural Humility is "a lifelong commitment to self-evaluation and critique, to redressing power imbalances… and to developing mutually beneficial and non-paternalistic partnerships with communities on behalf of individuals and defined populations" (Tervalon & Murray-Garcia, 1998, p. 123).

Culture Conserve is another term invented by Moreno. It indicates a phenomenon that has been locked into a cultural framework and no longer carries the spontaneity as it may have had in its origination. As Moreno writes, "The problem [is] to replace an outworn, antiquated system of values, the culture conserve, with a new system of values in better accord with the emergencies of our time – the spontaneity–creativity complex" (1946, p. 108).

Dance Movement Therapy "usually referred to simply as dance therapy or DMT, is a type of therapy that uses movement to help individuals achieve emotional, cognitive, physical, and social integration. Beneficial for both physical and mental health, dance therapy can be used for stress reduction, disease prevention, and mood management. In addition, DMT's physical component offers increased muscular strength, coordination, mobility, and decreased muscular tension. Dance/movement therapy can be used with all populations and with individuals, couples, families, or groups. In general, dance therapy promotes self-awareness, self-esteem, and a safe space for the expression of feelings." "GoodTherapy," (2021) (see also American Dance Therapy Association at adta.org).

Deception is "the act of causing someone to accept as true or valid what is false or invalid; the act of deceiving." (M-W.com). In the context of an ethics review, it indicates that the researcher is hiding some aspect of the research from the awareness of the subject.

Distancing is a term related to the emotional experience of the client. Are they in a state of being emotionally overwhelmed (underdistanced) or in a state of intellectual defensiveness (overdistanced)? Techniques in drama therapy can be used to promote either of these states and to bring the client into proper balance, known as "aesthetic distance." Some view the essence of drama therapy as being the art of manipulating distance (see Landy, 1996).

Doubling is a technique in psychodrama in which an Auxiliary stands to the side of the Protagonist and becomes their inner voice. The Auxiliary intuits what is really going on in the Protagonist's psyche and says what the Protagonist is not able to voice. The Protagonist, then, either rejects this hypothetical statement or expands on it. There are many forms of "Doubling" (see Leveton, 1992).

Down's Syndrome: "a congenital condition characterized especially by developmental delays, usually mild to moderate impairment in cognitive functioning, short stature, upward slanting eyes, a flattened nasal bridge, broad hands with short fingers, decreased muscle tone, and by trisomy of the human chromosome numbered 21 — called also *trisomy 21*." (M-W.com)

Drama Therapy is the intentional and systematic adaptation of theatre and drama processes for the purpose of psychotherapy, using such media as role-play, storytelling, mime, puppets, masks, and video (see also the North American Drama Therapy Association at www.nadta.org).

Dramatic Reality is a term used to differentiate the embodied imaginal world of dramatic enactment from ordinary reality. It has been especially well articulated by drama therapist Susana Pendzik in her work on assessment in drama therapy (Pendzik in Johnson, Pendzik & Snow, 2012).

Epilepsy: "a group of chronic brain disorders associated with disturbances in the electrical discharges of brain cells and characterized by recurrent seizures, with or without clouding or loss of consciousness." (APA-DPsy)

Ethics Certificate: once a researcher or research team has passed its ethics review, then they will receive an "Ethics Certificate" that usually is dated for a specific period of time. Each year during that period they will need to submit an "Annual Report." When that time is up, they will likely have to file a "Final Report" or reapply for the certificate, if the research is ongoing. When human subjects are involved, this certificate may read something like: "Certification of Ethical Acceptability for Research Involving Human Subjects."

Ethics Review: when applying for grant funding to support a research project or simply for approval, whether to a university's ethics board or a government agency's ethics committee, the applicant must undergo a very thorough ethics review that evaluates the risks and benefits of the project, as well as its value to the institution, the country and the international field of study. This often requires filling out a long form; usually, today, online (see Summary Protocol Form).

Future Projection is a technique used in both drama therapy and psychodrama. The client is asked to enter an imagined future time and space to see what it would be like in relation to their present condition. An embodied scene can be created in this future in order to concretize the experience for the client.

Ideal Speech Situation is a term coined by the German philosopher and sociologist Jürgen Habermas. This "ideal situation" is the goal of his communicative action method, wherein a group can dialogue in truthfulness, without exercising pressures of ideology or neurosis on the facts of the debate. Argumentation is based on validated facts and mutual respect, with a consensus on the truth being the ultimate outcome of the communicative process (see Habermas, 1990).

Informed Consent indicates "a person's voluntary agreement to participate in a procedure on the basis of his or her understanding of its nature, its potential benefits and possible risks, and available alternatives." (APA-DPsy)

Living History Theatre is a methodology that integrates life review, oral history and theatre practice to provide seniors the opportunity to share their unique life experiences with others through theatrical productions. It was developed at Elders Share the Arts, an agency advocating for the arts in the lives of elders, by Susan Perlstein, its founder (see Charnow et al., 1988).

Living Museum designates a historical museum site where historical figures are portrayed by costumed enactors who learn the historical and cultural backgrounds of the personages they portray, even the dialect of the place and times, and, either in first person or third person, tell the stories of the life of this person and their times. Plimoth Plantation and Colonial Williamsburg are good examples of this genre.

Life Review is a therapeutic method for the elderly to help them process their life's experience in the final stages of life. It can be done through storytelling, art works and dramatic embodiment. It allows full emotional expression of what can be remembered. It was developed by the psychiatrist Robert Butler (see Butler, 1963).

Likert Scale is a scale in which respondents indicate their level of agreement with statements that express a favorable or unfavorable attitude toward a concept. A typical Likert scale would provide a statement such as "I feel good about myself" and then ask the subject to answer whether they: (1) strongly agree; (2) agree; (3) disagree; (4) strongly disagree.

Music Therapy is the clinical use of music and musical elements by a certified music therapist to address therapeutic goals that promote growth, health and well-being, mentally, emotionally, physically and spiritually for individuals, families and groups (see also the American Music Therapy Association at www.musictherapy.org).

Noosphere is "a philosophical concept developed and popularized by the Russian and Ukrainian biogeochemist Vladimir Vernadsky, and the French philosopher and Jesuit priest Pierre Teilhard de Chardin. Vernadsky defined the noosphere as the new state of the biosphere and described as the planetary "sphere of reason." The noosphere represents the highest stage of biospheric development, its defining factor being the development of humankind's rational activities. The word is derived from the Greek νόος ("mind," "reason") and σφαῖρα ("sphere"), in lexical analogy to "atmosphere" and "biosphere." The concept, however, cannot be accredited to a single author. The founding authors Vernadsky and de Chardin developed two related but starkly different concepts, the former being grounded in the geological sciences, and the latter in theology. Both conceptions of the noosphere share the common thesis that together human reason and the scientific thought has created, and will continue to create, the next evolutionary geological layer. This geological layer is part of the evolutionary chain. Second generation authors, predominantly of Russian origin, have further developed the Vernadskian concept, creating the related concepts: noocenosis and noocenology" ("Noosphere," 2021, Wikipedia).

Oral History is "the collection and study of historical information about individuals, families, important events, or everyday life using audiotapes, videotapes or transcriptions of planned interviews. These interviews are conducted with people who participated in or observed past events and whose memories and perceptions of these are to be preserved as an aural record for future generations" ("Oral History," Wikipedia, 2021).

Paranoid Schizophrenia in *DSM–IV–TR*, "is a subtype of schizophrenia, often with a later onset than other types, characterized by prominent delusions or auditory hallucinations. Delusions are typically persecutory, grandiose, or both; hallucinations are typically related to the content of the delusional theme. Cognitive functioning and mood are affected to a much lesser degree than in other types of schizophrenia. This subtype has been eliminated from *DSM–5*." (APA-DPsy)

"p < .05" signifies that the result is statistically significant at the .05 level, meaning that there is a low probability (less than 5%) that the same outcome would occur if the null hypothesis were true (that is, if there were no systematic patterning in the data). When the outcome is "p < .05," by convention researchers often conclude that the result can be accepted as statistically reliable.

Participant observation is the primary approach to data collection in ethnography. The researcher immerses him or herself in the culture-sharing group and becomes a participant within the setting. Observations are recorded in field notes. In this way, the researcher sustains both an objective and subjective framework for the research endeavor.

Participatory Action Research (PAR) defines an approach to research where all involved are co-researchers. Both members of the community being studied and the research team undertaking the investigation are stakeholders in the project and constantly dialogue on the goals, methods and outcomes of research. It represents a kind of democracy-in-action where everyone has a voice in what is done and how to do it in regard to the research process.

Performance Ethnography was first implemented in the 1980s when social scientists began to turn their field notes into performances and people in theatre and performance studies started to adapt ethnographies for the purpose of performance. A succinct definition comes from one of the major scholars in this field, explaining how this discipline "uses performance as a method of investigation, as a way of doing ethnography, and as a method of understanding, a way of collaboratively engaging in meanings of experience" (Denzin, 2003, p. 31).

Performing Ethnography has to be distinguished from "Performance Ethnography," per se, as it was invented by one individual, anthropologist Victor Turner, as a way of teaching anthropology through the performance of ethnographic texts. It is based on the idea that "Anthropological literature is full of accounts of dramatic episodes which vividly manifest the key values of specific cultures" (Turner & Turner, 1986, p. 139). Performing such material can bring the human experience of culture alive for students.

Performance Studies "is an interdisciplinary academic field that uses performance as a lens and a tool to study the world. The term *performance* is broad, and can include artistic and aesthetic performances like concerts, theatrical events, and performance art; sporting events; social, political and religious events like rituals, ceremonies, proclamations and public decisions; certain kinds of language use; and those components of identity which require someone to do, rather than just be, something" ("Performance Studies," Wikipedia, 2021).

Performance Theory is a multidisciplinary approach to creating theories around all aspect of performance, including ritual, drama, theatre, politics, sports and everyday life. A good example of a classic work in the field is Richard Schechner's *Essays in Performance Theory, 1970–1976* (Drama Book Specialists, 1977).

Perseveration in neuropsychology, the inappropriate repetition of behavior that is often associated with damage to the frontal lobe of the brain. (APA-DPsy)

Playback Theatre is a form of improvisational theatre created by Jonathan Fox. Audience members come onto the stage were actors and musicians sit. They are guided in telling their personal story by a person called the Conductor. When ready, the actors and musicians re-create or "playback" the Teller's Story. This form of theatre is done all over the world today (see www.playbackcentre.org/affiliate-schools/current-affiliate-schools/).

Playspace is a term used in drama therapy to delineate the boundary between everyday living and entering a realm of spontaneous play. Sometimes the boundary is established as an imaginary curtain through which participants enter into the domain of play. The terminology is especially used in the method of "Developmental Tranformations" created by David Read Johnson (Johnson in Johnson & Emunah, 2009).

Prader-Willi-Lockhart syndrome: "a genetic disorder characterized especially by short stature, intellectual disability, hypotonia, functionally deficient gonads, and uncontrolled appetite leading to extreme obesity." (M-W.com)

Psychodrama is to be differentiated from drama therapy, as it was founded by one individual, Jacob Levy Moreno, and has its own philosophy, training programs and professional association. It is also an action-based therapy, and utilizes role-playing, role reversal and auxiliary actors to assist an individual in reenacting real life experiences and imaginary ones as well (see also the American Society for Group Psychotherapy and Psychodrama @ASGPP).

Role Reversal is one of the most used techniques in psychodrama. It is exactly as it says, switching one's role with some else. For instance, if one was doing a psychodrama about an issue with one's mother, one could switch into the role of mother and the mother could become one's self. This can allow for a deep experience of empathy by, holding, for a moment, someone else's point of view. The technique is often used to train Auxiliaries how to play a role in the Protagonist's drama. The Protagonist will role reverse, by steppng into the Auxiliary's role to show him/her how to play it.

Sandplay Therapy was developed by Dora Kalff in Switzerland in the 1950s and 1960s. Her approach was based on her studies at the C. G. Jung Institute, Zurich, and her training with Margaret Lowenfeld in England and her exploration of Tibetan Buddhism. In this approach, individuals, both children and adults, are invited to play in sand trays of wet or dry sand, sculpting the sand and positioning miniature figures and objects to create three-dimensional scenes or designs that express their inner worlds. Such depictions in the sand tray can also be used to psychologically assess the individual (see also Sandplay Therapists of Amercia at www.sandplay.org).

Schizophrenia is defined "by abnormalities in one or more of the following five domains: delusions, hallucinations, disorganized thinking (speech), grossly disorganized or abnormal motor behavior (including catatonia), and negative symptoms." (DSM-V, p. 87)

Selective Mutism: "an anxiety disorder of childhood characterized by consistent failure to speak in specific social settings (as at school) despite having the ability to speak normally in other settings (as at home)." (M-W.com)

Self-image: "one's conception of oneself or of one's role." (M-W.com)

Self-perception: "*n.* a person's view of his or her self or of any of the mental or physical attributes that constitute the self. Such a view may involve genuine self-knowledge or varying degrees of distortion." (APA-DPsy.com)

Self-Revelatory Performance (also known as Self-Rev) is a synthesized form of performance that combines deep self-exploration, drama therapy and theatrical performance. It was developed by drama therapist Renée Emunah. As she writes: "Some people hold the notion that if art is intentionally therapeutic, it cannot be truly art, but Self-Rev breaks that myth. Self-Rev manages to hold the tension between art and therapy. Neither component is sacrificed; rather, both are amplified" (Emunah, 2015, p. 81).

Social Activism "consists of efforts to promote, impede, direct, or intervene in social, political, economic, or environmental reform with the desire to make changes in society toward a perceived greater good. Forms of activism range from mandate building in the community (including writing letters to newspapers), petitioning elected officials, running or contributing to a political campaign, preferential patronage (or boycott) of businesses, and demonstrative forms of activism like rallies, street marches, strikes, sit-ins, or hunger strikes ("Social Activism," Wikipedia, 2021).

Social Justice "is the relation of balance between individuals and society measured by comparing distribution of wealth differences, from personal liberties to fair privilege opportunities. In Western as well as in older Asian cultures, the concept of social justice has often referred to the process of ensuring that individuals fulfill their societal roles and receive what was their due from society. In the current global grassroots movements for social justice, the emphasis has been on the breaking of barriers for social mobility, the creation of safety nets and economic justice" ("Social Justice," Wikipedia, 2021).

Sociodrama is another form of improvisational role-playing invented by J. L. Moreno. In this case, it focuses on collective roles and the purpose is more educational than therapeutic. A group of enactors create a fictional scenario around a social issue, then enact and discuss it. Some of the same techniques of psychodrama are used to process the creation of the performance and discussion (see Sternberg & Garcia, 1989).

Sociometry is a nexus of techniques created by Moreno to both measure the interconnections in a group and to promote group coherency in his various methods, including psychodrama, sociodrama, ethnodrama and axiodrama (for more information, contact the American Society for Group Psychotherapy and Psychodrama @ASGPP).

Spearman rho is a correlation coefficient based on the rank order of items rather than on their absolute values.

STD: "the term sexually transmitted disease (STD) is used to refer to a condition passed from one person to another through sexual contact. A person can contract an STD by having unprotected vaginal, anal, or oral sex with someone who has the STD. An STD may also be called a sexually transmitted infection (STI) or venereal disease (VD)." (www.healthline.com/health/sexually-transmitted-diseases)

Subscales: A subscale is a set of items within a larger test or scale that addresses one particular aspect of the construct targeted by the larger scale.

For example, an attitude scale or test may have subscales that address particular components of attitude.

Summary Protocol Form (SPF) is the term used for the form that an applicant for an ethics review must fill out in order to apply for certification from an ethics board. If human subjects are involved, this board or committee may be called a "Human Research Ethics Committee (HREC)." This application form will require summarized descriptions of the whole project, timelines, researchers, research participants, recruitment methods, etc. It will especially focus on "Research Concerns," such as informed consent, deception, risks, confidentiality and the handling of data. It is always a major undertaking to complete this document.

Surplus Reality is a concept invented by Moreno to define an imaginal "reality" where things can take place in the past, present or future that never really happened before. They are not in the outside world of reality, but in the "reality" of the imagined world, and can be acted upon "as if" they were real.

Synaesthetic Spontaniety is a term coined by the author. It indicates a simultaneous experience of different art forms – music, dance, poetry, visual art, drama and ritual – that are taking place in an improvisational process of creative exploration. All the senses are potentially opened in this context of play and improvisation.

Therapeutic Theatre denotes the use of theatrical performance, including rehearsals, the performance, itself, and post-performance processing, as a vehicle for therapy. Participants are clients who are actually undergoing a therapy process. Relevant therapeutic goals are developed for each participant. The whole process is similar to group therapy, and the director, as well other staff, are trained therapists, usually drama therapists or creative arts therapists.

Tourette's syndrome: "a familial neurological disorder of variable expression that is characterized by recurrent involuntary tics involving body movements (such as eye blinks or grimaces) and vocalizations (such as grunts or utterance of inappropriate words." (M-W.com)

Walk and Talk is a method in psychodrama in which the Director takes the Protagonist for a walk around the circumference of the stage and has sensitive discussion, often to set the therapeutic contract for what the Protagonist would like to get out of the session. It can also be used during the session to clarify the process, check-in with how the *Protagonist* is doing, or even to create some distance for an overwhelming moment in the process.

Warm-up is a term used in drama therapy, psychodrama and theatre. It essentially means stimulating the whole self on the psychosomatic level in order to be ready to enter into an activity. In drama therapy, it signifies the preparation to enter the *Play Space* and participate in *Dramatic Reality*. In psychodrama, it indicates both preparing the group to choose a protagonist and readying the *Protagonist* and *Auxiliaries* for the engagement in the psychodrama. One will often hear in such contexts, comments like "the client was not warmed-up enough." In theatre it is the prelude to performing or getting into one's role, an idea made famous by Stanislavski's *An Actor Prepares* (1963).

Williams Syndrome: "a rare genetic disorder marked especially by hypercalcemia of infants, heart defects, characteristic facial abnormalities, and mild to moderate intellectual disability but a high verbal aptitude." (M-W.com)

Youth Protection is a government agency in Québec which becomes involved when a child's safety or development is in danger due to physical, sexual, psychological or other forms of abuse. The agency runs centres across Québec where youth can be housed in safety, with educational services and care.

References

American Psychiatric Association. (2013). *Diagnostic and statistical manual of mental disorders* (5th ed.). Retrieved from https://doi.org/10.1176/appi.books.9780890425596.

American Psychological Association. (n.d.). Self-perception. In APA *dictionary of psychology*. Retrieved from https://dictionary.apa.org/just-world-hypothesis.

Butler, R. (1963). The life review: An interpretation of reminiscence in the aged. *Psychiatry, 26*(1), 65–76.

Charnow, S., Nash, E., & Perlstein, S. (1988). *Life review training manual.* Elders Share the Arts, Brooklyn, NY.

Denzin, N. (2003). *Performance ethnography: Critical pedagogy and the politics of culture.* Sage Publications.

Emunah, R. (2015). Self-revelatory performance: A form of drama therapy and theatre. *Drama Therapy Review, 1*(1), 71–85.

GoodTherapy (2021, July 19). Retrieved from www.goodtherapy.org/learn-about-therapy/types/dance-movement-therapy.

Habermas, J. (1990). *Moral consciousness and communicative action*. The MIT press.

Johnson, D. R (2009). Developmental transformations: Towards the body as presence. In D. R. Johnson & R. Emunah (Eds.), *Current approaches in drama therapy* (2nd ed., pp. 89–116). C. C. Thomas Publisher.

Landy. R. (1996). *Essays on drama therapy: The double life*. Jessica Kingsley.

Leveton, E. (1992). *A clinician's guide to psychodrama*. Springer.

Merriam-Webster. (n.d.). In *Merriam-Webster.com dictionary*. Retrieved from www.merriam-webster.com/dictionary/semantics.

Moreno, J.L. (1946). *Psychodrama, First Volume* (2nd ed). Beacon House.

Pendzik, S. (2012). The 6-key model: An integrative assessment approach. In D. R. Johnson, S. Pendzik & S. Snow (Eds.), Assessment in drama therapy (pp. 197–222). C. C. Thomas Publisher.

Schechner, R (1977). *Essays in Performance Theory, 1970–1976*. Drama Book Specialists.

Scheff, T. J. (1979). *Catharsis in healing, ritual and drama*. University of California Press.

Stanislavski, C. (1963). *An actor prepares* (E. R. Hapgood, Trans.). Theatre Arts Books.

Sternberg, P., & Garcia, A. (1989). *Sociodrama: Who's in your shoes?* Praeger.

Tervalon, M., Murray-Garcia, J. (1998). Cultural humility versus cultural competence: A critical distinction in defining physician training outcomes in multicultural education. *Journal of Health Care for the Poor and Underserved*, 9, 117–125.

Turner, V., & Turner, E. (1986). Performing ethnography. In V. Turner, *The anthropology of performance* (pp. 139–156). PAJ Publications.

Wikipedia.org. (2021). https://en.wikipedia.org/wiki/.

Index

Note: **Bold** page numbers refer to tables, *italic* page numbers refer to figures and page numbers followed by "n" refer to end notes.